Lessons from the
GRAND ROUNDS 2

Lessons from the
GRAND ROUNDS 2
Options in Rational Management

Third Edition

YK Amdekar MD DCH
Senior Faculty
SRCC Children's Hospital, Mumbai
Retired Professor of Pediatrics
Grant Medical College, Sir JJ Group of Hospitals
Mumbai, Maharashtra, India

RD Khare MD DCH
Senior Consultant
Holy Family Hospital, Mumbai
Former Professor
KJ Somaiya Medical College
Mumbai, Maharashtra, India

RR Chokhani MD DCH
Consultant
PD Hinduja Hospital
Mumbai, Maharashtra, India

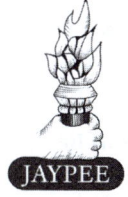

JAYPEE BROTHERS MEDICAL PUBLISHERS
The Health Sciences Publisher
New Delhi | London

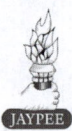 **Jaypee Brothers Medical Publishers (P) Ltd**

Headquarters
Jaypee Brothers Medical Publishers (P) Ltd
EMCA House, 23/23-B
Ansari Road, Daryaganj
New Delhi 110 002, India
Landline: +91-11-23272143, +91-11-23272703
+91-11-23282021, +91-11-23245672
Email: jaypee@jaypeebrothers.com

Corporate Office
Jaypee Brothers Medical Publishers (P) Ltd
4838/24, Ansari Road, Daryaganj
New Delhi 110 002, India
Phone: +91-11-43574357
Fax: +91-11-43574314
Email: jaypee@jaypeebrothers.com

Overseas Office
JP Medical Ltd
83 Victoria Street, London
SW1H 0HW (UK)
Phone: +44 20 3170 8910
Fax: +44 (0)20 3008 6180
Email: info@jpmedpub.com

Website: www.jaypeebrothers.com
Website: www.jaypeedigital.com

© 2024, Jaypee Brothers Medical Publishers

The views and opinions expressed in this book are solely those of the original contributor(s)/author(s) and do not necessarily represent those of editor(s) or publisher of the book.

All rights reserved. No part of this publication may be reproduced, stored or transmitted in any form or by any means, electronic, mechanical, photocopying, recording or otherwise, without the prior permission in writing of the publishers.

All brand names and product names used in this book are trade names, service marks, trademarks or registered trademarks of their respective owners. The publisher is not associated with any product or vendor mentioned in this book.

Medical knowledge and practice change constantly. This book is designed to provide accurate, authoritative information about the subject matter in question. However, readers are advised to check the most current information available on procedures included and check information from the manufacturer of each product to be administered, to verify the recommended dose, formula, method and duration of administration, adverse effects and contra-indications. It is the responsibility of the practitioner to take all appropriate safety precautions. Neither the publisher nor the author(s)/editor(s) assume any liability for any injury and/or damage to persons or property arising from or related to use of material in this book.

This book is sold on the understanding that the publisher is not engaged in providing professional medical services. If such advice or services are required, the services of a competent medical professional should be sought.

Every effort has been made where necessary to contact holders of copyright to obtain permission to reproduce copyright material. If any have been inadvertently overlooked, the publisher will be pleased to make the necessary arrangements at the first opportunity.

Inquiries for bulk sales may be solicited at: jaypee@jaypeebrothers.com

Lessons from the Grand Rounds 2: Options in Rational Management

First Edition: 2011
Second Edition: 2018
Third Edition: **2024**

ISBN: 978-93-5696-634-5

Printed at Rajkamal Electric Press, Kundli, Haryana.

Dedicated to
*The children who suffered
from whom we learnt a lot.*

PREFACE TO THE THIRD EDITION

The continued demand for our book suggests that readers find them useful and identify with the cases discussed—both in content and in style. This has encouraged us to bring out another edition of the same. Since the content matter in our book is largely clinical, not much has 'changed'—the clinical approach remains the same. Nevertheless, we have made some revisions, mainly in the form of additions to some sections. These are in the form of additional discussion on 'treatment' and some newer cases in some sections. We trust that our readers will find these new additions equally useful.

YK Amdekar
RD Khare
RR Chokhani

PREFACE TO THE FIRST EDITION

Encouraged by the overwhelming response that we got for our first book Lessons from the Grand Rounds, we decided to once again share the lessons that we have learned from our patients. Last time, the focus was on the power of clinical analysis to help reach an accurate diagnosis. We now try to build on the foundations that were laid last time and venture into some other areas of interest. There are four sections to this book.

The first section reiterates the value of a painstakingly detailed history and a meticulous clinical examination. It illustrates how short cuts that bypass these fundamental steps often end up in confusion. It is only after retracing one's steps and falling back on these basics that one can extricate oneself from a maze of investigations that seem to lead to nowhere. In other words, this section reinforces the lesson that there is no point in trying to save time by bypassing what has stood the test of time. A few cases of this section were originally included in our first book. Since they almost symbolize the magic of clinical medicine, we have intentionally overlooked their repetition.

In the second section, we continue this process of clinical analysis and step beyond, into the realms of management. Management includes the establishment of a provisional diagnosis, with the help of the planned investigations, if necessary, before proceeding with specific treatment. Partially treated cases are often difficult mysteries to solve, since the telltale fingerprints have been either wiped off or have been smudged. It is not easy to pick up the loose ends and reconstruct the true story. Typically, these are areas of clinical medicine where there may be more than one management option—some are more correct than the others. We have picked up a few such situations and a few others, commonly encountered in office practice, where we present our views on the principles that guide the choice of the correct management option.

This is followed by a section on a few commonly encountered recurrent problems in clinical practice. Recurrent problems may have a totally different diagnostic and therapeutic implication, as against a one-time occurrence of the same problem. Illustrative cases drive home the lessons to be learned in this section.

Last, but not least, is the section on tuberculosis. Understanding tuberculosis has never been easy. As a result, a lot has already been written on various aspects of tuberculosis. We are all aware that the causation of disease depends on the interrelationship between the agent, host and environment. Over the years, a lot of advances have been made in defining the etiological agents of various diseases. A lot of efforts have gone into studying the 'behavioral' characteristics of individual 'agents', including Mycobacterium tuberculosis. But, in the bargain, the host and the (internal) environment, which seem to possess the power to modify this 'behavior', have been probably relegated to the backseat. As a result, when the same disease behaves differently in different hosts under different circumstances, it is considered perplexing and adds to the clinical difficulties in diagnosis, management, assessment of response to therapy, etc.

We believe that the explanations to such vagaries probably lie in understanding the host responses and the body milieu, i.e., the internal environment. We have tried to bring out this aspect of tuberculosis and put forth our views on the same.

Each section does not claim to be exhaustive, and therefore, does not cover each and every subtopic or every conceivable situation. We have tried to include prototypes of those cases that are commonly encountered in day-to-day practice. If an occasional relatively uncommon case has been included, it is only because of the interest it generates. A few cases figure in more than one section. This is so, because the same case conveys different messages, when looked at from different perspectives. Purists may not find 'evidence' in current medical literature in favor of some of the hypotheses put forth by us. However, at this point in time, we believe this is a rational conjecture.

All the material is derived from cases that have been actually seen by us; largely in our personal practice, but sometimes as a part of some academic group discussion with close colleagues. In other words, we have learned our lessons from our patients, and the experience so gained has been further enriched by our regular interactions with students and colleagues. Therefore, we are indebted not only to our patients, but also our students and colleagues. We wish to share these experiences with others, because, after all, the benefits of such exchanges are mutual. It has been well said, "Man is always learning; the day he stops learning, he becomes old."

We also sincerely thank our family and friends for all their support and encouragement.

YK Amdekar
RD Khare
RR Chokhani

CONTENTS

Section 1: Time Tested Hypothesis

CASE 1	'Patient' Hearing a Must	4
CASE 2	History Begins with Age. How 'Old' are You?	6
CASE 3	History Begins with Age	8
CASE 4	Respect Chief Complaints	9
CASE 5	Respect Chief Complaints	10
CASE 6	Origin Matters	12
CASE 7	Origin Matters	14
CASE 8	Do not Ignore Clinical Setting	15
CASE 9	Do not Ignore Clinical Setting	16
CASE 10	Duration is Important	17
CASE 11	Caution against Unexpected Progress	19
CASE 12	Sudden Improvement may be Ominous	20
CASE 13	Beware of Partial Improvement	21
CASE 14	Monitor Progress of Fever: Biphasic Fever	23
CASE 15	Past—A Lead for the Future	25
CASE 16	Attention to Personal History	26
CASE 17	First Impression	28
CASE 18	General Examination is Special	30
CASE 19	Correlate Temperature, Pulse and Respiration (TPR)	31
CASE 20	Observe Pattern of Breathing	32
CASE 21	Listen to the Sounds that Breathing Makes	33
CASE 22	Nail Down the Diagnosis	34
CASE 23	Stick Out the Neck	35
CASE 24	Stretch your Imagination	36
CASE 25	Head Start	37

Section 2: Management Dilemmas in Office Practice

CASE 26	Viral Fever	42
CASE 27	Enteric Fever	45
CASE 28	Enteric Fever	48
CASE 29	Enteric Fever	51
CASE 30	Frequent Illnesses Diagnosed as Primary Complex Twice	53
CASE 31	Short Stature due to IUGR with Malpositioned Kidney	56
CASE 32	Breastfed Baby with Intermittent Blood in Stools	58
CASE 33	Breastfed Baby with Suspected GI Infection Who Recovered Fast	61
CASE 34	Empyema	63
CASE 35	Empyema Who was Given Steroids	66
CASE 36	Rheumatic Fever	69
CASE 37	UTI—1st Episode at 4-year of Age	72
CASE 38	Constipation	75
CASE 39	Nephrotic Syndrome	77
CASE 40	Immune Thrombocytopenic Purpura	79
CASE 41	Reactive Arthritis Secondary to Mediastinal Malignancy	82
CASE 42	Mismanaged Gastroenteritis	86
CASE 43	Inadequate Feeding Investigated for Failure to Thrive	90
CASE 44	Infant with Atypical Kawasaki Disease	93
CASE 45	Fungal Pneumonia	96
CASE 46	Palatopharyngeal Incompetence	101
CASE 47	Hemophagocytic Syndrome	104
CASE 48	Leukemia Presenting as Scurvy	107
CASE 49	Poststreptococcal Reactive Arthritis	110
CASE 50	Suspected Kawasaki Disease Presenting in 2nd Week	112
CASE 51	Galactosemia	115
CASE 52	Mismanaged UTI Presenting as Breathlessness	118
CASE 53	Gaucher Disease	120
CASE 54	Autoimmune Disorder	121
CASE 55	Idiopathic Thrombocytopenic Purpura	123

CASE 56	Sudden Falls in a 12-year-old	125
CASE 57	Dengue Shock Syndrome	127
CASE 58	*Capillaria Hepatica*	129
	Fever with Skin Rash	**131**
CASE 59	Systemic Inflammatory Disorder	133
CASE 60	Meningococcemia	135
CASE 61	Stevens–Johnson Syndrome	137
CASE 62	Dengue Shock Syndrome	138
CASE 63	Rickettsial Disease	139
CASE 64	Severe Combined Immunodeficiency	140
CASE 65	Streptococcal Infection	141
CASE 66	Hodgkin's Lymphoma	142
	Inborn Errors of Metabolism	**144**
CASE 67	Metabolic Disorder Presenting as Complication of Diarrhea	146
CASE 68	Metabolic Disorder Presenting as Unexplained Encephalopathy	148
CASE 69	Urea Cycle Defect	149
CASE 70	Galactosemia	151
CASE 71	Phenylketonuria	152
CASE 72	Mitochondrial Encephalopathy with Lactic Acidosis	153
CASE 73	Metabolic Disorder with Cardiomyopathy	154
CASE 74	Ataxia Presenting as Metabolic Disorder	155

Section 3: Recurrent Problems

	An Approach to Recurrent/Persistent Pneumonia	160
CASE 75	Clinical Recovery, Radiological Persistence	164
CASE 76	Clinical Recovery, Radiological Persistence	166
CASE 77	Clinical Recovery, Radiological Persistence	167
CASE 78	Clinical and Radiological Persistence	169
CASE 79	Clinical Persistence, Radiological Recovery	171
CASE 80	Recurrent Pneumonia at the Same Site	174
CASE 81	Subacute Pneumonia	176
CASE 82	Nonbacterial Etiology	177

CASE 83	Complication	179
CASE 84	Complication	180
CASE 85	True Recurrence	182
CASE 86	True Recurrence	184

Recurrent Cough With or Without Wheezing 186

CASE 87	Wheeze Associated Lower Respiratory Infection	187
CASE 88	Gastroesophageal Reflux Disease (GERD)	189
CASE 89	Achalasia Cardia	191
CASE 90	Coarctation of Aorta	193
CASE 91	Cystic Fibrosis	195
CASE 92	Foreign Body	196
CASE 93	Miliary Tuberculosis	197

Recurrent Cough, Cold and Fever in Office Practice 198

CASE 94	Frequent Viral Infections	199
CASE 95	Asthma	200
CASE 96	Bacterial Infection Secondary to Adenoid Hypertrophy	201
CASE 97	Recurrent Cold and Fever	203

Recurrent Abdominal Pain 204

CASE 98	Habitual Constipation	205
CASE 99	Meckel's Diverticulum	207
CASE 100	Dyspepsia	209
CASE 101	Functional Abdominal Pain	210
CASE 102	Inflammatory Bowel Disease	211
CASE 103	Irritable Bowel Syndrome	212

Recurrent Diarrhea 213

CASE 104	Recurrent GI Infection	214
CASE 105	HIV Infection	215
CASE 106	Gluten Induced Enteropathy	216
CASE 107	Chronic Giardiasis	218

Miscellaneous 219

| CASE 108 | Recurrent Swelling around Angle of Mandible | 219 |

Section 4: Vagaries in Tuberculosis

Host Chooses Pathology and Decides the Outcome 223

CASE 109	Lobar Emphysema as a Presentation of Large Mediastinal Lymph Node 237
CASE 110	Missed Mediastinal Lymph Node Enlargement on Routine Chest X-ray 239
CASE 111	Missed Mediastinal Lymph Node Enlargement on Routine Chest X-ray 240
CASE 112	Acute Onset Pleural Effusion that was TB 242
CASE 113	Localized Pleural Effusion 243
CASE 114	Tuberculous Empyema 245
CASE 115	Bilateral Pleural Effusion 246
CASE 116	Subacute Pneumonia Missed as Acute Bacterial Pneumonia 248
CASE 117	Mediastinal Lymph Node, Cavity and Miliary Lesion in Same Child at a Time 250
CASE 118	Fever, Cough, Breathlessness (TB Lymph Node and Miliary) 254
CASE 119	Recurrent Arthritis as an Immune-mediated Manifestation of TB 256
CASE 120	Persistence of Fever for Months in Spite of Radiological Improvement 258
CASE 121	Suspected MDR TB 260
CASE 122	MDR TB 262
CASE 123	Extensive Tuberculosis in Infant Poorly Responsive to Treatment 264
CASE 124	Worsening Mediastinal Lymph Node Enlargement on Recovery of Primary Complex 267
CASE 125	Development of Cervical Lymph Node on Recovery of TB Pneumonia 270
CASE 126	Recurrence of Meningitis on Compliant Anti-TB Therapy 271
CASE 127	Development of Tuberculoma on Recovery of TBM 272
CASE 128	BCG Lymphadenitis 273
CASE 129	Flaring of BCG Scar as a Manifestation of Immune Disorder 274
CASE 130	Psoriatic Arthritis Mistaken for TB 275
CASE 131	Suspected Abdominal TB 277
CASE 132	Multiple Recovering Bony Lesions of Hodgkin's Mistaken as TB 279
CASE 133	TB Lymphadenitis Which was Lymphoma 281

Index *283*

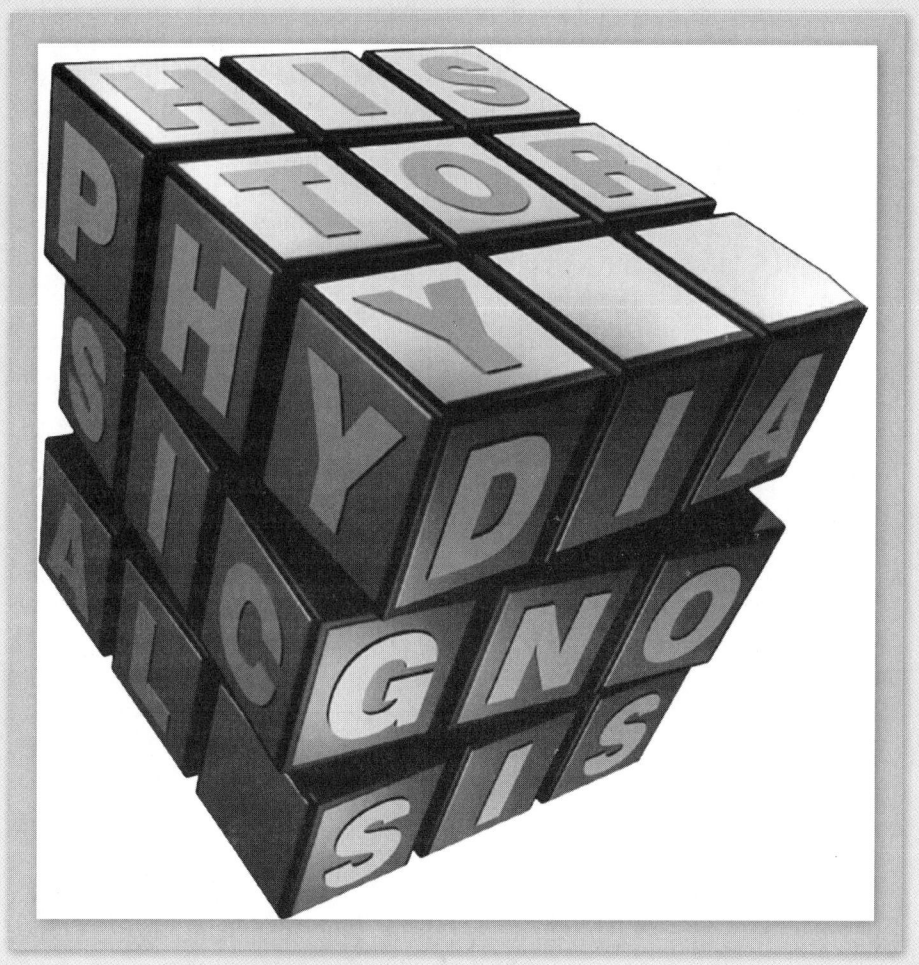

SECTION 1

Time Tested Hypothesis

Ever since time immemorial, much before investigatory facilities were available, clinicians depended heavily on analysis of history and interpretation of physical findings, in order to reach a correct diagnosis. The earliest generation of physicians practiced the art and science of medicine, and thereby laid down the format of history taking and systematic physical examination. It is that pattern which we all have learnt during our undergraduate training. However, over the years, with the development of modern techniques of investigations, the newer generation of physicians started ignoring this art, least realizing that this was a time-tested hypothesis which guaranteed results. Modern laboratory techniques may have surely led to the more frequent diagnosis of rare conditions. However, extreme reliance on these techniques has occasionally delayed the diagnosis of common conditions; at times, they have even been missed.

It is worth reiterating that the standard format of history taking and physical examination, that we recommend, should be followed at all levels of medical practice. The first step is to be a **'patient'** listener to the patient. History begins with the name and age and then proceeds sequentially with the chief complaints, origin, duration, and progress, past, personal, family, socioeconomic, birth and developmental history. History is not 'his story'. History taking is a "thought in action". It means that the answer to the first question should guide the next question. It is possible only when a physician develops a thought process after listening to each answer and formulates an interpretation in the mind. It continues throughout the entire inquiry. Thus, at the end of such "thought in action" history, we can arrive at a provisional diagnosis in most cases. This facilitates anticipating abnormal physical findings and adds value to the physical examination with a proper focus on such expected findings.

Physical examination begins with the 'appearance' of the patient at first glance, and then proceeds sequentially with the detailed general examination followed by systemic examination. The physical examination must be conducted in a systematic standard way irrespective of individual experience and confidence. The clues to the diagnosis could be hiding in any small part of the body and hence a thorough examination is a need, lest one may miss the diagnosis. It is obvious that there is no place for a shortcut in history taking and physical examination. Such an approach helps in arriving at a near-final diagnosis and only after that, specific minimal tests can be ordered to confirm the clinical diagnosis, if necessary. Eliciting the history and physical findings is an art—the skill that one acquires through observation, repetitive practice and experience.

This section illustrates actual cases that we encountered, where such time-tested methods saved the day and clinched the correct diagnosis, even when, at times, modern investigatory techniques had failed.

CASE 1

■ 'Patient' Hearing a Must

Events...

A 4-year-old child was referred for failure to reach the diagnosis in spite of several investigations and trial of therapy for various diseases. This child started with fever and cough for which he consulted his doctor. A chest X-ray was ordered which showed an ill-defined radiological lesion on the left side. Considering it to be pneumonia, he was treated with amoxicillin. While the child had recovered symptomatically within a couple of days, a repeat chest X-ray continued to be abnormal. This time it was interpreted as pneumatoceles following the bacterial pneumonia, and Cefotaxime was added. Over the next few days, the child continued to be asymptomatic, but a repeat chest X-ray suggested multiple cavities. On the basis of this, a diagnosis of cavitary tuberculosis was considered and the child was put on anti-TB treatment. At this point, they went for a second opinion; fresh X-rays were asked for, and a differential diagnosis of hydatid cysts vs. multiple lung cysts emerged. Another possibility that was considered was congenital cystic adenomatoid malformation, in view of the lesions being persistent. As the child remained asymptomatic, it was decided to observe the child without any treatment. However, the chest X-ray was repeated after a few weeks and this time, it showed an air-fluid level in the pleural cavity; therefore, a hydropneumothorax was diagnosed. A pleural tap was attempted, which yielded some milky fluid; as a result, further tests were now done for chylothorax. All along, the child remained well without any symptoms and grew well.

Explanation...

The parents were quite upset because none of the doctors were ready to listen to their views about the child's illness. They insisted that their child's problem was related to the abdomen and not the chest; so much, that they repeatedly pleaded for an abdominal X-ray. However, their pleas fell on deaf ears.

At this center, when the parents were probed as to why they thought the problem was related to abdomen, they gave a clue to the diagnosis. They felt that even after a meal their child's abdomen never looked protuberant or full; it was always sunken. They were giving a clue to the diagnosis of **diaphragmatic hernia**. Depending upon the contents of the hernia in the chest, the shadows varied each time an X-ray was ordered. The 'pleural tap' that suggested a chylothorax was actually a tap in the stomach that happened to lie in the chest at that time.

Experience gained...

> Clinicians must be 'patient' to listen to a patient. It has been noticed on numerous occasions that the observations of the child patient's mother offer vital clues, only if we clinicians recognize the power of such observations. This is true even if it comes from an apparently illiterate mother; obviously, experienced clinicians would know when to ignore and when not to.
>
> This case also illustrates how physicians (and radiologists) read radiographs casually and 'jump' at the obvious. They then compound the error by continuing to toe the same line, in total disregard of the patient's clinical condition and parental views.

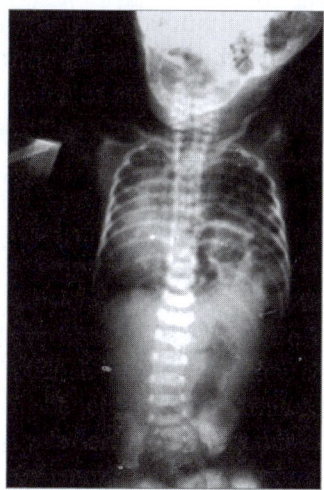

Congenital diaphragmatic hernia.

CASE 2

■ History Begins with Age. How 'Old' are You?

Events...

A 2-month-old infant presented with pallor that was noticed by the parents over the last two weeks. There was no other complaint. The child was born after a full term and through a normal delivery. The parents were known to carry the thalassemia gene with both of them being thalassemia minor. Antenatal screening had been done during this pregnancy and thalassemia major had been ruled out.

Physical examination revealed significant pallor with hepatosplenomegaly. Considering the possibility of thalassemia major, certain laboratory tests were ordered. They revealed marked anemia with reticulocytosis, and the fetal hemoglobin was 25%. It was inferred that an error had been made in the antenatal diagnosis, and this was indeed thalassemia major. So, this was the diagnosis that was announced, to the utter dismay of the parents.

Explanation...

When both the parents are thalassemia minor, it is quite likely that the baby could be thalassemia major, but such an infant would not *present so early* at two months of age. Therefore, other probabilities, such as disseminated infections (like TB, malaria, and torch group of infections) must be considered. Usually, torch group of infections would present with a low birth weight and hence are unlikely in this child. Storage disorders could present in a similar way but at a later age. On the other hand, malaria is likely, since pallor is the main presenting feature. Even though there was no fever and no maternal history of recent malaria, it was considered as a possibility since the *clinical manifestations* in this infant were *only hematological*. Such a presentation of malaria is known in early infancy; even the malarial parasite could be absent on the peripheral smear.

This infant was treated with antimalarial drugs. On further follow-up, investigations were repeated and were found to be normal.

The initial detection of 25% fetal hemoglobin was a part of the normally decreasing fetal hemoglobin at that age. Marked anemia with reticulocytosis was due to neonatal malaria.

In this infant, even if thalassemia major were to be confirmed on investigations, it would have meant a coincidental detection, in an infant who has presented with malaria.

At times, a disease may manifest at an unusual age. In such cases, other simulating conditions should be ruled out first.

Experience gained...

One should carefully consider the age at presentation as some conditions can be ruled out simply on this basis. In this case, it was obviously overlooked that thalassemia major never presents at two months of age. Even if thalassemia major were to be confirmed in this child on investigations, it would have meant a coincidental detection, in an infant who presented with malaria.

Other such examples include:
- The first episode of simple febrile seizure does not occur in early infancy or late childhood.
- Tuberculous pleural effusion does not occur in infancy and preschoolers.

CASE 3

■ History Begins with Age

Events...

An 8-month-old infant presented with recurrent episodes of cough and wheezing for the last three months. There was no history of any associated fever or cold. Nor was there any history of vomiting or choking preceding any of the episodes. Each episode took about two weeks to settle down; usually the infant was nebulized with bronchodilators and administered steroids. The father was an asthmatic. There was no history of atopic dermatitis in infant so far. After the third attack of wheezing, the infant was put on inhaled steroids, but the episodes continued in spite of compliant therapy.

Explanation...

Early onset asthma is known, but it is a diagnosis of exclusion in infancy. Aspiration syndromes due to various etiologies, hyper-reactive airways (in preterm babies and in those who suffered lung damage in the neonatal period), inhaled foreign body and congenital heart defects must be ruled out before one label an infant as asthmatic. Further, a poor response to bronchodilators in any case of suspected asthma in an infant, should alert us to these other possibilities. Since the diagnosis of asthma is basically a clinical diagnosis, investigations (for asthma) play a limited role in helping to confirm the diagnosis in the above situation; if the serum IgE is raised, it just helps indirectly by providing supportive evidence. Knowing that what looks like asthma in an infant, may not be so, an esophagogram was done in this infant, which revealed **esophageal stenosis**. When it was treated with repeated dilatation, the infant's 'asthma' disappeared. This esophageal stenosis must have resulted from an undiagnosed GER in early infancy.

Experience gained...

> Cough with wheeze in infancy must not be taken as asthma till other causes are ruled out, such as aspiration syndrome. Such infants may not necessarily vomit or give a history of choking episodes. Therefore, even in the absence of symptoms suggestive of aspiration syndrome, investigations must be planned to rule out GER, upper GI anomalies or palatopharyngeal incoordination, before labeling an infant as asthmatic.

CASE 4

■ Respect Chief Complaints

Events...

An 8-year-old child presented with an acute onset of severe abdominal pain. He had passed a few loose stools and had vomited once. There was no history of fever. He was diagnosed as acute gastroenteritis and treated accordingly. However, his condition worsened over the next day. Though he had not passed any more stools, he became toxic and had vomited a few times more. Subsequently he was diagnosed as **acute appendicitis** and was operated on in an emergency.

Explanation...

Whenever the patient presents with multiple symptoms, one needs to assign relative importance to each symptom. This child's chief complaint was severe abdominal pain and not loose stools or vomiting. However, more attention was focused on the loose stools, which retrospectively, was just an accompanying symptom due to irritation of the intestines because of an inflammatory pathology around. The initial symptom complex suggested a GI infection at first glance but the loose stools did not continue as expected, instead the chief complaint continued to be pain, so the alternative diagnosis of appendicitis was reached. To further elaborate the point, for example, acute hepatitis, acute gastroenteritis, and acute appendicitis may all present with the symptom complex of fever, vomiting and abdominal pain. However, in acute gastroenteritis, the chief complaint is diarrhea or vomiting and not abdominal pain, while in appendicitis, the pain dominates. Fever may often be an accompanying symptom of acute bacillary dysentery, while fever is uncommon in acute appendicitis. On the other hand, vomiting and nausea may be the *predominant* symptoms in hepatitis and not abdominal pain.

Experience gained...

> In case of multiple symptoms that the patient may complain of, while we do take into consideration the other symptoms, the chief complaint needs to be addressed properly. It often provides clues to the correct diagnosis.

CASE 5

■ Respect Chief Complaints
Events...

A 2-year-old child presented with recurrent bouts of severe cough for the last one year. Every time, the episode would start with a cold and cough, followed only at times by fever. The fever used to be mild and short lasting, but the cough was severe and often ended up with vomiting. It would last for a few weeks and would not settle down with antibiotics. Though the antibiotics were often changed, they did not work, and the episodes would recur. Clinical examination did not reveal any significant positive findings. Laboratory tests, whenever ordered, did not give any clues though the chest X-ray at times was reported as 'pneumonitis'; however, there was never a significant patch of haziness or infiltrates.

This child was investigated for recurrent respiratory tract infections and tests for tuberculosis were also carried out. In spite of the tuberculin test being negative, in view of the recurrent episodes, anti-TB drugs were tried, but without any benefit.

Explanation...

This child's most predominant complaint was severe cough, which meant an airway disease. Airway disease, especially lower airway involvement, is rarely due to bacterial infection. Therefore, it is no surprise that there was no response to antibiotics. Repeated viral infections may present as repeated cough and cold, but with fever on each occasion. Since fever was never a significant complaint in this child, viral infections are also ruled out. Cough is rarely a major symptom of childhood tuberculosis (exceptions being fibrocaseous cavitary tuberculosis and occasionally, a large paratracheal lymph node pressing over the airways). So, this is a noninfective condition. The most common noninfective airway disease is asthma. Details of the personal history or a family history of atopy may add to the possibility of asthma in this child. However, absence of such a history does not take us away from asthma in an appropriate clinical setting. It is worth noting that even if there is no apparent family history of atopy or asthma, *a history of recurrent respiratory complaints in the adult members of the family almost always indicates atopy*. It is well-known that asthma being episodic (and in cough equivalent asthma), there may not be any rhonchi at the time of clinical examination. Therefore, in such cases, the diagnosis is based purely on history. The X-ray being reported as 'pneumonitis' is quite common in such cases; these are areas of atelectasis or increased bronchovascular markings that are reported as pneumonitis.

Experience gained...

In case of multiple symptoms that the patient may complain of, while we do take into consideration the other symptoms, the chief complaint needs to be addressed properly. It often provides clues to the correct diagnosis.

For a clinician, the history of fever can often be misleading because it seems to suggest infection, though there may be none. It is important to realize that fever is a nonspecific symptom that can also represent noninfective inflammation or even noninflammatory conditions such as drug fever, heat fever, dehydration fever, thyrotoxicosis, and 'central' fever. In noninfective inflammatory conditions, the degree of fever correlates with the degree of inflammation. Thus, in asthma which is an allergic inflammatory disease, the patient often reports mild fever. On the other hand, in collagen vascular disorders, the fever can be quite high.

CASE 6

■ Origin Matters

Events...

An 8-year-old healthy child presented with an acute onset of high fever in the evening; by the next morning, he was breathless. Over the next 12 hours, the breathlessness increased considerably so that he had to get hospitalized. He was noted to have developed a large pleural effusion that was confirmed by a chest X-ray. The CBC showed a marked neutrophilic leukocytosis and the pleural fluid also demonstrated significant neutrophilia. Considering the diagnosis of an acute bacterial infection based on the acute onset of symptoms and neutrophilic leukocytosis, he was prescribed IV antibiotics after tapping the pleural cavity dry. At this point, an X-ray was repeated which did not show any underlying lung lesion. However, over the next two days, there was no response in the fever and the pleural fluid had collected again, sufficient to make him breathless again. So it was decided to put in a continuous intercostal drain and the antibiotics were continued. By now, the pleural fluid that had been cultured was reported as 'no growth'. However, with no change in the condition of the child in spite of an adequate draining system, the antibiotics were changed; but there was no benefit. It was at this point that he was shifted to a tertiary care center for further management of what looked like an unresolving empyema.

Explanation...

Empyema is a complication of an improperly treated bacterial pneumonia. In a healthy child of 8 years, it would have developed only after a few days of a poorly treated pneumonia. In this child, a pleural effusion (large enough to cause breathlessness) had developed within 24 hours of the onset of fever. Such a fluid collection, without an underlying lung lesion, favors the diagnosis of tuberculosis. If this fluid collection had developed over 4 or 5 days, it could have been an empyema, provided there was an underlying lung lesion. Thus, even in the presence of neutrophilic leukocytosis, this cannot be an empyema. Neutrophilic leukocytosis just indicates an acute inflammation, which is commonly due to a bacterial infection. However, inflammation may also be due to allergy or hypersensitivity, as it is seen in tuberculosis and collagen vascular disease. Conventional cytology and protein estimation may not always help to differentiate between the causes of a pleural effusion; other tests like pH, lactate, glucose, specific gravity and LDH may be necessary. An acute onset of pleural fluid collection may be traumatic, vascular (as in capillary leak), or allergic in origin. In this case, there was no history of trauma. Capillary leak syndrome is accompanied by signs of intravascular contraction and often, fluid collection is seen elsewhere in the body also. Hence, this is likely to be an allergic manifestation of an infection like tuberculosis. Once this child was started on anti-TB treatment, he showed improvement over the next two weeks.

Experience gained...

It is important to consider the origin of clinical symptomatology. The pathogenesis of symptoms that begin suddenly, is often traumatic, allergic, vascular, or neurogenic.

The clinical symptoms of any *infection* usually evolve over a few days; they do not start abruptly (except, may be in neonates or young infants). However, *complications of infections* may develop suddenly. This child presented abruptly with a complication of his primary infection (tuberculosis). The infection itself had remained undetected so far, because its symptoms were too subtle to be even noticed.

CASE 7

■ Origin Matters

Events...

A 6-year-old child presented with a moderate degree of fever and mild cough over the last four days. Initially, he was treated symptomatically but on the fourth day of persistence of symptoms, he was investigated. The CBC showed mild neutrophilic leukocytosis, and the chest X-ray was normal. He was put on amoxicillin considering it to be an acute respiratory infection. As there was no response after five days of antibiotic therapy, the tests were repeated. The CBC showed no change, while the chest X-ray, this time showed a middle lobe pneumonia on the right side. Considering it to be an amoxicillin-resistant pneumonia, the antibiotic was changed to IV Cefotaxime. However, a week passed without any significant response though there was no deterioration either. At this point, he was referred for a 'persistent pneumonia'.

Explanation...

What was overlooked was the fact that the first chest X-ray, done at the end of four days of onset of symptoms, was normal. In other words, till then, this child had not developed pneumonia. It was only by day nine of the illness, that a repeat chest X-ray revealed a pneumonia. This meant that the pneumonia in this child had developed over nine days. Clinical and radiological diagnosis of acute bacterial pneumonia is almost always evident within the first few days of onset of fever, more so when not treated with antibiotics during these first few days. Even though this child had been treated with antibiotics from day one, administration of oral antibiotics may influence (limit) the spread (extent) or complications of pneumonia; however, it cannot completely mask the presence of the pneumonia itself. Therefore, this was not acute bacterial pneumonia and hence there was a poor response to antibiotics. Thus, this was considered to be due to a subacute infection, such as tuberculosis. This was confirmed by a positive tuberculin test, and a CT scan which revealed a mediastinal lymphadenopathy with caseation along with the middle lobe pneumonia. Since, this was a slowly developing pneumonia due to tuberculosis, the child did not deteriorate in spite of improper treatment.

Experience gained...

> In this child, the subacute origin of the disease prompted the search for an alternative diagnosis, i.e., tuberculous pneumonia.

CASE 8

■ Do not Ignore Clinical Setting

Events...

A 10-year-old child presented with severe backache, following a fall while playing on the ground. Immediately after the fall, he could not get up. He was found to have a vertebral crack fracture, for which he was put in a plaster cast. He was noticed to have developed fever within a few hours of this incidence and was initially treated with paracetamol. As the fever continued over the next few days, it was thought that the fracture site might have got infected; so, IV antibiotics were prescribed. As the fever still did not subside, the plaster cast was removed to examine the wound. There was no evidence of local infection. So he was referred for a second opinion to find the cause of fever.

Explanation...

What was missed, was the fact that the fall was too trivial for a fracture to have occurred in a healthy child with no local bony abnormality or generalized bony disease. Further, a closed fracture can get infected only if the child is bacteremic at the time of trauma. In clinical practice, it sometimes 'appears' that trauma has precipitated an infection (if there is a local dormant infection as is sometimes seen in TBM, which seems to have been triggered off by a head injury). Even then, it will take at least 2–4 days for the clinical manifestations of the infection to develop; this child developed fever within a few hours of the fracture. Thus, both the occurrence of the fracture and the subsequent fever were unusual. Further laboratory tests revealed marked lymphocytic leukocytosis that strongly called for a bone marrow examination; it clinched the diagnosis of acute lymphocytic leukemia.

Experience gained...

> This child suffered from trauma that was too trivial to account for his fracture, i.e., it was a pathological fracture. Since there was neither any local abnormality nor a generalized bony demineralization, it became mandatory to search for a systemic disease. Thus, it is very important to consider the clinical setting in which the disease occurs; it may offer a clue to the hidden underlying problem.

CASE 9

■ Do not Ignore Clinical Setting

Events...

A 2-month-old infant presented with loose stools for the last two weeks. He had been on exclusive breastfeeding. The infant looked in good health and happy. He had gained adequate weight in spite of the frequent loose stools. He was investigated for probable infection. Routine stool microscopy did show a few pus cells and the stool culture grew *E. coli* sensitive to all the antibiotics. The infant continued to pass loose stools in spite of antibiotic therapy and hence was referred for further evaluation.

Explanation...

Exclusive breastfeeding cannot be a source of any infection and obviously this infant has been too healthy and normal in spite of his frequent loose stools. This does not need any investigations nor any therapy. The parents need to be reassured about this being normal for this infant. Though this 2-month-old baby complained of loose stools only since the last two weeks, it is well-known that in breastfed babies, the stool pattern may be extremely variable, both between two babies and in the same baby over time. In fact, an exclusively breastfed baby is well-protected against any serious infection; therefore, if such an infection does occur, it could prompt the search for an underlying defect, such as immune deficiency or cystic fibrosis. (Of course, in such cases there would also be failure to thrive, overtime). Sometimes, in the above setting, a history of occasional feeds of water is taken as supportive evidence in favor of an infection; however, such a history by itself should not necessarily suggest the diagnosis of a GI infection. The presence of a few pus cells in the stool does not suggest an infection. *E. coli* that was isolated from the stools may be a commensal.

Experience gained...

> The clinical setting of exclusive breastfeeding should alert the physician against the diagnosis of an intestinal infection. Moreover, the behavior of an infant is a fairly good marker to denote infection or otherwise.

CASE 10

■ Duration is Important

Events...

A 9-year-old child presented with fever for the last one year. There have been no other significant symptoms. The fever has been confirmed by recording the temperature. It has been erratic, not responding to antipyretics, but self-limiting. He has been otherwise maintaining normal health. Physical examination has never revealed any abnormality. He has undergone several investigations to rule out infections, collagen vascular disorders and malignancy. Factitious fever and drug fever were also considered and ruled out.

Explanation...

What was ignored in this child was the long duration of fever that had not disturbed the well-being of the child and had not led to any other symptoms or physical signs. The duration of fever really takes us away from infections which should have localized by now. The relative well-being of the child almost rules out any major illness; in fact, factitious fever is quite likely. However, in this child the fever has been confirmed and factitious causes ruled out. The non-response (absence of sweating) of the fever to antipyretics gives a clue to its 'central' nature characteristically central fever does not respond to antipyretics, i.e., there is no sweating. This is different from the lack of response typically encountered in the first two or three days of any acute febrile illness especially due to acute bacterial infection. Riley-Day syndrome may also present with undiagnosed fever; in these cases, absence of sweating and tears may offer a clue to the diagnosis. Ectodermal dysplasia may also present similarly; hair growth in such children is affected.

This turned out to be a hypothalamic tumor that resulted in a disturbance of the temperature regulating mechanism, leading to fever. Hypothalamic tumors are known to present in diverse manners, depending upon which area of the hypothalamic-pituitary axis is involved. Thus, they may present with endocrine manifestations, vision problems, or increased intracranial tension.

Experience gained...

> The duration of symptoms often gives a clue to the probable diagnosis as in this child. At the least, it helps to rule out certain conditions that may not last that long.
>
> The duration of a symptom often helps in assessing its probable cause. When a symptom persists for a long time, it offers an insight into the longitudinal progress of the underlying condition. In general, the longer the duration of symptoms in a child who has remained reasonably well, lesser is the chance of it being a serious problem. This is true especially in the case of a single isolated symptom. For example, abdominal pain for many months or years without any other significant symptom would suggest a functional disorder and in such a case, investigations are unlikely to help in the diagnosis of the condition. Similarly, an isolated symptom of headache for a long duration without any other disturbance is likely to be a benign problem. However, documented fever is an exception to this rule as we found in this case of hypothalamic tumor.

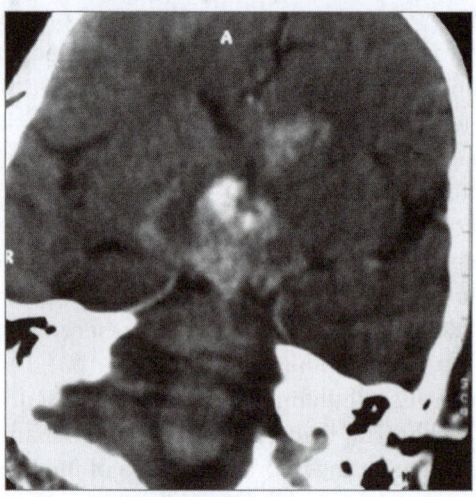

Hypothalamic tumor.

CASE 11

■ Caution against Unexpected Progress

Events...

A 5-year-old child presented with high fever and mild cough for the last four days. Physical examination showed signs of a pneumonia on the right side, that was confirmed radiologically. The CBC showed a marked neutrophilic leukocytosis. So the child was put on IV Augmentin. Since there was no response even after four days of IV antibiotic therapy, the investigations were repeated. There was a further increase in the leukocyte counts, with thrombocytosis. However, the chest X-ray surprisingly demonstrated resolution of the right-sided pneumonia, but a small patch of pneumonia had now appeared on the left side. The treating physician considered a change of antibiotics, which produced no benefit. Repeat tests showed worsening counts as well as increasing haziness on the left side.

Explanation...

This child apparently had a quickly resolving pneumonia on the right side and a newly developing pneumonia on the left side, *while on the same given line of treatment*. This is most unexpected, since a bacterial pneumonia is normally expected to show symptomatic improvement within a few days, but may take two weeks or more to resolve radiologically. Development of another pneumonia on the other side, later, is also rare in bacterial infections. While this child continued to be highly febrile, his original lung lesion on the right side had disappeared. Therefore, there seemed to be a radiological clearance before even symptomatic improvement. This suggested that the pneumonia could have been an inflammatory lesion that was noninfective. Lesions that appear acutely and also disappear quickly, only to reappear again, could be allergic phenomena. Thus, this child was diagnosed to have Wegener granulomatosis.

Experience gained...

> An unanticipated progress of the disease, which may otherwise be easily misinterpreted, offers a clue to the final diagnosis.

CASE 12

■ Sudden Improvement may be Ominous

Events...

An 8-month-old infant presented with diarrhea for the last 3 days. He was seen by the family doctor who prescribed symptomatic therapy. The diarrhea came under control abruptly. The parents were happy, though the infant continued to be irritable. Over the next few hours, he started vomiting and had developed abdominal distention. These symptoms were ascribed to crying and aerophagy. It was only later that it was realized that he had developed intestinal obstruction due to **intussusception**.

Explanation...

Frequency of stools in a diarrheal disease diminishes gradually and never abruptly. Such a sudden change may signify a complication such as paralytic ileus or a more serious underlying disorder as in this case. Sudden improvement may occasionally be seen in a self-limiting disease but in that case the patient is doing well in all the parameters. Moreover, vomiting is often reported at the *onset* of a diarrheal disease, often before the appearance of loose stools and it is usually relieved within a short period. In this infant, not only did the diarrhea stop abruptly, but the vomiting also started later in the course of events, thereby offering vital clues.

Experience gained...

> Sudden abrupt improvement is rare in clinical practice and must be considered as a sign of complication rather than quick improvement. The sequence of improvement in the various symptoms and clinical parameters is usually quite typical for a given condition. In case of an atypical sequence in an apparently improving situation, close observation is mandatory for any unusual complications.

CASE 13

■ Beware of Partial Improvement

Events...

A 2-month-old infant presented with fever for two days. There were no other significant symptoms. He was seen by the family doctor who prescribed amoxicillin. Over the next two days, the fever reduced, though the infant was irritable. The same line of treatment was continued, and then suddenly by the 5th day of the illness, he was found to be deteriorating, with a higher degree of fever—he looked very sick. At this stage, the antibiotic was changed to IV cefotaxime. However, the next day, he developed a generalized seizure that lasted for more than an hour. He was hospitalized, where he was diagnosed to have **multiple brain abscesses** with bacterial meningitis.

Explanation...

In any illness, particularly at two months of age, behavior is very important—undue lethargy, undue irritability, poor feeding, etc. cannot be ignored. Irritability is a common symptom in many pediatric illnesses; however, one needs to distinguish between *'pathological irritability'* and *'irritability as a logical fallout of the illness'*. So in this infant, even though the fever did reduce for two days, the behavior of the infant should have warned the physician against recovery, prompting urgent evaluation and intervention. Further, since the fever returned in spite of continued treatment, it was a clear indication that something was amiss. It obviously suggested that a partially suppressed infection had come back with a vengeance, probably with a serious complication.

Experience gained...

Partial improvement in this child was considered to be a favorable sign because it always offers hopes of a successful outcome by continuing with the same strategy; however, this may turn out to be fallacious and dangerous, as in this case. An erroneous interpretation of partial improvement delayed the diagnosis in this child, leaving behind permanent brain damage.

This illustration also emphasizes the risk of empirical antibiotic therapy, especially in young infants. This infant would have been saved from permanent neurological damage, even if antibiotic therapy had been delayed by a day or two and started only after relevant investigations.

At this point, it is worth noting that in case of a routine viral infection in an older child, the fever generally disappears within 3–4 days. But following that, generalized weakness may often be complained of, which in fact, was not appreciated so much even at the peak of the illness. This may be especially related to low body potassium as a result of poor intake, in the face of continued excretion of potassium by the renal tubules. This leads to muscle weakness.

Our cultural practice of drinking coconut water during the recovery phase of an illness has a sound basis!

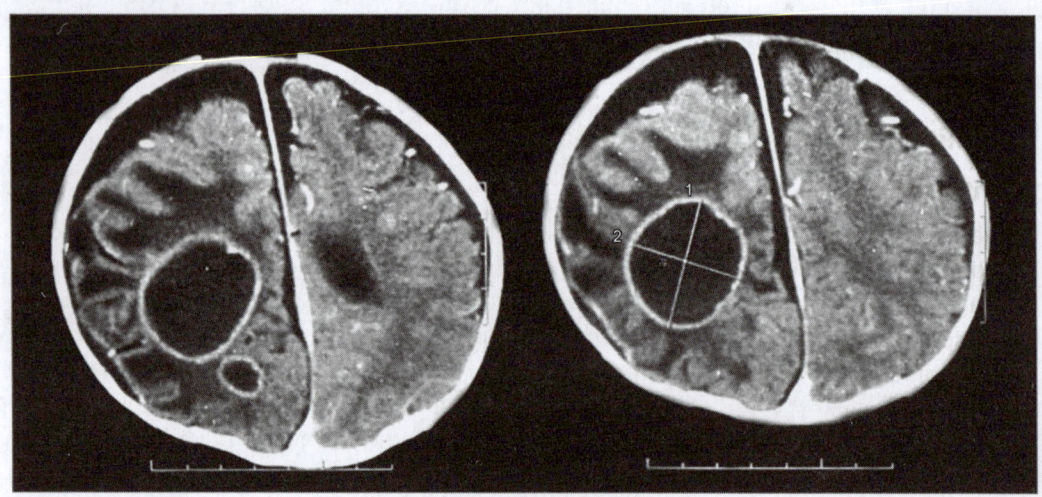

Multiple brain abscesses.

CASE 14A to C

■ Monitor Progress of Fever: Biphasic Fever

Events... (A)

A 2-year-old presented with high fever and a cold for two days. He was diagnosed to have a viral infection and treated symptomatically. Fever subsided after another two days and returned after a gap of a day. However, the fever was moderate this time and lasted for just two days before settling down by itself.

This was typically a viral infection with biphasic fever in which the second part of fever was milder and shorter.

Events... (B)

A 10-year-old child presented with moderate fever, cold and a mild cough for the last two days. He was diagnosed to have a viral infection and prescribed symptomatic therapy. The fever subsided over the next 2 days, only to return after a gap of another 2 days. Considering it to be a secondary bacterial infection, an antibiotic was started. However, the fever continued to be high, and he developed a seizure after six days of onset of the second bout of fever. Spinal tap done at that time showed only a few lymphocytes without any other abnormality. The culture did not grow any organism. Subsequently, this child was confirmed to be a case of leptospirosis.

Events... (C)

A 2-year-old child presented with fever, cold and mild cough for two days. Considering it to be a viral infection, he was treated symptomatically. He developed a macular skin rash following which the fever subsided. It appeared that the illness was over, and the parents were reassured accordingly. However, by the next day, he was looking drowsy, though there was no fever or any other symptoms reported by the parents. Physical examination revealed signs of shock and the child required a large amount of IV fluids for adequate resuscitation. This was dengue shock syndrome. In such cases, symptoms of circulatory failure are often picked up by a change in behavior and reduced urine output.

Explanation...

The first two children (cases 14A and B) both had a biphasic fever. Such biphasic fevers can be viral, or due to infections known to have a secondary immune phase. The first child (14A) typically had a viral infection. Though his fever was biphasic, the second phase of fever was milder and shorter. As against this, the second child (14B) had a biphasic fever with a short lasting, self-limiting first phase, followed by a prolonged and complicated second phase. Viral fevers are self-limiting, whereas in this child, the fever continued and was more prolonged and severe, thereby suggesting immune mediated complications following a primary infection that may have already subsided.

Further, if a secondary bacterial infection is suspected in a viral fever, it should be clinically localized to a specific anatomical site/organ. Such secondary bacterial infection in a primary viral infection is rare, except in severe viral infections like measles. Also, failure to respond to an antibiotic in a reasonable time should have prompted a review.

Clinically, the third child (case 14C) also had a viral fever. However, just as he seemed to have almost recovered from his fever, he suddenly ran into a serious life-threatening complication and was luckily saved.

Experience gained...

> The above three cases emphasize the need to 'announce' a cure only after sustained improvement for a certain length of time. Such an observation period varies from illness to illness. For a viral fever, it is important to follow a child for 3–4 days even after the illness seems to be over. Capillary leak syndrome in Dengue fever may typically occur at the defervescence of fever and may catch the physicians by surprise and may endanger life. On the other hand, if the fever turns out to be a biphasic fever, it is important to follow the progress of the second phase of the febrile episode. If it is shorter and milder, no action is necessary. This is not uncommon in influenza and parainfluenza. One just needs to reassure the parents. However, if it is severe and prolonged, one needs to watch for organ involvement and dysfunction; it may suggest an immune-mediated complication of the primary illness.

CASE 15

Past—A Lead for the Future

Events...

An 8-year-old child presented with high fever for the last six days. There were no other significant symptoms, except that he had developed a skin rash after 2 days of fever. At that time, though there was no clinical localization of any infection, laboratory tests showed neutrophilic leukocytosis while urinalysis and X-ray chest were normal. Hence, an antibiotic was arbitrarily started; however, there was no response. In view of the skin rash and the neutrophilic leukocytosis, the differential diagnosis of bacterial infections with a skin rash was reviewed. Since a broad-spectrum antibiotic had already failed, a drug-resistant streptococcal infection or a rickettsial infection was considered and the patient started on tetracycline. However, there was still no response, so the patient was sent for a second opinion.

When asked about a history of any major illness in the past, the parents reported a pneumonia at four years of age, an episode of arthritis a year later (which was investigated for rheumatic fever, but the reports were normal and the child had recovered), and an admission for nephritis last year, which recovered after a few months.

Explanation...

When any child reports three major illnesses in the past, it is likely that they are the manifestations of the same disease process rather than a chance occurrence of different diseases. Since different organs have been involved, it appears to be a multisystem disease. However, these illnesses involving different organs have occurred over a few years, at different times. Therefore, conditions like a disseminated infection, storage disorders or immune deficiency are unlikely. In other words, this history suggested the possibility of a **collagen vascular disease** involving multiple organs. This was subsequently confirmed by relevant tests. Normally, on the 6th day of any febrile illness, it is not easy to suspect collagen vascular disease and one would logically keep chasing an infection. However, this past history of major illnesses helps to suspect collagen vascular disease at such an early stage of the fever. Unfortunately, in day-to-day practice, one often skips the past history while evaluating for what looks like a small acute illness.

Experience gained...

As a part of our basic undergraduate training, it has been standard teaching to enquire about a past history of similar illness or any major illness. If these basic protocols are skipped, one may miss important leads to the diagnosis. Thus, the past history may lead to the correct diagnosis of the present illness, even when the current illness manifests quite differently and therefore, may apparently seem to be unrelated. There are other subtle physical signs of collagen vascular disorders that one must keep in mind and they include mouth ulcers, nail abnormalities and alopecia. A direct enquiry about such symptoms in the past may be important to diagnose the present illness.

CASE 16

■ Attention to Personal History
Events...

An 8-month-old infant presented with vomiting for the last two months. There were no other symptoms reported by the parents. Physical examination did not reveal any abnormality. So this was initially considered as forced feeding and the parents were reassured. However, on persistence of the complaints, the infant was thoroughly investigated for gastrointestinal, hepatic, renal and central nervous system disease but all the tests were negative. Symptomatic treatment did not give any relief either. He was referred for psychological assessment, but that was also noncontributory.

Explanation...

Since there was no clue to the possible diagnosis based on the presenting complaints and the physical examination, it was imperative to look beyond and get into the details of other parts of the history. When enquired about his personal history, it came to be known that this infant had marked anorexia, constipation, polyuria, and irritability besides vomiting. He had obviously failed to thrive though that was ascribed to persistent vomiting. Neither parents nor doctors had concentrated on personal history; instead, vomiting was considered to be the sole symptom. Anorexia was attributed to the primary disease process, but the disease itself was elusive since anorexia does not have a localizing value. Constipation was explained on the lack of intake and therefore not given much importance. Irritability was ascribed to his prolonged illness, which had resulted in near starvation and lots of medical intervention. Normally one would miss asking for the history of urination as part of the personal history; here, when the mother was asked about urination (partly to judge the adequacy of hydration) she surprisingly came out with polyuria. This was really the clue when taken as a constellation of symptoms along with constipation, anorexia, and irritability. This led to the suspicion of a diagnosis of **idiopathic hypercalcemia**. Serum calcium was 16 mg%. The infant was treated with steroids and recovered within a few days.

Based on the complaint of vomiting and the history of polyuria, one could also have considered chronic renal failure; however, this infant was absolutely normal till 6 months of age; further, the blood urea and serum creatinine done as part of the multiple investigations for vomiting were also normal.

Chronic adrenal failure (Addison's disease) can also present with vomiting and lethargy; however, this is per se an uncommon disease, more so, rare at this age. Further, polyuria is not a feature.

Inborn errors of metabolism could also present with persistent vomiting. However, they would usually present earlier in infancy and would be progressive, i.e., they would result in additional clinical features such as convulsions, mental retardation, or organomegaly.

Experience gained...

This case illustrates the importance of detailed history taking, particularly when there is no clue to the diagnosis, and when laboratory tests have also failed. But for personal history, this infant's diagnosis was elusive even after several laboratory tests were carried out. In a case of persistent vomiting, routinely one is unlikely to ask for calcium studies; unless of course, one is prompted by the history of polyuria.

CASE 17

■ First Impression

Events…

An 8-year-old child presented with fever and increasing breathlessness over the last four days. Physical examination revealed a massive pleural effusion. Pleural tap showed hemorrhagic fluid. Since pleural effusion that develops acutely is often tuberculous, and since hemorrhagic effusions are known in TB, he was started on anti-TB treatment. But over the next few days the child kept on deteriorating.

What was missed in this child was the fact that he looked pale and very sick in spite of drainage of the pleural fluid. This was obviously overlooked. A CT scan of the chest showed a large mass that was proved to be a **pleural endothelioma** that had led to the hemorrhagic pleural effusion. A child with tuberculous pleural effusion may be breathless but does not appear pale and sick and becomes reasonably comfortable after drainage of the pleural fluid.

Explanation…

First impression is also described as appearance, which is evaluated while evaluating the ABC of any child presenting to the emergency department. In this, we primarily evaluate whether the child is sick or not sick. Later, all through the steps of diagnosis and management, one would keep concentrating on the specific clinical findings and sideline the relevance of this overall general impression (of sick or not sick).

It is worth noting that as against a TB pleural effusion, a child with empyema would also look sick and pale; in this case, the hemorrhagic fluid ruled it out.

If we look at all TB pleural effusions, only a few of them are hemorrhagic. However, if we look at all hemorrhagic pleural effusions, TB may be a cause, besides malignancy and pancreatic disorders. Therefore, it is not surprising that a TB effusion was thought of. It is also worth noting that when, there is a *massive* unilateral hemorrhagic effusion, malignancy has to be a close differential. The plain X-ray just showed the massive effusion and did not show the mass hiding under the fluid. Therefore, the AKT could have dragged on for some more time, but for these considerations prompting the search for an alternative diagnosis. It is also worth looking for subtle clues like rib erosion in such a plain X-ray which could point to malignancies like Ewing's sarcoma.

Occasionally, the first impression can be deceptive, as when a child is seen in high fever; he may look sick at the peak of fever but may look different when the fever subsides temporarily following an antipyretic.

Experience gained...

A mere look at the patient from a distance (the first impression), may offer an important clue to a probable diagnosis, and is certainly a parameter to go by when considering the need for urgent intervention.

Other examples where the 'look' of the child helps in the diagnosis include:
- Acute onset purpura with a sick look (leukemia) as against not sick (ITP)
- Generalized edema with a sick look (CCF, liver disease, hypoproteinemia) as against a happy child (nephrotic syndrome)
- Nephrotic syndrome with a sick look (infection)
- A 'confused state' suggesting hypoxia in a child with pneumonia
- 'Extreme irritability' in a child with diarrhea suggesting hypernatremia.

Similarly, a lot of information can be derived by a 'first look' at the posture or gait of a child. It can help in the evaluation of the motor system as one can assess power, tone, coordination and abnormal movements.

Observing an infant play with a toy can provide similar information.

'First look' may not be restricted to acutely ill children.

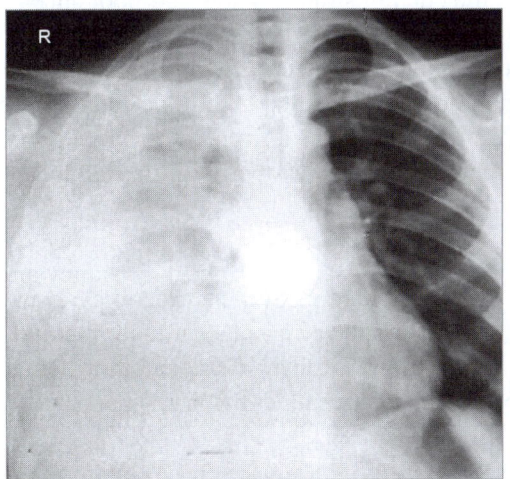

Massive pleural effusion.

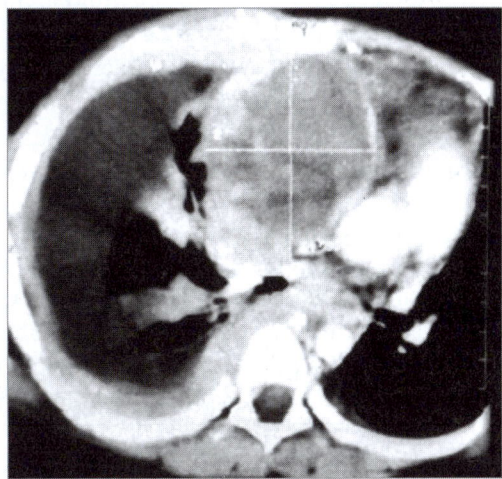

CT scan showing pleural endothelioma.

CASE 18

■ General Examination is Special

Events...

A 1-day-old neonate was referred for lethargy and poor sucking noticed at 12 hours after birth. The baby was hypothermic but did not improve even after thermal control. Considering it to be early sepsis, a septic screen was ordered, and IV antibiotics were started. The septic screen came negative and there was no response to antibiotics. However, there was no deterioration either. At this point, a metabolic screen was also negative (specifically, hypoglycemia had also been ruled out). So he was referred for an opinion.

Explanation...

General examination revealed significant bradycardia, quite contrary to the expectation of tachycardia due to probable sepsis. Once bradyarrhythmia was ruled out, this gave a clue to the diagnosis of **hypothyroidism**. It was confirmed by hormonal assessment. In fact, the USG demonstrated a complete absence of the thyroid gland; this could probably explain such an early presentation. Usually, hypothyroid infants may demonstrate lethargy and poor sucking *after a few days* of birth, *not on D1*.

Bradycardia could be a late sign of sepsis; in this infant, early sepsis was being suspected, and in fact, over time, there was no deterioration either. Congenital heart block could have been a possibility; but if such a patient was symptomatic (in the form of lethargy and poor sucking as in this case), there would have been other findings suggestive of cardiac failure.

Experience gained...

> It was simply the basics of general examination that guided us to the correct diagnosis. There are many other similar examples of how a systematic physical examination could have saved the day. Not palpating the peripheral pulses have led to many a coarctation being missed. Not taking blood pressure has led to many encephalopathies being mismanaged.

CASE 19

■ Correlate Temperature, Pulse and Respiration (TPR)

Events...

A 6-month-old infant presented with acute onset of breathlessness over a day. He had minimal cold but no cough. Physical examination revealed a heart rate of 160/min, respiratory rate of 80/min, with a normal body temperature and hepatomegaly. There was a doubtful soft systolic murmur; in this setting, it prompted the treating doctor to consider the possibility of a congenital heart defect leading to cardiac failure. An echocardiogram was asked for, that turned out to be normal. Considering it to be early myocarditis, the infant was digitalized. However, he suddenly improved unexpectedly within the next two days. He had suffered from acute viral bronchiolitis.

Explanation...

It should have been evident that his respiratory rate was relatively much faster than his heart rate, with a ratio of 1:2. It spelt a primary respiratory problem rather than a cardiac problem. In normal infants, the ratio of the respiratory rate to the heart rate is around 1:3, which gradually shifts to the adult ratio of 1:4 overtime. Unexplained, but proportionate (i.e., with their relative ratio maintained) tachypnea and tachycardia, in a clinical situation of fever and leukocytosis may spell early sepsis. A disproportionate increase in any one of the parameters helps in deciding the primary problem.

In infants with fever, the heart rate may increase disproportionately because the cardiac output can largely be increased only by increasing the heart rate; the stroke volume cannot be changed significantly. On the other hand, the respiratory rate does not increase to the same extent, because partial compensation can also be achieved by increasing the depth of respiration. Similarly, in the presence of therapeutic interventions (which may upset this ratio), a cautious interpretation is advisable. Lastly, all this is more relevant at the onset of the disease as the disease progresses compensatory phenomena and secondary metabolic derangements may alter the proportions of respiratory and cardiac rate.

Experience gained...

> Correlating the TPR parameters with one another often gives a proper direction to the primary problem.

CASE 20

■ Observe Pattern of Breathing

Events...

A 4-week-old infant presented with 'breathlessness' as reported by the parents. They noticed it over the last two days. There were no other significant symptoms reported by them; however, on direct questioning they thought that the baby was lethargic and feeding poorly. He had a respiratory rate of 60/min and a heart rate of 145/min with a normal body temperature. The systemic examination was essentially normal. He was suspected to have early sepsis, and was investigated and treated accordingly. The septic screen was normal, while the chest X-ray showed a doubtful collection of a small amount of air in the pleural cavity. An attempt to drain the air from the pleural cavity failed.

Explanation...

What was not observed, was the breathing pattern. This infant had no dyspnea as evident by absence of chest retractions; it was tachypnea without dyspnea. His breathing was deep and rapid. So this was neither a respiratory nor a cardiac problem. It was metabolic acidosis. There was no air in the pleural cavity; sometimes, such areas of hyperlucency are erroneously imagined/suspected. Anyway, a small amount of air in the pleural cavity could not have explained the tachypnea. This turned out to be **renal tubular acidosis**.

If an ABG would have been done, it would have shown metabolic acidosis, which at first glance would appear to be consistent with sepsis; however, on studying the anion gap, the cause could have been differentiated. Also, the severity of the acidosis would have been disproportionate to the degree of circulatory compromise.

When an infant is brought for sepsis, 'breathlessness' is not *complained* of; tachypnea is just noted by the doctor. The parents are more likely to complain of fever, lethargy, poor feeding. In this case, these were elicited on direct questioning, whereas the chief complaint was 'breathlessness'.

Experience gained...

> The pattern of breathing must be observed; it may offer a clue to the site of disease.

CASE 21

■ Listen to the Sounds that Breathing Makes

Events...

An 8-month-old *undernourished* infant presented with diarrhea for three days prior to hospitalization. He was referred as he had developed tachypnea. Since he did not have any chest retractions, it was considered to be metabolic acidosis, and fluid resuscitation was carried out. However, though the hydration improved, the respiratory rate did not improve. At this stage renal tubular acidosis was considered, and pending laboratory results, a trial of therapy with soda-bicarb was instituted; but it failed.

Explanation...

What was missed in this infant was the fact that this infant had lost his voice, and the breathing was shallow. It was voiceless breathlessness. Most of the infants with breathlessness are irritable; in fact, crying may be one way of manifestation of breathlessness in an infant. Obviously, this infant had a respiratory muscle weakness which was due to marked **hypokalemia**. It was also noticed that he had a paucity of limb movements.

It is well known that the 'sounds' generated during breathing lead to the localization of the disease, but usually a lack of voice is missed. Stridor indicates upper airway inspiratory obstruction, wheeze denotes a lower airway expiratory obstruction and a grunt indicates lung parenchymal involvement and an attempt to increase end-expiratory pressure—it may suggest impending respiratory failure. On the other hand, absence of voice suggests respiratory muscle weakness. It may result from respiratory muscle paralysis as in poliomyelitis or GBS, though in this child it was due to severe hypokalemia.

Similarly, in a case of respiratory distress, one often thinks of metabolic causes in addition to respiratory and cardiac; however, a neuroparalytic cause is often not thought of.

Experience gained...

> Observation of the pattern of breathing and listening to the noise produced during respiration helps to localize the anatomical site of disease and is an important part of physical examination.

CASE 22

■ Nail Down the Diagnosis

Events...

An 8-year-old child was noticed to have mild cyanosis on cursory examination by the primary doctor who saw him for a mild viral respiratory infection. Knowing that cyanosis was not due to the viral infection, he rightly suggested a specialist's opinion. The child was referred to a cardiologist his asymptomatic cyanosis. The cardiologist found nothing abnormal on physical examination, and the chest X-ray, ECG and echocardiogram were also normal. Considering it to be a probable case of pulmonary arteriovenous fistula that can be missed by routine investigational modalities, he planned a pulmonary angiogram and a radionuclide scan; both these tests ruled out any such anomaly. At this point, he was referred for a pediatric opinion.

Explanation...

Though this child had a mild central cyanosis, there was no clubbing of nails. This suggested that that the cyanosis must have appeared recently. On physical examination, it was clear that this child was stunted and had failed to thrive. On direct questioning, the parents said that this child always liked to sit and play as he would complain of tiredness even on routine walking, and over the years this complaint had been getting worse. This gave the clue to a chronic respiratory disease with a gradually developing respiratory failure in this child, and it was proved to be due to **chronic interstitial lung disease**. He was in a state of compensated respiratory failure for a long time though over the last few months, he had gone into a decompensated phase and that is when he presented with mild cyanosis.

Experience gained...

> Cyanosis without clubbing suggests cyanosis of recent onset and this fact was totally overlooked by even a super-specialist who searched for a nonexistent cardiovascular defect.

CASE 23

■ Stick Out the Neck

Events...

An 8-year-old child presented with abdominal distention noticed over the last two months. There were no other significant symptoms. Physical examination revealed marked abdominal distention with a firm hepatomegaly without splenomegaly or jaundice. This was considered to be compensated cirrhosis without liver cell failure. Liver function tests showed a mild increase in the liver enzymes, with normal proteins and other parameters. A liver biopsy was planned, but the parents refused and opted for another opinion.

Explanation...

What looked superficially like a cirrhotic liver disease was in fact, a case of **constrictive pericarditis**. This child had engorged neck veins without a hepatojugular reflux, and this had been missed.

Experience gained...

> It is important to look at the neck veins especially in a child with hepatomegaly. Any congested liver may result in a mild elevation of the liver enzymes. This may further confuse the clinician as to it being a primary liver disease.

CASE 24

■ Stretch your Imagination
Events...

A 4-year-old child presented with a gradually increasing abdominal distention over the last one year. The mother did notice the protuberant abdomen ever since the age of one year, but her doctor reassured her that this was normal for an infant and a toddler. As the child was otherwise normal, his mother accepted her doctor's view, though with a bit of suspicion. However, over the last one year, she was sure that the abdomen was getting more distended. So she insisted on an abdominal ultrasound. It was reported as localized ascites. Considering this to be the result of a chronic infection, the child was investigated for tuberculosis. The Mantoux test led to an induration of 8 mm and the chest X-ray was normal. Nevertheless, he was put on anti-TB therapy. After two months of compliant therapy, the abdominal ultrasound was repeated, only to find that the localized ascites had increased in size. This made the treating physician consider a diagnosis of multidrug resistant tuberculosis, and second-line anti-TB drugs were prescribed. At this stage, the parents sought another opinion.

Explanation...

Physical examination revealed an umbilicus that was unilaterally stretched. This led to a clinical diagnosis of a localized collection of fluid, without any systemic symptoms and hence this was considered to be a cyst. It was proved to be a **mesenteric cyst** that was subsequently operated.

Experience gained...

> The simple observation of a unilaterally stretched umbilicus was good enough to suggest the correct diagnosis. We are all aware of a 'smiling umbilicus' and this was half smiling.

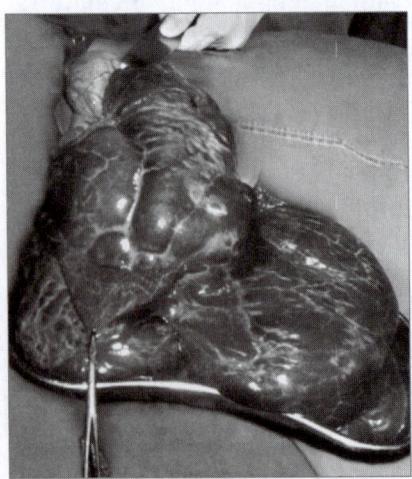

Mesenteric cyst removed surgically.

CASE 25

■ Head Start

Events...

An 8-month-old infant presented with high fever for the last one month. There were no other significant symptoms. Physical examination did not reveal anything significant. Several tests were ordered, but there was no clue to the diagnosis. Trials with various antibiotics had also failed. The infant was getting more and more sick and irritable and had started failing to thrive. The fever continued to be high. At this stage, the child was referred for an opinion.

Moving the hand over the head of the infant, as is often a reflex with most pediatricians while beginning their examination, it was realized that there was a small lump on the scalp. That led to the diagnosis of neuroblastoma with secondary deposits over the scalp.

Experience gained...

> Examination of the head should be a reflex and may offer important clues to the diagnosis.

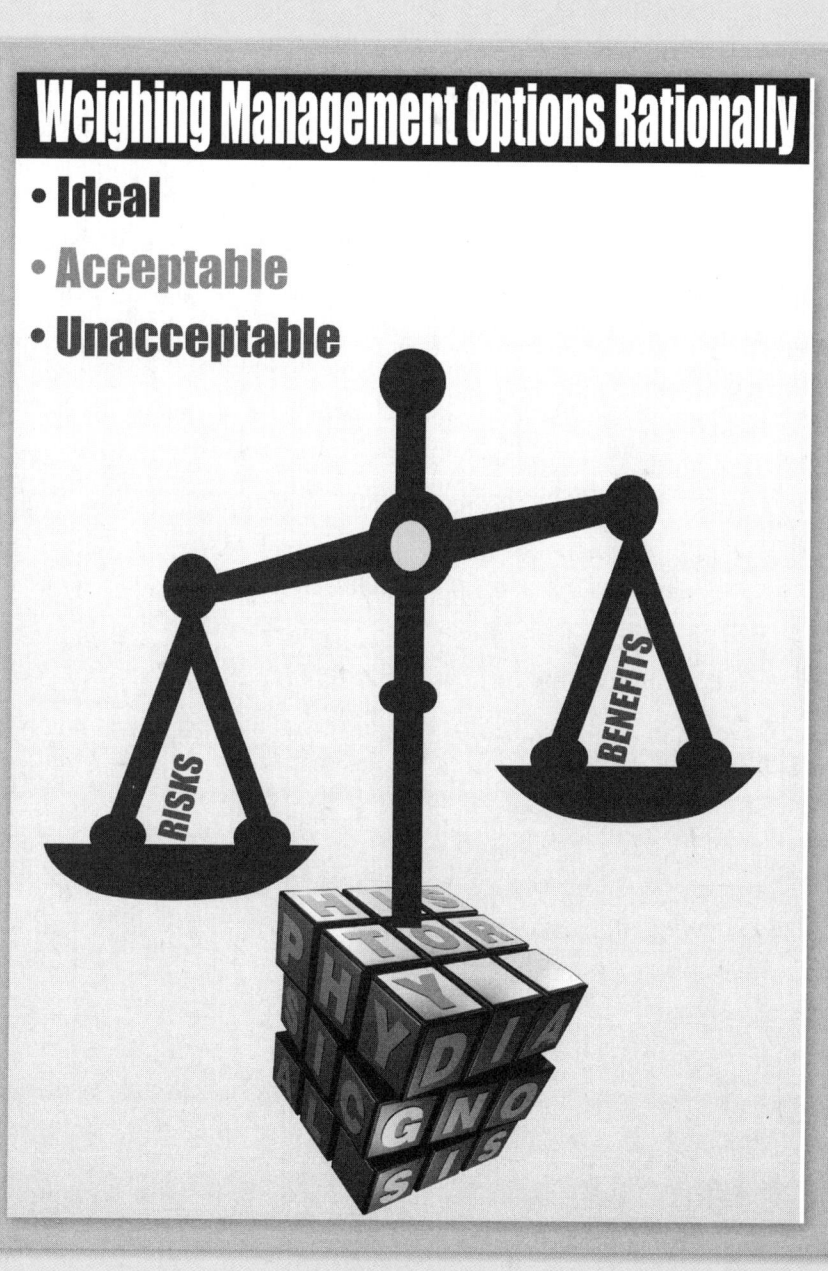

SECTION 2

Management Dilemmas in Office Practice

■ Management Dilemmas in Office Practice

Having reached a diagnosis, there could be different ways of managing the same illness. The various options may apparently look similar. However, a particular option may actually be more correct than the others. Obviously, one would like to choose the **ideal option**. But, if for some reason, such an option is not available, one would accept the next best alternative—**acceptable** option. As against this, certain management options may be scientifically **unacceptable**.

In order to be able to take the right decision and choose the correct action, one must have a probable clinical diagnosis. This, in turn, heavily depends on a detailed history followed by a thorough clinical examination. Once a provisional diagnosis is made, one needs to define the anticipated course of events in the next few days. The options discussed are based on the provisional diagnosis as on initial assessment and the anticipated course of events. In case of any deviation from the expected, the options will change.

While deciding the management options that are ideal or acceptable, one has to take into account two things. The first is the risk of morbidity and mortality, in case the action chosen initially turns out to be wrong. Secondly, one has to also consider the increased difficulty in subsequent assessment that may be created by such an action. For example, prior antibiotic therapy may viciate subsequent bacteriological diagnosis. Similarly, the use of potent antipyretics like nimesulide may interfere with subsequent clinical monitoring of the patient.

These above-mentioned steps are applicable to every subsequent case regarding management issues that is discussed in the following pages.

CASE 26

Viral Fever

Events...

A 4-year-old child presented with fever, cough, cold and headache for two days. He was seen by a pediatrician, diagnosed as throat infection, and started on oral cefadroxil and nimesulide. Fever subsided within a day of starting therapy but recurred after an interval of two days in spite of continued therapy.

What are the options for further management?

In order to be able to take the right decision and choose the correct action, one must have a probable clinical diagnosis, for which many more details in the history need to be known. This history is too inadequate for proper analysis. This should be followed by a thorough clinical examination.

In direct questioning, the following details were available:

The fever was moderate to high in intensity right at the onset and responded temporarily to antipyretics. The child looked normal during the period when he was afebrile. There was a significant cold and cough accompanying the fever, while the child had a headache only at the peak of fever. There were no other symptoms. He did not suffer from repeated colds and cough in the past. Another sibling in the family suffered from a similar illness a few days ago.

The clinical examination revealed a mildly congested throat. The rest of the examination was normal.

Analysis

Analysis of the history suggests a *probable viral infection* in view of the sudden onset of moderate to high fever (which responds temporarily to antipyretics), the accompanying symptoms of significant cold and cough, the biphasic pattern of fever (common viral infections may have a biphasic pattern of fever with the second phase of fever being short) and the absence of response to an antibiotic (the lack of response cannot mean a resistant bacterial infection, since the child was afebrile in between). Headache occurring only at the peak of fever rules out intracranial infection. Any other serious infection is less likely. In this child, it is expected that the fever will subside shortly.

While deciding the management options that are ideal or acceptable, one has to take into account two things. The first is the risk of morbidity and mortality, in case the action chosen initially, turns out to be wrong. Secondly, one has to also consider the increased difficulty in subsequent assessment that may be created, by such an action. For example, prior antibiotic therapy may viciate subsequent bacteriological diagnosis. Similarly, the use of potent antipyretics like nimesulide may interfere with subsequent clinical monitoring of the patient.

These above-mentioned steps are applicable to every subsequent case regarding management issues that is discussed in the following pages.

Ideal Option—Stopping Antibiotic

Since the provisional diagnosis is a viral infection, stopping Cefadroxil is acceptable. Anyway, it is clear that this antibiotic has not worked in this child, because the fever recurred in spite of the antibiotic being continued. Such an action is also safe, since the child is stable, and the clinical examination is essentially normal. Even if one is worried about a partially treated respiratory bacterial infection, it is safe to wait and review, as the subsequent action can be more specific. As mentioned earlier, it is anticipated that this child's fever will subside shortly. If it does not, it is mandatory to review the child. In fact, this review is the safeguard against any catastrophe. Therefore, stopping the antibiotic and following up the child is not only acceptable and safe, but also it is the *ideal and the only acceptable option* at this point.

Unacceptable Option—Continue Antibiotic or Change Antibiotic

Continuing the same antibiotic has no rationale in this child as fever did recur in spite of the antibiotic being continued and that clearly denotes failure of Cefadroxil. Change of antibiotic is totally irrational since, as of now, there is no probability of it being a bacterial infection. Even if one considers a probable bacterial infection, it may be best to define the site and etiology of infection before choosing another antibiotic. A common excuse used to change/continue antibiotics is the alleged inaccessibility of the patient to further follow-up. In fact, if this is so, it is all the more dangerous to continue antibiotics in the absence of a clear diagnosis.

Case Progression

If the fever does not subside in the next two days...

It is important to repeat a *thorough physical examination.* It is possible that physical signs of an infection which had been inadvertently partially treated, or which has now evolved and localized, may be now apparent. If so, the patient needs to be accordingly treated, with or without appropriate confirmatory investigations, as needed. However, if one is confident about the absence of physical signs suggestive of a bacterial infection in this child, one may continue to observe the child without any laboratory tests. In that case, it is mandatory to *review the progress within the next 24 hours.* If fever shows a downward trend, no further action may be called. However, if fever continues the same way, since a viral fever should have improved by now, *repeat careful physical examination and laboratory tests* are necessary. Cold and cough being such common symptoms in the population, it may now be necessary to consider them to be unrelated to the present disease.

If laboratory tests suggest the possibility of a bacterial respiratory infection which has not clearly localized clinically, the choice of another antibiotic should be based on the probable etiology. In this child with a respiratory infection, it is safe to presume that this is a community-acquired infection in an otherwise normal immune host. Hence, it is unlikely to be a drug resistant infection. If such an infection has not responded to Cefadroxil, it is likely to be due to intracellular organisms such as *Mycoplasma* and hence hypothetical change of antibiotic may be a macrolide and not merely the latest broad-spectrum antibiotic.

On the other hand, if tests suggest a possibility of typhoid or UTI, it should be dealt with accordingly.

Final Outcome

This child was examined thoroughly, and a clinical diagnosis of probable viral infection was made. As the child was accessible for a review again, it was decided to observe him without any laboratory tests. Fever showed a downward trend, and he got better within the next two days.

Experience gained...

1. Analysis of a detailed history and thorough physical examination are prerequisites for rational action.
2. Periodic reassessment with detailed physical examination is a must, especially if rational judgment demands that the child be observed without investigations.
3. If serious infections are ruled out by a proper history and physical examination, delay in institution of specific therapy is harmless, till a specific diagnosis is made based on clinical judgment and relevant laboratory tests.
4. Prescribing an antibiotic without a probable diagnosis may lead to a difficulty in planning further action, with the result that the course of disease may get prolonged and the outcome serious.
5. Nimesulide is not an ideal antipyretic, as it may bring down the fever but hide serious underlying infection that may surface too late. Fever is a protective mechanism and is useful within limits. An ideal antipyretic is one that controls fever to a safe level but may not bring down the body temperature to normal. Paracetamol or ibuprofen are rational antipyretics of choice. However, a combination of these two drugs is not necessary and irrational.

Treatment of Viral Infection

Most viral infections settle by themselves within a few days without specific therapy. Specific antiviral drugs are available for the treatment of a few viral infections such as herpes group of viruses, CMV, influenza, HCV and HBV, HIV and COVID-19. For acute viral infections specific therapy is most useful if started early in the course of infection but confirmation of such a diagnosis is not possible unless confirmative tests are ordered during the first 1–2 days. It may not be cost-effective. Thus, the hypothetical use of antiviral drugs in acute viral infections should be restricted to emergency situations such as acute viral encephalitis or viral infection in an immunocompromised patient. At times, they may be considered in children at increased risk of complications due to an underlying disorder, on the basis of local epidemiology. Routine use of specific antiviral drugs is fraught with the risk of developing resistance. Acyclovir or ganciclovir is used for Herpes group and CMV, oseltamivir or zanamivir for influenza and remdesivir for COVID-19 infection.

Chronic viral infections such as HBV, HCV, HIV can also be treated with specific drugs in combination. Such drugs include DAA direct-acting antiviral drugs for HCV, adefovir, tenofovir for HBV and anti-retroviral drugs—NRTI (nucleotide reverse transcriptase inhibitor)—Zidovudine, lamivudine, tenofovir, NNRTI (Non-nucleotide transcriptase inhibitor) efavirenz, nevirapine, PI (protease inhibitor) ritonavir. However, treatment of such chronic viral infections is best left to specialists.

CASE 27

■ Enteric Fever

Events...

A 10-year-old child presented with fever for last 12 days. He started with a moderate fever that increased in intensity over the next two days. There were no other symptoms. He was seen by a pediatrician on D3 because of high fever and was prescribed oral amoxicillin. After four days of therapy, as there was no improvement, the CBC and urinalysis were ordered. Urinalysis was normal and the CBC showed the following:

Hb 11 g%   WBC 4,200/mm^3 P 40 L 56 E 0 M 4   Platelets 1.4 lac/mm^3

Considering the CBC reports to be in favor of typhoid fever, he was prescribed oral cefixime in a dose of 20 mg/kg/day, given in two divided doses. At the end of another six days of cefixime therapy, fever continued, so the child was referred for further management. No clinical notes were recorded through the last 10 days that the pediatrician was treating.

What are the options for further management?

In order to be able to take the right decision and choose the correct action, one must have a probable clinical diagnosis, for which a detailed history should be followed by a thorough clinical examination.

Physical Examination

Fairly built and nourished child—   Weight 31 kg;   Height 135 cm
Febrile, not toxic or ill, comfortable
No significant abnormality on general examination
Liver just palpable, not tender;   Spleen not palpable
Rest of the systemic examination—normal

Ideal Option—Order Blood Culture and Change Antibiotic to Ceftriaxone

Considering the absence of localizing physical signs even at the end of 12 days of fever and the CBC showing leukopenia, lymphocytosis, eosinopenia and mild thrombocytopenia, it is likely that this child is suffering from typhoid fever. While antibiotics have failed to control disease, the child has not deteriorated either; hence, it is possible that the organism may have been partially resistant. Thus, it may be acceptable to order a blood culture for *S. typhi* along with the CBC and chest X-ray and consider intravenous ceftriaxone as an alternative antibiotic. The CBC is likely to be useful from the diagnostic point of view, if the results show a marked variation from the earlier values in the form of a significant increase or decrease in hemoglobin, leukocyte or platelet counts. It may also offer a clue to an improving trend, if eosinophils appear (that were absent earlier). The chest X-ray may rule out any respiratory infection that is clinically not obvious.

The blood culture may grow *S. typhi* over the next few days and/or the child may respond to IV ceftriaxone. In either case, it may be best to continue ceftriaxone for a period of seven days after defervescence. However, if the blood culture is negative and fever does not respond after four days of this treatment, it may be best to stop the antibiotic and observe the child. Repeated physical examination is mandatory to diagnose an evolving uncommon infection, collagen vascular disease or malignancy.

Acceptable Option—Stop Antibiotic and Observe for Next 2 or 3 Days

In spite of using two antibiotics, fever has continued for 12 days without any localizing signs. In the absence of neutrophilic leukocytosis, acute bacterial infections, such as meningitis, pneumonia or UTI are unlikely. As the child is comfortable and not sick looking, in this situation it is safe to discontinue cefixime and observe for next 2 or 3 days. It is likely that fever may subside, in which case, one may not know the correct diagnosis but all the same, the child has got better, and hence there is no immediate issue. In this event, one is not sure whether disease will relapse; if it does, one should not use an antibiotic without relevant laboratory tests.

However, if the fever continues, thorough physical examination and immediate laboratory tests are mandatory and they should include CBC, blood culture and chest X-ray.

Unacceptable Option—Try Other Antibiotics without Investigations

In general, hypothetical antibiotic therapy without clinical diagnosis and/or relevant laboratory investigations is not acceptable. Further it is our observation that, if two antibiotics fail, diagnosis of common community acquired bacterial infection is most unlikely and laboratory investigations are mandatory. The choice of antibiotic always depends upon whether suspected etiological agents are gram-positive or gram-negative; this can only be guessed after localizing the site of infection. In absence of such knowledge, the proper antibiotic cannot be selected. If change of antibiotic is considered, one must choose an antibiotic that would act on organisms not covered by the previous antibiotic. Routinely, one should not be considering drug-resistant infections unless the epidemiology of that particular infection demands such an action (as in case of multidrug resistant typhoid fever, malaria or tuberculosis). Even, if one has to consider a drug-resistant infection (like typhoid in this case), such infections are difficult to treat, but easy to confirm and every attempt must be made to confirm such an infection by blood culture.

Final Outcome

A blood culture was asked for and this child was started on IV ceftriaxone. Blood culture grew *S. typhi* and the child showed an improvement over four days. The antibiotic was continued for a period of seven days after defervescence.

Experience gained...

1. Hypothetical antibiotic therapy may result in the correct diagnosis being missed and may lead to prolongation of disease, serious complications or sequelae.
2. Change of antibiotic therapy must be based on a logical consideration of the site and type of infection.
3. Discontinuing an antibiotic that has failed, is often the best alternative, especially, if the child is not toxic or ill. Of course, repeated thorough physical examination is important to pick up clues, if any.

Treatment of Enteric Fever

Irrational use of antibiotics without confirmation of the etiology has led to increasing resistance to antibiotics and is seen even in community-acquired infections such as typhoid fever. In a fresh case of fever, diagnosis of typhoid may be suspected only by D3-4 and in case of a strong suspicion, one can start an antibiotic but only after sending out the sample for blood culture and CBC. It is easy to culture *Salmonella* in a laboratory and so, it should be a routine before an antibiotic is administered in a suspected case of typhoid fever. Moreover, it is safe to wait without an antibiotic till D3-4 of fever when "seriousness" is clinically ruled out.

An ideal antibiotic is best decided by local epidemiology. In general, third generation cephalosporins are the drugs of choice such as ceftriaxone or cefixime.

In this child, amoxicillin was started in the first place without a diagnosis. Though it may be effective in typhoid in general, it failed in this child, possibly because of partial resistance—it is best reserved for acute respiratory infections. In fact, this child also received cefixime which failed—possibly the dose of cefixime fell short because the routine dose of cefixime is half of that used in typhoid. Besides, there could be issues such as vomiting out the drug, incorrect measurement of drug dosage, etc. At times, the immune response to *Salmonella* may prolong fever in spite of the drug-sensitive bacteria. In such cases, general improvement is seen in terms of appetite and well-being though fever may continue (see next case). Such a situation does not suggest antibiotic resistance and there is no need for upgrading an antibiotic or adding another one.

Ceftriaxone may be switched to oral cefixime once early signs of recovery are evident. In general, the drug is continued for at least 4–5 days after the defervescence of fever. These early signs are improvement in appetite and general well-being; the fever responds later. At times, the fever continues beyond an expected period of time well after other symptoms and signs improve. Chloromycetin was widely used a few decades ago; its irrational use resulted in drug resistance. Besides this drug had a risk of serious side effects such as bone marrow suppression, and hence with the availability of safer drugs, it is not used anymore, even though it has regained its sensitivity against *Salmonella*. Azithromycin is another drug effective against typhoid fever—it shows a post-antibiotic effect that lasts for a few days after stopping the drug. However, in practice, it is often started without a diagnosis in an undifferentiated fever, and hence typhoid may be inadvertently treated, often partially, which confuses matters. Once a diagnosis of typhoid is suspected/confirmed, one would rather choose a cephalosporin than azithromycin. A combination of cephalosporin and azithromycin is not routinely necessary and should be avoided.

CASE 28

■ Enteric Fever

Events...

A 7-year-old boy presented with a continuous fever for last six days, with a rising trend over the last three days, with the fever now touching 105°F every 4 or 5 hours. There were no other localizing symptoms or any abnormal physical signs. He was initially treated with only antipyretics and a CBC was done on D4 of the illness, which showed a total count of $4300/mm^3$ N 64 L 30 E 0 M 6. At that time, the pediatrician found the abdomen to be somewhat tumid, suspected enteric fever, ordered a blood culture, and then started the child on IV ceftriaxone. After another 48 hours, he found hepatosplenomegaly on clinical examination, the abdomen was definitely tumid by now, and the blood culture had grown *S. typhi* sensitive to all except cotrimoxazole and nalidixic acid. IV ceftriaxone was continued, but on D5 of the treatment (and D9 of the illness) the fever continued to be in the range of 104° to 105°F.

What are the options for further management?

In order to be able to take the right decision and choose the correct action, one must have a probable clinical diagnosis.

Analysis

Since this child has been systematically managed right from the beginning, the diagnosis is quite clear. This child is definitely suffering from typhoid fever, correctly diagnosed clinically and confirmed by a positive blood culture. In typhoid fever, the first sign of a response to treatment is often seen in terms of subjective improvement. The child appears less toxic and is generally feeling better. His appetite may improve. Physical examination may demonstrate an improvement in the feel of the abdomen, as it now feels soft and not distended. Though fever may continue, the interval between two spikes of fever starts increasing, the fever seems to respond better and faster to antipyretics, and the peaks of fever spikes may be lower. On direct questioning, this is exactly what was happening in this child.

Ideal Option—Continue with the Same Antibiotic

In view of a clearly established diagnosis, in view of the organisms being sensitive to the drug used, and if one is confident of the early signs of a response in terms of subjective improvement, it is acceptable to continue the same antibiotic and wait for a further response. At the same time, one may consider repeating CBC to look for the reappearance of eosinophils that may herald recovery.

Acceptable Option—Continue with the Same Antibiotic, but Investigate Further

It may not be totally unacceptable, if one wants to play safe and investigate further at this point. The investigations will be directed mainly towards establishing an additional illness. Therefore, an X-ray chest, urine-routine and culture, smear for malarial parasite, and a Mantoux test may be called for. Acute bacterial pneumonia would have been clinically obvious by now; further, the original CBC was not in favor of pneumonia. Once the patient is on antibiotics, urinalysis and urine culture have their limitations; further the same antibiotic is quite likely to be effective even in a UTI. Though the pattern of fever is not suggestive of malaria, if one does pick up a malarial parasite, it would explain the persistence of fever.

Unacceptable Option—Change/Add Antibiotics, or Start Empirical ATT

There is no rationale for changing or adding an antibiotic; the culture report clearly shows the sensitivity of the antibiotic being currently used. If credence is given to the fact that *in vitro* and *in vivo* sensitivity may differ, then changing or adding an antibiotic would be based purely on guesswork and not on scientific logic. In routine clinical practice, this difference in sensitivity is relevant only in selected situations. A combination of two antibiotics is generally not advocated in such patients. In fact, it is reserved only for serious infections with a high chance of drug resistance that may endanger life. Though typhoid fever is often caused by drug resistant organisms, mortality has been extremely low and so we do not recommend a combination of antibiotics to preempt drug resistance. Similarly, in the absence of any diagnostic pointers in favor of TB, empirical anti-TB treatment is also not justified.

Case Progression

The treating pediatrician continued ceftriaxone, the range of fever reduced partially, the child became absolutely nontoxic, eating well, looking cheerful, but even after 14 days of IV ceftriaxone, the fever continued to be 101°F once a day.

What are the options for further management?
Ideal Option—Stop Antibiotic and Observe

Host responses do vary, and it may not be easy to differentiate between persistence of infection resulting in continuation of fever, and control of infection but persistence of fever due to toxemia. As this child has improved in all other parameters except fever, it is reasonable to conclude that the drug has worked. One may confirm the clearance of bacteria from blood by way of a blood culture, though it is not routinely required. In typhoid, fever may be due to toxins produced by *Salmonella* and may not necessarily mean persistence of infection. If toxemia is the cause of persistence of fever, it may take its own course and eventually get better. However, in such a situation, if one is sure of the diagnosis and drug sensitivity, as is so in this child, one may consider a short course of prednisolone that will suppress the fever. However, it is *mandatory* that one be sure of the diagnosis and drug sensitivity; even then, one must restrict this short course to just a day or two.

Acceptable Option—Continue Antibiotic for Another 5 to 7 Days

As hosts vary in their response to drug therapy, one may continue the drug for another few days in the hope that fever subsides. As it is safe to continue the drug for some more time, it may be an acceptable option. However, if fever continues beyond another few days in spite of continuing the same antibiotic, one must stop the antibiotic and just observe further progress.

Unacceptable Option—Change or Add Antibiotic

Since this child has shown subjective improvement, the organisms cannot be totally drug resistant; hence, changing the antibiotic is not rational at all. One may argue in favor of adding an antibiotic. However, it is impossible to decide on clinical grounds which antibiotic would be sensitive *in vivo* as well, for sure. Since the blood culture has isolated a drug sensitive organism, drug should not be blamed for the continuation of fever. Multiple antibiotics may result in drug interactions about which our knowledge is limited. So, it is best to avoid a combination of antibiotics in this situation.

Final Outcome

It was decided to stop the antibiotic and use a short course of prednisolone and within the next two days, the fever subsided completely.

Experience gained...

> In typhoid fever, steroids are not indicated routinely. But in exceptional situations, as happened in this case, steroids may be just the right drug to use. However, this option should be considered only when the diagnosis and the drug sensitivity have been bacteriologically proved.
>
> Fever is a cytokine-induced phenomenon, triggered by infections as well as noninfective factors, such as toxins, as in this case.

CASE 29

Enteric Fever

Events...

A 5-year-old child presented with fever for last 12 days. The fever was high grade and with chills. After symptomatic therapy for the first three days, CBC showed leukopenia, lymphocytosis, and thrombocytopenia and the Widal test was positive. Therefore, oral cefixime was started with a provisional diagnosis of typhoid fever. However, even after five days of antibiotic therapy, as fever did not subside, the parents stopped the drug and tried alternative system of medicine. After another four days, as the fever continued, he was hospitalized on the advice of the family physician. On admission, this child was febrile but not sick looking, and had no positive findings on general or systemic examination.

What are the options for further management?

Ideal Option—Investigate and Observe

As this child has been off an antibiotic for the last four days, it may be best at this stage to send the blood for culture and repeat CBC and Widal test in view of a probable diagnosis of typhoid fever. As far as possible, the diagnosis of any infection must be backed by bacteriological proof, which is the gold standard of diagnosis. This is especially so, when the collection of a sample does not involve invasive procedures and the disease may have a serious outcome. Typhoid fever satisfies these criteria, and hence, one must always attempt to send blood for culture. Ideally, this should be done before starting an antibiotic, but it is worth trying even, if the patient is already on antibiotic therapy, as there is always a chance of proving the diagnosis. Further, *Salmonella typhi* is not a fastidious organism and is quite easy to culture, unlike *Haemophilus influenzae*. For diagnosing typhoid, Widal test alone may not be dependable, since many children may have had a previous exposure to *Salmonella* either through natural sources or through prior vaccination. However, in this child, since it has already been done, if a fourfold rise can now be demonstrated, it will support the diagnosis of typhoid. It is important to note that the Widal test does not assess Vi antibodies. Hence, it may be falsely positive only after the classical TA vaccine but not after the Vi antigen vaccine.

Though this child does not have a past history of UTI, urinalysis and urine culture should also be ordered, as fever without an obvious focus can also be due to urinary tract infection. Since this child does not appear sick, it is acceptable to wait for the preliminary results of CBC, routine urine and Widal test before starting an antibiotic.

Acceptable Option—Investigate and Start IV Ceftriaxone

In view of a probable diagnosis of typhoid fever in this child, it may be acceptable to investigate as mentioned above and simultaneously start IV ceftriaxone, without waiting for the reports, so as to not waste time. Further, if blood culture fails to grow any organism because this child is partially treated, one may anyway have to go by the clinical possibility of typhoid fever and start IV ceftriaxone.

Unacceptable Option—Start Another Antibiotic without Investigations

It is irrational to start another antibiotic without investigations. No doubt, a fever of 12 days duration without any clinical localization, in a child who is not so sick, is quite likely to be typhoid in our epidemiology. No doubt, there are limitations to the yield of investigations in partially treated patients. However, these considerations do not justify empirical treatment with antibiotics without investigations. If such a treatment fails, the diagnostic difficulties will only be compounded.

Case Progression

In this child, the first (ideal) option was chosen, and while waiting for the results of CBC, urinalysis and Widal test, his fever subsided. So, it was decided to wait for the blood culture report. It reported a growth of *Salmonella typhi* within the next 48 hours.

What are the options for further management?

Ideal Option—Wait and Observe without Antibiotic

Since there was no fever, it was considered rational to wait without an antibiotic, even when the blood culture had grown *Salmonella typhi*. One may note that prior to the antibiotic era, some patients did get better with symptomatic treatment alone, though many others must have succumbed. Thus, immunity of the host may be good enough to cure the disease without specific therapy and on the other hand, one may occasionally find a child who does not improve even with an antibiotic, in spite of the diagnosis being correct and the organism being drug sensitive. As this child was available for proper follow-up, it was decided to wait without an antibiotic and not treat the laboratory report alone.

Acceptable Option—Treat with Antibiotic

As this child had been running fever for a long time and was haphazardly treated, now that the diagnosis had been proved by culture, it would be best to treat with an oral antibiotic and ensure complete cure to avoid a relapse. More so, because typhoid fever is known to relapse, if not completely cured.

Final Outcome

It was decided to follow the ideal option. So, he was observed without antibiotic therapy. He remained well for the next five days and then returned with high fever again. At that time, there was no new focus of infection, repeat blood culture was positive for *S. typhi* again, and he recovered on oral cefixime.

Experience gained…

1. Starting a broad-spectrum antibiotic early in the course of an illness, in the absence of an urgent need to start treatment, can seriously jeopardize subsequent diagnosis and management.
2. Fever with chills or rigors is not specific to malaria; in fact, it is quite common in enteric fever and of course may suggest UTI or any other disease as well.

CASE 30

■ Frequent Illnesses Diagnosed as Primary Complex Twice

Events...

A 4-year-old boy presented with recurrent episodes of fever, cold and cough for last two years and not growing well almost since birth. Each episode was treated with antibiotics, and he would be alright for a few weeks till the next episode occurred.

Because of recurrent febrile illnesses and malnutrition, he was investigated. Results of the tests were as follows:

Hb 11 g%   WBC 14,300/mm^3 P 35 L 62 E 3   ESR 48 mm at the end of one hour
Mt test 10 mm   Chest X-ray - ? hilar prominence

Based on these results, he was diagnosed as primary complex and advised ATT. He did well during the course of ATT and had no recurrence of his previous complaints. He had gained 500 g in weight and 3 cm in height. However, after completion of ATT for six months, he again started getting recurrent fever with cold and cough.

He was advised to repeat a Mantoux test and chest X-ray. The results were identical to the earlier reports. He was, therefore, advised to restart ATT. At this time, he was referred for further advice.

What are the options for further management?

In order to be able to take the right decision and choose the correct action, one must have a probable clinical diagnosis, for which, many more details in the history need to be known.

On detailed enquiry, it was noted that he was an IUGR baby with a birth weight of 2.2 kg. He was bottle-fed for the first two years and had two episodes of diarrhea, one of which required hospitalization. He weighed 7.2 kg at 1 year of age. He did not eat well and had to be force-fed. At two years of age, he joined playschool and thereafter, started getting recurrent respiratory infections. Physical examination revealed that his weight was 12 kg, height 97 cm, and he had mild pallor. There were no other positive findings.

Analysis

This child has gained 10 kg in weight over last 4 years. Considering that he was an IUGR baby, who was bottle-fed with two episodes of diarrhea in infancy, and poor eating, this weight gain is reasonable. Again, considering his IUGR status at birth, a height of 97 cm is good for this age. Thus, this child has done reasonably well under the circumstances and cannot be considered to have failed to grow, contrary to the parental complaints. Further, recurrent fever with cold and cough are anyway not the symptoms of tuberculosis. As this child was getting better each time and remained well in between episodes, it does not suggest a chronic disease. Thus, a search for tuberculosis was not justified. Moreover, the results of the tests were not conclusive of tuberculosis either. Lymphocytosis with a moderate increase in ESR are nonspecific indicators. Mantoux test that is 10 mm positive may not necessarily mean active disease at this age and the chest X-ray showing a suspicious hilar adenopathy was not adequate in this scenario to consider a diagnosis of tuberculosis.

This child's symptoms suggest recurrent upper respiratory infections. They could be either viral or bacterial. Recurrent bacterial infections necessitate investigations for the background cause while recurrent viral infections result from environmental exposure. Just because the child remained well during ATT, it cannot be inferred that he did suffer from tuberculosis. It is possible that continued antibiotics such as rifampicin kept recurrences of bacterial URTI under control, and as soon as ATT was stopped, infections recurred.

Ideal Option—Reassure Parents, Follow-up the Child and Investigate SOS

Not only was this child's original diagnosis of tuberculosis suspect, there was no need for repeat Mantoux test and chest X-ray. It is important to realize that investigations for tuberculosis must be ordered only on clinical suspicion of the disease and laboratory test results must be interpreted in the light of clinical profile. Therefore, the correct option is to merely counsel the parents and advise regular follow-up. The recurrent respiratory infections in this child could be attributed to viral infections as a result of exposure to such infections in nursery. However, if one considers recurrent bacterial infections in this child (in view of child remaining well during ATT), a search for background cause such as enlarged adenoids or sinusitis would be mandatory. The need for this could be decided based on the follow-up.

If there are still some concerns about the possibility of tuberculosis, one must consider close clinical observations for a few weeks without specific therapy. Of course it is important to ensure the safety of waiting without any specific therapy. Infancy and adolescence would be considered high-risk situations, but in this child it would be safe to observe without specific therapy.

Unacceptable Option—Restart ATT

It has been discussed above that this child did not justify repeat tests for tuberculosis at all. Mantoux test once positive is likely to remain positive subsequently. Repeat chest X-ray again showing a suspicious hilar lymphadenopathy is inconclusive. Such vague reports need careful interpretation. It is worth noting that, even if the child did have a primary complex the first time, recurrence of tuberculosis will not present as a primary complex again. In other words, there cannot be 'primary' infections twice! Thus, there is no justification in restarting ATT again.

Experience gained...

> This child suffered from trauma that was too trivial to account for his fracture, i.e., it was a pathological fracture. Since, there was neither any local abnormality nor a generalized bony demineralization, it became mandatory to search for a systemic disease. Thus, it is very important to consider the clinical setting in which the disease occurs; it may offer a clue to the hidden underlying problem.
>
> Investigations for tuberculosis must be ordered only on clinical suspicion of the disease and laboratory test results must be interpreted in the light of clinical profile. A primary complex can never recur; if tuberculosis does recur, it is post-primary tuberculosis with different clinical manifestations.

Treatment of Tuberculosis

It is extremely important to confirm the diagnosis by asking for easily available microbiological tests before embarking on therapy. Generally, there are no emergency situations in tuberculosis that justify empirical therapy in a hurry. However, if a sincere attempt at confirmation of diagnosis fails, and the clinical suspicion is strong, one may be forced to call it "clinically diagnosed" tuberculosis. This course of action should only be used if one is forced to do so and it is ideal to ask for an expert opinion before starting therapy in such a case. Standard guidelines must be followed in the diagnosis of tuberculosis. Clinical suspicion is based on fever and/or cough of recent origin >2 weeks or weight loss of >5% or no gain in weight for previous 3 months without any other cause with or without Tb contact. Chest X-ray can often strengthen clinical suspicion more so if it shows miliary shadows, fibrocaseous lesions or mediastinal lymph nodes. In the case of nonspecific shadows, a trial with amoxicillin for a week may be attempted but it is best to order laboratory tests for confirmation. CBNATT or GeneXpert is an ideal test with or without liquid culture (BACTEC or MGIT). GeneXpert-ultra or GeneXpert XDR is not necessary upfront. Line probe assay (LPA) is used for the detection of MDR, only on culture +ve samples. Second-line LPA is used to detect second-line drug resistance.

Treatment is of two types—RS-TB (R sensitive) and RR-TB (R resistant). In clinically diagnosed TB, start RS-TB regimen—2HRZE/2HRE. In the case of neuro and spine TB, extend the continuation phase till 10 months. HRZE: 10–15—35–20 mg/kg/day in single dose. Pediatric fixed drug combinations are available. FDC-P has H50, R75, Z150 which is a dispersible tablet + E as a separate tablet for IP and H50-R75 dispersible tablet for CP in addition to E as separate tablet. For older children and adults, H75, R150, Z400, E275 a single non-dispersible tablet for IP and H75 R150 E275 single tablet for CP. A combination of pediatric and older children/adult tablets can be used as per the dosage required for age groups 25-30 years, 3P+3E+1A, and for 31-40 age, 2P+2E+2A.

- H-monoresistance is treated with 6LfxRZE (levofloxacin containing uniphasic regimen).
- MDR >5 years for localized pulmonary lesions
  4-6Lfx+Cfz clofazimine + bedaquiline + Eto-ethionamide + Hh + Z + E as IP followed by 5 Lfx+Cfz+ZE as CP
- MDR <5 years for localized pulmonary lesions
  4-6Mfx + Cfz + Km/Am (kanamycin or amikacin IM) + Eto + Hh + ZE as IP, 5 Mfx + Cfz + Z + E

CASE 31

■ Short Stature due to IUGR with Malpositioned Kidney

Events...

An 8-year-old female child was referred for growth failure. She had an acute attack of UTI two weeks ago, at which time, she was thoroughly investigated. Her urine culture had grown *E.coli* with the colony count being significant. She was treated successfully with antibiotics and was cured. Abdominal USG done after the control of infection showed malpositioning of one kidney but no other abnormality. VUR was also ruled out. Considering that a chronic renal problem could be the probable cause of her growth failure, she was evaluated further. While chronic renal disease was ruled out on investigation, her tuberculin test was positive and anti-tuberculosis IgM antibodies were also borderline positive. Though her chest X-ray was normal, she was advised anti-TB treatment in view of these test results and her growth failure. Since her renal function tests turned out to be normal, she was also advised further tests to evaluate any other causes that may be contributing to her growth failure At this point, she came for a second opinion.

What are the options for further management?

In order to be able to take the right decision and choose the correct action, one must have a probable clinical diagnosis.

Physical examination revealed an active, happy child with no evidence of any chronic disease. She weighed 21 kg and her height was 114 cm. She was not pale, and her blood pressure was normal. She had no other abnormality on clinical assessment.

Analysis

As this child is clinically so normal, we need to first establish the claim of growth failure. On detailed enquiry, it was noted that she was an IUGR baby with a weight of 2.1 kg and a length of 46 cm. Her parents had recorded a few growth measurements at periodic intervals. After constructing her growth chart, it was realized that she was always at about the 5th centile, and she had maintained the same centile curve throughout her life. So, there was in effect no growth failure at all and therefore, there is no question of ascribing it to chronic renal disease. Further, she does not even have a chronic renal problem. The mere finding of a malpositioned kidney does not entail any risk to her life. In fact, this was her first episode of UTI, and at this age, she does not qualify for any further tests to evaluate an underlying cause.

Ideal Option—Reassure Parents, no Investigations or Treatment

Since this child has not really failed to grow, she does not need any medical intervention in the form of diagnosis or treatment. All that needs to be done is to reassure the parents and explain to them that her health is normal, even if she happens to be the shortest and the thinnest amongst her classmates.

Unacceptable Option—Start ATT, and/or Investigate Further

Though this child's Mantoux test is positive, tuberculosis is certainly not the cause of her short stature. Her problem of so called 'growth failure' has been a long-standing one and that cannot be explained on the basis of tuberculosis now, and that too tuberculosis that is not evident either symptomatically, clinically or radiologically. Therefore, there is no question of starting ATT. Further, since there is no growth failure at all as discussed above, investigating further to search for a cause for the same, becomes superfluous.

Final Outcome

The parents were reassured. On further enquiry, it was noted that her father also had a similar stature throughout childhood, and it was only later in adulthood that he had gained weight. So she also had another factor responsible for her low velocity of growth.

Experience gained...

> Growth is best evaluated longitudinally and only then can one judge the real picture. Otherwise, one proceeds along the wrong path and tries to find some cause for the problem that really does not exist.

CASE 32

■ Breastfed Baby with Intermittent Blood in Stools

Events...

A 2-month-old infant presented with fresh blood in stools noticed intermittently from D15 of life. Apart from this, the infant was happy, playful, feeding well and there were no other symptoms reported by the mother. The infant was born of a full-term normal delivery with a birth weight of 3.2 kg and was exclusively breastfed.

The pediatrician considered it to be a GI infection and prescribed oral Walamycin for five days. There was no improvement in the complaint. Stool microscopy showed the presence of RBCs. Considering drug resistance, IV amikacin was administered for the next seven days; however, the intermittent fresh blood continued. The CBC showed a Hb of 11.5 g%, and was otherwise normal. At this juncture, stool culture was ordered; meanwhile, a trial with metronidazole and probiotics was attempted. Stool culture showed *E.coli* sensitive to all antibiotics. As there was no improvement, substitution of breastfeeds with soya formula was advised but mother refused to stop breastfeeding and called for another opinion.

What are the options for further management?

In order to be able to take the right decision and choose the correct action, one must have a probable clinical diagnosis.

Physical Examination

Comfortable happy infant, not sick
Weight 5.4 kg   Length 58 cm
No pallor   No other abnormality

Analysis

This infant is being treated as suspected GI infection. However, he has gained excellent weight and is active, playful and feeding well. This signifies that there is no infection at all, nor any other serious illness. In fact, exclusively breastfed infants cannot develop GI infection at all. If they do develop a bacterial infection anywhere in the body, some underlying cause such as immune deficiency or cystic fibrosis may have to be seriously considered. The results of investigations have also been quite nonspecific. Stool culture in general is of limited use and should be reserved for protracted diarrhea in a malnourished child. Most of the laboratories are not able to subtype *E. coli* and hence, merely reporting *E. coli* in stool has no significance.

Since there is no pallor and the hemoglobin is 11.5 g%, it signifies that the bleeding has been minimal.

Noninfective conditions that can lead to blood in stools include a bleeding disorder, hemangiomatous malformations or protein allergy (due to maternal exposure to foreign protein in her diet which would lead to microscopic blood in stools). It is unlikely to be a bleeding disorder as there is no evidence of bleeding from any other site.

Ideal Option—Continue Breastfeeding, no Further Intervention

As discussed above, there is no evidence of any infection in this infant. The other noninfective causes are difficult to prove even by laboratory tests and may not need intervention unless the infant gets sick. Hence, it may be safe to observe the child with exclusive breastfeeding and unless bleeding disturbs the well-being of the child or leads to significant anemia, no further intervention is called for.

Unacceptable Options—Invasive Investigations, Stop Breastfeeding, Further Drug Treatment

This infant has so far been managed quite irrationally. Hypothetical antibiotic therapy without an attempt to diagnose the condition is dangerous, particularly in infants.

Further, administration of oral antibiotics to treat acute bacterial infections in neonates or young infants is irrational; IV antibiotics are mandatory. Metronidazole is irrational as amebiasis is most unlikely at this age. Indications for probiotic and prebiotic are far and few and these drugs are not routinely required. In the absence of any likelihood of infection, all this intervention has been unnecessary.

Even though clinically, there is no clue to the probable source of bleeding, investigations, such as colonoscopy are not easy at this age. Nor is there any other modality of investigation that may conclusively diagnose the cause of bleeding. Since, the bleeding is minimal and does not disturb the well-being of the infant, it may be sensible to avoid any invasive investigations at this stage.

Obviously, there is no need to stop breastfeeding, even if one considers this to be an effect of some maternal food ingestion. Similarly, further drug treatment is also not necessary.

Case Progression

The child gained further 600 g in two weeks on exclusive breastfeeding and had no blood in stools thereafter.

Experience gained...

1. Well-being of infant or child is a strong indicator of absence of at least serious disease and hence close observation without any intervention is rational.
2. Exclusively breastfed infant is most unlikely to harbor bacterial infection unless there exists serious underlying disease.
3. Empirical antibiotic therapy is dangerous in infants in particular.
4. Stool culture is reserved only for selective situations.

Comment

Blood in stools in a breastfed infant is a tricky situation to deal with as clinical diagnosis is often not possible and the decision to order tests—often invasive is not so easy, especially if an infant looks fine. Surely, if such an infant is significantly pale, there would be a need to rule out vitamin K deficiency (mostly gastric bleeding) or an intestinal bleeder. Cow's milk protein allergy is known to cause blood in stools even in exclusively breastfed infant as the antigen may pass through breast milk from the mother. However, in routine practice, it should not be considered unless breastfed infant fails to gain adequate weight, Routine stool examination will confirm the presence of fresh or altered blood and further endoscopic evaluation can be planned accordingly. In the absence of significant pallor, if an infant is happy and gaining weight well, one may consider a "wait and watch" policy with close monitoring. It must be supported by detailed communication and counseling with the parents but often pressure from parents and considering an evidence-based era in modern medicine, we are likely to order tests that are usually negative. Self-limiting small undetected bleeder is not rare and needs to be followed up.

CASE 33

Breastfed Baby with Suspected GI Infection Who Recovered Fast

Events…

A one-month-old exclusively breastfed infant developed high fever for a day, followed by loose motions without blood. There was no history of vomiting or refusal to feed. He had gained one kilogram in weight since birth. On examination, he was febrile but not sick looking, had no localizing signs, and was not dehydrated. Standard protocol demanded that this child be hospitalized, and after ordering relevant tests, immediately started on combination antibiotics. This was done promptly. Investigations were sent and IV ceftriaxone and amikacin were started. The investigation results were as follows:

WBC 12,000/mm^3 P 34 L 63 E 2 M 1   CRP >250

Stool microscopy—30 to 40 pus cells, 20 to 30 RBCs and few macrophages.

Stool culture grew *E. coli* sensitive to imipenem and vancomycin but resistant to other antibiotics. Meanwhile the infant improved; he was afebrile and his stools were normal.

What are the options for further management?

In order to be able to take the right decision and choose the correct action, one must have a probable clinical diagnosis.

Analysis

This infant never looked sick, though the action taken initially was justified at this age. That he would improve so dramatically was unexpected; retrospectively, this may have been a self-limiting viral infection. It would be worthwhile enquiring whether any close family member had suffered from a similar illness, which would support this diagnosis. This infant's stool culture report seemed to be very unusual in that the organism grown, i.e., *E. coli*, was resistant to most of the antibiotics and sensitive only to imipenem and vancomycin. It is difficult to accept the isolation of such an organism from an infant who is exclusively breastfed and is living in a hygienic home environment. Therefore, this sample could have been contaminated. Since this infant recovered within a day, one could ignore such a report.

Ideal Option—Continue the Same Antibiotics

Since this was an infant who presented with high fever, it should be taken as a bacterial infection. Thus, starting two antibiotics was justified. Just because he improved within a day, though unexpected, it could be risky to withdraw antibiotics at this stage even when repeat tests are within normal limits. However, there is no need to change antibiotics on the basis of stool culture report. Considering such a quick improvement, antibiotics could be stopped after a week, once the infant remained well.

Less Acceptable Option—Observe Infant Carefully and Decide Further Management

Since, this infant may need antibiotics for at least 10 to 14 days, if he is diagnosed to have a bacterial infection, it is necessary to define the diagnosis as objectively as possible. However, it is not easy to do so, since there seemed to be a disparity between the results of investigations done earlier and the speed with which this infant recovered. Repeating the investigations that were abnormal to begin with, may also not help. If the CRP has normalized, it was expected to do so, on successful treatment. On the other hand, even if the CRP continues to be high, treatment cannot be based on CRP alone, disregarding the clinical status. Similarly, whether the stool routine or culture turns out to be normal or abnormal, it cannot guide us now whether there was a bacterial infection or not. Therefore, it is difficult to decide whether this infant did have a bacterial infection or not. If there is a definite history of a viral infection in a close family member, and if one is confident of closely following up the infant clinically, one may stop the antibiotics and observe. If the fever recurs after stopping the antibiotic, one should thoroughly investigate (CBC, blood culture, CSF routine and culture, urine routine and culture, chest X-ray), and start the same antibiotic to which the infant had earlier responded so well.

Unacceptable Option—Change Antibiotic to Imipenem and Vancomycin

This is certainly not called for as this infant had improved clinically. Therefore, an isolated laboratory report should not guide therapy. Laboratory reports should be respected, but not allowed to override clinical judgment.

Final Outcome

This infant was treated for a week, and he remained well on close follow-up.

Experience gained…

> It is safe to presume acute bacterial infection in a young infant with high fever, even if there is no localization of disease.
>
> In rare situations, such a fever may be a viral infection. However, this should be entertained only in a breastfed baby, who is not looking sick and is feeding well, with a definite contact with a close family member suffering from a viral infection. Even then, this infant should be closely followed up, at least 12 hourly.

CASE 34

■ Empyema

Events...

A 1-year-old child presented with high fever for 15 days, breathlessness for 10 days and cough for four days. Initially, he was seen by his family physician, who treated him with amoxicillin. At the end of five days, as he was not improving, chest X-ray was ordered that showed fluid in the pleural cavity on the left side. He was hospitalized for the same. A diagnostic tap confirmed the diagnosis of empyema, and an intercostal drain was instituted. Simultaneously, he was started on a combination of amoxicillin and clavulinic acid intravenously. Initially the drainage from the intercostal tube was continuous and looked like thin pus. However, subsequently there was no drainage from the tube in spite of it not being blocked. Meanwhile, the child had not improved much and fever and mild breathlessness continued. At this point, an HRCT was ordered that showed loculated fluid in the pleural cavity along with pleural thickening. There was also a collapse consolidation of the left lower lobe. Based on this report, the intercostal drain was adjusted accordingly, to drain the loculated fluid and the antibiotic therapy was continued. As a result, there was some further improvement, but the parents decided to take another opinion.

What are the options for further management?

Physical Examination

Comfortable, not appearing 'sick'
Afebrile   RR—40/min   moderate pallor
RS—Breath sounds diminished on left lower zone; scattered crepitations.

Investigations

Hb—9 g%   WBC count—normal
Chest X-ray—left sided haziness with obliteration of costophrenic angle
USG—loculated small collection of pleural fluid

Acceptable Option—Continue Conservative Management

Though this child has presented to us 15 days after the onset of symptoms, he is afebrile and comfortable at present. Since this child's fever seems to have just settled, it is acceptable to manage him conservatively at present, continue the antibiotic, and follow his progress. If this child continues to remain afebrile and steadily improves constitutionally in terms of appetite and general well-being, we could continue the antibiotic for a week more, and institute chest physiotherapy and breathing exercises. In that event, there may be a good chance that the damaged lung recovers completely. If conservative management does succeed, he will have to be followed up periodically, for the next three months, to assess his respiratory status. If the lung remains collapsed in spite of his being asymptomatic, he may need planned surgery at a later date.

On the other hand, if the fever persists and there is no constitutional improvement, conservative management needs to be abandoned and one should opt for further surgical intervention.

Alternate Acceptable Option—Surgical Intervention

In view of the likelihood of the underlying lung getting irreversibly damaged, it may be acceptable to undertake surgical intervention. If this child had been seen early in the course of his disease, shortly after his empyema was diagnosed, it would have been ideal to opt for endoscopic surgery—video assisted thoracoscopic surgery (VATS). This would have not only prevented long-term damage to the lung, it would also have eliminated the need for major surgical intervention later, in an attempt to salvage the lung. At this stage, VATS could be attempted, failing which, the surgeon may have to explore, in addition.

The final choice between the above two acceptable options should be left to the parents after a detailed discussion about the pros and cons of both the options. The first option offers a chance to avoid immediate surgery; whether surgery can be totally avoided, or it will be required at a later date, can only be decided on follow-up.

Unacceptable Option—Attempt to Treat with only Additional Antibiotics

Once an empyema is diagnosed, it is mandatory to ensure adequate drainage; continuation of antibiotic therapy takes a backseat. If this step is not ensured, any amount of additional antibiotic therapy is unlikely to produce the desired results.

Final Outcome

This child fared well over the next three months, and repeat chest X-ray then, showed that both the pleural and the lung lesion had cleared. Eventually surgery was avoided in this child by patient observation. To emphasize a point again, one would not have waited, if the child had presented early in the course of illness, because at that time, one does not want to take any chances (of suffering irreversible lung damage); instead, one wants to offer a definite cure.

Experience gained...

> After instituting an ICD in a case of empyema, if the ICD drainage is less than 30 mL/day, and yet the child continues to run fever, is not constitutionally better, and imaging reveals pleural loculation, it is necessary to go for VATS/Thoracostomy. These were exactly the conditions two days prior to this child coming to us, and therefore, at that point, surgery was justified. So, had this child come to us two days prior, we would also have gone ahead with surgery. However, it so happened that when this child had come to us two days later, and we reviewed his clinical condition, we noted that he had just become afebrile, he was getting constitutionally better, and had only a pleural lesion. When such a situation is encountered, the child often improves on conservative management alone.

Treatment of Empyema

Early detection of empyema is important to prevent permanent damage to the pleura and underlying lung. In the case of acute bacterial community-acquired pneumonia in an infant <6 months, there is a significant risk of developing empyema and it is ideal to order USG of the chest early, to pick up a collection in the pleural cavity. In the case of acute bacterial pneumonia in older children, failure of response to an ideal antibiotic should suggest the need to exclude empyema. The antibiotic choice in most cases is ceftriaxone with or without amoxiclav and in suspected MRSA, vancomycin may be considered or clindamycin that takes care of MRSA and MSSA. Antibiotics need to be continued for four weeks or longer in case of MRSA. Linezolid should be a "reserve" antibiotic used ideally only when gram +ve bacterial infection is confirmed, and is resistant to other antibiotics. It has significant side effects that may be irreversible. In addition to antibiotic therapy, interventions including one-time drainage, or continuous tube drainage or VATS are necessary as guided by the stage of empyema.

CASE 35

■ Empyema Who was Given Steroids

Events...

A 10-year-old girl presented with a history of high fever that started 15 days ago, followed by chest pain on the right side that lasted for two days. Thereafter, she became breathless over the next two days, and was therefore, investigated. The CBC showed marked neutrophilic leukocytosis and chest X-ray showed a large right-sided pleural effusion. She was treated by her family physician with some medications, but she did not improve. As a result, she sought treatment from another doctor. After another five days of this treatment, her fever subsided but mild breathlessness continued. Repeat chest X-ray showed no change in the pleural effusion; the entire right hemithorax was hazy, and there was a mediastinal shift. As chest X-ray had not shown any improvement and she was mildly breathless, she was sent for another opinion.

What are the options for further management?

One may have to consider provisional diagnosis before embarking on options of management.

Physical Examination

Comfortable, afebrile
RS— dull note on percussion, complete absence of breath sounds on entire right side anteriorly as well as posteriorly
— mediastinal shift to left
Liver 2 cm, soft
Other systems—normal

Investigations

CBC—normal
Chest X-ray—complete haziness on right side of chest.

Analysis

This child had an acute onset of pleuropneumonia that developed into a pleural effusion. She has improved in terms of fever and does not appear to be acutely sick, but continues to demonstrate a persistent large pleural effusion and mild breathlessness. This clinical profile is typical of empyema, but persistence of a large pleural collection should have been accompanied with high spiking fever and also, leukocytosis. On the other hand, a tuberculous effusion which is large enough to cause breathlessness, would have presented acutely within the first 24–48 hours of onset of the illness, and the child would have been in acute respiratory distress till the pleural fluid was drained out. In fact, as pleural effusion in tuberculosis is due to allergy, it presents acutely, even more acutely than empyema. Even if she had received anti-TB treatment, her breathlessness would not get relieved unless the fluid was tapped.

In tuberculosis, a small effusion can develop over a few days, but would not lead to breathlessness. So analysis of history and physical findings does not guide us to a provisional diagnosis though it rests between empyema and tuberculous effusion, both conditions not fitting well.

Ideal Option—Investigate, and then Decide Further Treatment

An USG should be able to detect whether there are any loculations with fibrous septae. If so, it would suggest a diagnosis of empyema. In case there are no loculations detected on USG, one may consider a CT scan of the chest to find out whether there is an underlying pneumonia. If there is one, it is a bacterial pneumonia with empyema. If there is no lung lesion, it is a tuberculous pleural effusion. Once that is clear, a diagnostic tap or an attempt at complete drainage would be in order. As this child is partially treated, pleural fluid cytology and biochemistry may not be interpretive, and bacteriological diagnosis may also be elusive. If one found pus, it could still be tubercular empyema and this differentiation would come through either a CT scan of the chest showing mediastinal lymphadenopathy or by histopathological evidence. There is no urgency for drug treatment in this child and if it is empyema, mere good drainage by surgical intervention would improve this child. Since antibiotics have been already used, this could be a sterile empyema, just like a sterile abscess and may not need further antibiotics.

Unacceptable Option—Intercostal Drain and/or Continue Antibiotics

This is not a candidate for intercostal drainage. Even if it is empyema, it is late enough in the course of the disease to anticipate multiple loculations that would not be drained by an intercostal drain. In which case, she would need thoracoscopy. Continuation of antibiotics alone, without any kind of surgical intervention, is just not justified. Further treatment with antibiotics should be considered only, if there is proof of infection or if there is a poor response to good drainage.

Final Outcome

USG showed a multiloculated collection of thick fluid. This meant that the diagnosis was acute bacterial pneumonia with empyema, and she would need surgical intervention. What was intriguing was her afebrile state, which prevented us from diagnosing this clinically. It was later found out that she had received steroids from the second doctor, as a result of which her fever subsided, and led to further problems.

Experience gained...

> Delay in the diagnosis of an empyema is commonly due to pursuing changing antibiotics in a case of unresolving pneumonia. However, in these children, as the fever persists, the diagnosis is at least finally made. But when steroids are added, fever may disappear, as happened in this case, but the child would deteriorate. This poses a bigger clinical challenge to the etiological diagnosis.

Extra...
Recommended protocol for the management of empyema
Depending upon the time of diagnosis in relation to the onset of disease, management differs. If the disease is diagnosed in the initial stages (generally within 3 or 4 days), intercostal drainage of pus usually suffices. If the disease is diagnosed 4 or 5 days after the onset of empyema, it is best to decide on the basis of a lateral decubitus film. If the thickness of fluid on such a film is less than 1 cm, mostly intercostal drainage would suffice. If the thickness gauged is more than 1 cm, mere intercostal drain may not cure the disease, but one needs endoscopic surgery. If the child presents much later, imaging should be used to detect multiloculated effusion. Now, if the child is afebrile and looking well, one may observe closely and decide later about surgery. However, if such a child is febrile and sick, he needs decortication.

CASE 36

■ Rheumatic Fever

Events...

An 8-year-old boy presented with the history of fever with joint pains for last two months. He was advised certain laboratory tests, wherein the ASO titer was reported to be 125 todd units, CRP was negative and ESR was 40 mm at the end of one hour; the CBC was within normal limits. So he was put on long-term penicillin prophylaxis. 2D echocardiogram was normal. Except the above-mentioned reports and a prescription of injection Penicillin, there were no other records available.

He has started taking the injections but has now come for a second opinion.

On physical examination, no abnormality was detected.

What are the options for further management?

In order to be able to take the right decision and choose the correct action, one must have a probable clinical diagnosis, for which many more details in the history need to be known. At present, since this child is completely normal, there are no abnormal physical findings to go by, that will help us to make a retrospective diagnosis of rheumatic fever. At this stage, laboratory tests may also not offer any definite clue to the diagnosis of rheumatic fever. Finally, one may have to weigh the probable need for long-acting penicillin prophylaxis against the risk involved in not giving it.

Ideal Option—Obtain a Detailed History and Decide

It is difficult to decide now whether this child did suffer from acute rheumatic fever in the past, in the absence of any detailed clinical records or notes. The diagnosis of acute rheumatic fever is based on clearly defined clinical manifestations, with supportive evidence of a recent streptococcal infection. While the latter is an absolute necessity to diagnose rheumatic fever, it is in conjunction with appropriate clinical manifestations. It is not rational to diagnose rheumatic fever only on the basis of evidence of recent streptococcal infection, in the absence of appropriate clinical features. The mere presence of ASO antibodies does not necessarily mean a recent streptococcal infection, though the higher the titer, more is the chance of it being a recent infection.

On trying to obtain a detailed history, the parents could not remember the events clearly but said that this child had high grade fever for 3 or 4 days, which was followed by pain in both the knees and ankles. The pain was apparently severe enough, so that the child could not walk for two days. On direct questioning, they said that there was minimal swelling of the joints. There was no clear history of the pain of being migratory in nature. The patient was prescribed ibuprofen along with an antibiotic and some other medications after which the pain and fever gradually subsided. There was some history of soreness of the throat, about three weeks prior to this event.

On analyzing the above history, while it seems reasonable to deduce that this child had an episode of polyarthritis, its migratory nature has not been established. If we ignore this and take the polyarthritis as a major criterion, and fever as one minor criterion, then the elevated ESR could be another minor criterion (though the CRP is negative), thereby suggesting the possibility of rheumatic fever. In that event, a positive ASO titer is significant. However, ASO titers have to be interpreted in the context of the prevailing baseline titers in the community. In about 15 to 20% of patients the ASO titer may not be high enough even in a genuine case of rheumatic fever. At such times, anti-DNAse B (whose positivity lasts longer), if positive, strengthens the case. A 2D echocardiogram may be repeated, and of course, if it is abnormal, retrospective diagnosis of rheumatic fever is confirmed.

Acceptable Option—When in Doubt Consider it to be Rheumatic Fever

If the history given by the parents convincingly refutes the diagnosis of rheumatic fever, and the laboratory evidence is flimsy, one may be bold enough to discontinue penicillin prophylaxis, since continuation of therapy has its own attendant problems. However, since the consequences of discontinuing penicillin prophylaxis could be disastrous in a genuine case of rheumatic fever, one may be compelled to continue when the doubts cannot be resolved clearly, one way or the other.

Unacceptable Option—Stop Penicillin Prophylaxis

Since the arthritis has not been documented, but is only inferred from the patients, version, and its migratory nature has not been established, the major criterion of migratory polyarthritis itself is not unequivocal. In that event, the minor criteria and the laboratory evidence cannot support the diagnosis by themselves. While a dramatic response to salicylates adds to the diagnosis of rheumatic fever, in this case the use of ibuprofen and an apparently gradual response confuses the issue. A close differential of the above situation would be reactive arthritis following a viral fever; clinical notes favoring the same would have been helpful. However, in the absence of medical records clearly denoting physical findings at the time of the acute illness, it would be unwise to rule out the diagnosis of rheumatic fever at this stage. One cannot even depend on the negative history given by the parents to refute the diagnosis of rheumatic fever. In this child, parents confirmed an acute onset of pain and swelling of the large joints that lasted for a short duration and recovered completely. Such statements can be consistent with the diagnosis of rheumatic fever, even though there was no history of fleeting joint involvement. If most of the statements suggest the diagnosis of rheumatic fever, one may have to give credence to the possibility of it being correct and advise long-term prophylaxis.

Experience gained…

> In illnesses characterized by short lasting clinical manifestations, when the patient is seen in the asymptomatic stage and does not have any residual physical signs to go by, it is impossible to come to a definitive diagnosis in the absence of observations recorded by a doctor. Thus, it is extremely vital to document clinical findings and the course of events, as they progress. If this is not done, there may be many situations in clinical medicine where one ends up with the proverbial difficult choice between the devil and the deep sea.

Rheumatic Fever

Diagnosis of acute rheumatic fever can be challenging, more so when there is a recurrence of rheumatic fever in a child with pre-existing valvular damage. For many years, we have been using Jones criteria for diagnosis—either two major or one major and two minor criteria along with evidence of recent streptococcal infection—either in the form of positive culture/antigen test or elevated or increasing antibody titer. However, we must understand some limitations. ASLO peaks in 3 weeks and starts coming down by 6 weeks or sometimes even longer. Minor criteria are non-specific and may even be seen in juvenile idiopathic arthritis. Early administration of aspirin/NSAIDs may not allow some criteria to clinically manifest sufficiently enough to justify the diagnosis. The presence of subcutaneous nodules generally seen on the extensor surface of upper limbs indicates active carditis but such nodules disappear within 2–3 weeks. Erythema marginatum has no relation to carditis.

The Jones criteria have been revised in 2015; the key changes are:
1. In moderate/high-risk populations, which is defined as ARF incidence >2 per 100,000 in school-age children per year, or all-age RHD prevalence of >1 per 1,000 population:
   a. Recurrent attack can be diagnosed if 2 major, or 1 major and 2 minor, or 3 minor criteria are present (plus evidence of recent GAS infection).
   b. Monoarthritis or polyarthralgia are also considered as a major criterion (as against the need for polyarthritis, which remains a requirement in low-risk populations).
   c. Monoarthralgia is a minor criterion (because polyarthralgia is now a major criterion); the others being fever of >38°C and ESR >30 mm/hr.
2. Carditis is now defined as clinical and/or subclinical; so echocardiographic valvulitis (with defined changes) is also a major criterion even in the absence of clinical signs of carditis.

Streptococcal reactive arthritis is different than acute rheumatic arthritis in that arthritis is non-migratory, often involves small and big joints, manifests within a week of streptococcal infection and is often prolonged with poor response to aspirin. It is due to different streptococcal strains. Treatment of acute arthritis/carditis without cardiomegaly or CCF consists of aspirin 75 mg/kg/day for 3–5 days followed by aspirin 50 mg/kg/day for 3–4 weeks, further by 25 mg/kg/day for another 3–4 weeks guided by ESR coming back to normal. Strenuous exercise should be avoided though routine movements in the house are fine. Carditis with cardiomegaly or CCF should be treated with prednisolone 2 mg/kg/day for 3–4 weeks followed by 1 mg/kg/day for another 3–4 weeks and then gradually taper prednisolone and add aspirin 50 mg/kg/day for next 6 weeks. Chorea is treated with haloperidol or phenobarbitone till control.

CASE 37

UTI—1st Episode at 4-year of Age

Events...

A 4-year-old female child presented with a history of high fever for three days without any focus of infection. After initial symptomatic treatment had failed, she underwent routine laboratory tests that showed neutrophilic leukocytosis and 40 to 50 pus cells per high power field in the urine. She was diagnosed to have a urinary tract infection and started on Norfloxacin. She recovered within the next four days and therapy was continued for a total of eight days.

What are the options for further management?

Ideal Option—Detailed History, Abdominal USG, DMSA Scan

It is important to confirm whether this was the first attack of UTI. This is not easy. She must have had episodes of fever in the past, and it is likely that she might have received antibiotics without a proper diagnosis, in which case one cannot be sure of the absence of urinary tract infection in the past. It makes sense to clearly define the status of the kidneys in terms of any scar due to previous infective episodes, instead of debating whether this was the first attack of UTI or otherwise. So even, if an abdominal USG is normal, it may be ideal to confirm normality on a DMSA scan, so as to not be in the dark. In case one picks up any abnormality on the DMSA scan, antibiotic prophylaxis may have to be considered for at least a year before reviewing the situation again. A close follow-up is mandatory in every case of UTI, irrespective of the plan of action.

Acceptable Option—Detailed History and Abdominal USG

If one is sure that this child has remained healthy all along, without any recurrent episodes of high fever since early infancy, it may mean that the present episode is the first attack of UTI. If her abdominal USG is normal and she has grown well (good height and weight), one may consider no further investigations, though one must follow her closely. Obviously, this decision may have to be subsequently modified, in case there is another attack of UTI. It goes without saying, that if the abdominal USG is abnormal, one would definitely order a DMSA scan.

Unacceptable Option—No Intervention

It is incorrect to merely follow her up, without even an abdominal USG. While there is a high chance of her being normal and this episode of UTI being an accident, it is worthwhile to do an abdominal USG to confirm the absence of any obvious defect that may result in recurrence of infection.

Experience gained...

It is not enough to diagnose UTI and treat it successfully with antibiotics. At the end of proper treatment, it must be followed by relevant laboratory and imaging studies to rule out any underlying abnormalities, and to assess the damage done already in terms of renal scarring.This has repercussions on subsequent renal function and the health of the child. Depending on the results of such investigations, antibiotic prophylaxis and careful follow-up is mandatory to ensure normal renal function in future.

In the case of a presumed first attck of UTI, when the patient is an infant or a young child, he/she obviously needs to be thoroughly investigated. These investigations are primarily aimed at detecting underlying abnormalities. Amongst these abnormalities, VUR usually resolves naturally by 5 years of age. So, when the patient is a child who is 5 years or older, one may attempt to minimize investigations (especially VCUG), if one can reasonably gauge the presence/absence of significant VUR (that needs antibiotic prophylaxis), by less invasive investigations. If the USG picks up a VUR, it implies that VUR is of a significant grade still, and therefore needs further investigation and management. On the other hand, if the USG is normal, even if the DMSA scan shows renal scarring, it may be reasonable to assume that VUR has nearly resolved, and therefore, does not need further investigations or management.

Needless to say, all such children require a close follow-up.

Urinary Tract Infection

Diagnosis of acute UTI is an emergency as delayed or irrational treatment runs the risk of permanent renal damage and more so in younger children. Acute onset of high fever in a sick-looking infant or young child demands ruling out UTI before starting an antibiotic.

Routine urinalysis showing >10 leukocytes or a centrifuged sample showing >5 leukocytes is suggestive of UTI. However, it must be confirmed by urine culture. If the culture grows organisms which are the normal periurethral flora (*Lactobacillus* in females and *Enterococci* in infants and toddlers) or if it grows multiple organisms it should be considered a contaminated sample. In a correctly collected sample, significant growth of *Klebsiella*, *Acinetobacter* or *Pseudomonas* even in the absence of pyuria should be considered as UTI, while the growth of other uropathogens in the culture without pyuria needs repeat tests to confirm the diagnosis. A urine dipstick test is acceptable for monitoring progress.

Every case of UTI in an infant must be investigated with USG at the time of diagnosis, MCU after 3-4 weeks and DMSA scan after 3-4 months to rule out any congenital malformations, VUR and renal scarring (if already developed). Between 1 and 5 years of age, USG and DMSA scan should be ordered and >5 years, only USG is adequate. Subsequent follow-up should include periodic growth chart and blood pressure monitoring, urinalysis during every non-localized febrile episode, irrespective of its probable etiology and eGFR if necessary to evaluate renal function. A rise in serum creatinine is a late biochemical sign of renal dysfunction.

Lower UTI is referred to as simple UTI and upper UTI as complicated UTI. Infant <3 months with simple UTI and complicated UTI at any age should be treated with IV ceftriaxone for 10-14 days and simple UTI in an infant/child >3 months of age may be treated with oral cotrimoxazole or cefpodoxime for 7 days. Prophylactic therapy with cephalexin or cotrimoxazole in a single morning dose is ideal for recurrent UTI and children with grade 1-2 VUR for one year and those with grade 3-4 VUR till 5 years of age.

CASE 38

Constipation

Case

A 2-year-old child presented with constipation since birth. He was born after full term with C-section delivery and birth weight of 3 kg. He was started on formula feeds at birth as mother reported lack of breast feeds. At present, he consumes fresh animal milk through bottle. He refuses to eat solid food; his intake is largely milk. He has been passing hard stools since early infancy and it is worsening over last one year, so much that he passes stool once in 4–5 days with great difficulty. He suppresses the urge as long as possible and then tries to pass the stool in a standing posture. There is no history of vomiting.

Physical Examination

Weight 10 kg, length 86 cm, normal development, generalized abdominal distension with palpable fecal masses. Other systems were normal.

Does this child need further investigations?

It is important to analyze the history to consider whether constipation in this child could be due to a pathological cause. As constipation has existed almost since birth, one must be cautious to rule out congenital megacolon, any other cause of intestinal obstruction and hypothyroidism. There is no information about the timing of passage of meconium. Delayed passage of meconium may have suggested congenital megacolon or hypothyroidism. However, since the growth has not been affected much in this child, both conditions are unlikely. Theoretically, ultra-small segment Hirschsprung's disease or mild degree of hypothyroidism may still be a possibility. Any other cause of intestinal obstruction can be definitely ruled out as constipation has been present for too long. Quantitative or qualitative nutritional deficiency may also cause constipation. While this child consumes enough calories, his intake is certainly qualitatively imbalanced in that he survives only on milk with much higher protein intake. His refusal to eat is due to bottle addiction. It is the fear of pain while passing stool that makes him suppress his urge and avoid passing stool; this leads to further hardening of stool, which makes it further difficult and more painful to pass, and this sets up a vicious cycle. So, it is best that these factors are corrected first before embarking on multiple tests.

How do you manage this child's constipation?

It is imperative that parents cooperate fully, and this will be possible only, if we communicate well with them and provide a detailed explanation of the problem. The first thing to change is to de-addict him from his bottle feeding and offer him milk in a glass or cup. This would automatically reduce his intake of milk and avoid feeding in sleep. In turn, the child would be hungry to accept anything other than milk. It would initiate him into normal eating habits. It takes patience on the part of parents to get rid of bottle feeding. Family food should be offered to him with particular emphasis on roughage and avoiding food items that may lead to constipation. Forced feeding should be avoided even at the expense of poor intake for a while. Eating willingly and happily is important to ensure ideal intake. Fear of getting hurt while passing stools needs to be addressed properly. Within limits, child should be left to handle this issue by himself and should not be forced to squat on a potty. Stool softeners, such as polyethylene glycol or lactulose help to pass stool easily, and this gradually allays the fear associated with the act of passing stool. Suppositories and enema are best avoided as they induce more fear; these should be reserved only for an emergency to relieve long-standing fecal masses. It is most important that stool must be passed each day with or without intervention. Otherwise, it may lead to undue stretching of rectal muscles that may result in permanent constipation due to loss of muscle tone. It takes quite some time for all these measures to take effect and relieve the constipation in such a child. Parents have to be both patient and persistent in their efforts.

Lessons Learnt

> Constipation is a common problem in children that is often ignored. It is often caused by diet related habits more than pathological conditions. Inculcating good eating and bowel habits is important in a toddler. Balanced food with enough roughage helps pass stool every day with ease. Persistent constipation is a semi-emergency because, if not tackled in time, it may lead to irreversible loss of rectal muscle tone resulting in permanent constipation.

CASE 39

■ Nephrotic Syndrome

Events...

A 4-year-old girl with steroid responsive nephrotic syndrome suffered from a relapse as her steroids were being tapered off. The relapse was precipitated by a respiratory infection which was controlled with amoxicillin. She became afebrile and was looking well, but her edema and ascites persisted. At this stage, she was hospitalized, prednisolone was reinstituted in appropriate doses and frusemide was added to allay her discomfort due to edema and ascites. However, there was no response even after four days of this treatment; in fact, her edema and ascites had increased. She was not dehydrated nor oliguric, and there was no evidence of infection clinically or on investigations. Peritoneal tap was not done.

What are the options for further management?

Ideal Option—Critically Review the Present Management

Routinely while the maximum focus is on the drug treatment of any illness, ancillary management is believed to play an insignificant role and is often sidelined. Further, the execution of this ancillary management is usually left to the parents and is often not monitored. As a result, in chronic illnesses, their enthusiasm to implement this part of the management tends to slacken with time. Nephrotic syndrome is one illness where this ancillary management, which includes regulated salt and fluid intake, is extremely important. Therefore, it makes sound clinical sense to review each and every aspect of the present management, including drug dosages and their compliance and the ancillary management, before planning additional investigations or therapy.

Acceptable Option—In Addition to the Above, Add Spironolactone

Secondary hyperaldosteronism is always associated with nephrotic syndrome and may contribute significantly to the vicious cycle of salt and water retention, thereby preventing the edema from resolving. To counteract this, one may add spironolactone.

Unacceptable Option—Add Broad-Spectrum Antibiotic without Investigations

Assuming an uncontrolled infection, which is the most common cause of failure to respond to steroids, one may wish to start higher antibiotics. However, without any proof of infection, this could be dangerous. At the least, a CBC, peritoneal tap, and urine culture should be asked for before taking this step.

Case Progression

It was decided to critically review the present management. Though this child was on a salt restricted diet, she was consuming a few biscuits daily, which contributed to her sodium intake.

Her fluid intake ranged between 1150 to 1750 mL while her urine output was between 950 to 1175 mL. Her salt restriction was strictly enforced, and her fluid intake was also restricted to 800 mL.

Final Outcome

From the next day, her urine output started increasing and went up to 3000 to 3500 mL/24 hours. Her edema and ascites decreased considerably in the next four days, and a week later she went into remission.

Experience gained...

> Maintaining a balance between the intake of fluids and the output, and salt restriction are two important interventions in a child with nephrotic syndrome. Especially in case of a therapeutic failure, these factors must be carefully managed. If a child with nephrotic syndrome has lost fluids due to diarrhea or vomiting and has thereby become oliguric, intravenous fluids may be necessary. However, in case of oliguria without loss of fluids, restriction of fluids is mandatory.

Nephrotic Syndrome

Generalized edema, proteinuria, and hypoalbuminemia are characteristic of this disease while hypercholesterolemia is not an essential part of the definition. Primary NS is most often due to minimal change disease but may also be due to many other pathologies. Congenital NS (Finnish type) presents early in infancy and does not respond to treatment. At times, NS may be secondary to infections such as HBV or HCV, *Plasmodium malariae* (not common in India), autoimmune disorders such as SLE or HSP and also due to lymphoma or leukemia. The pathophysiology of edema is ascribed to either low osmotic pressure (underfill theory) or to primary sodium retention (overfill theory)—the latter explaining some patients of NS who present without oliguria.

Standard treatment consists of prednisolone 2 mg/kg/day for 6 weeks followed by 1.5 mg/kg alternate morning in a single dose for another 6 weeks. Relapse is treated with prednisolone 2 mg/kg/day till remission is achieved followed by 1.5 mg/kg/day alternate morning dose for 4 weeks. Steroid-dependent NS is treated with the least possible steroid dose that can maintain remission and if this dose happens to be more than 0.5 mg/kg or in case of toxicity, other drugs are used such as levamisole, mycophenolate, cyclophosphamide, cyclosporine, tacrolimus or rituximab. Both steroid-dependent and steroid-resistant nephrotic syndromes are best treated by specialists. Infections and hypercoagulable states are likely complications of nephrotic syndrome.

CASE 40

■ Immune Thrombocytopenic Purpura

Events...

A 4-year-old healthy girl presented with a sudden onset of a petechial rash all over the body over a period of three days. She also developed epistaxis and bleeding from the gums. There was no history of fever, and she was active and playful. There was no history of recent drug use. On examination, there was no pallor or hepatosplenomegaly. She was diagnosed to have Immune (idiopathic) thrombocytopenic purpura (ITP), with her platelet count being $8000/mm^3$.

What are the options for further management?

Such a child, who has been correctly diagnosed as ITP, can be managed in different ways; there may not be any difference in the final outcome, anyway. However, one may have to justify the particular option chosen.

Ideal Option—Hospitalize the Child and Start Steroids

The logic behind admitting a child with ITP with a platelet count of $8000/mm^3$ could possibly be:
- Keeping the child under close observation for symptoms and signs of intracranial hemorrhage, which is a potentially life-threatening complication of ITP at these platelet counts.
- Medicolegal implications of not admitting such a child and
- Enforce rest thereby minimizing chances of injury.

Steroid therapy appears to induce a more rapid rise in platelet counts than in untreated patients and may therefore be justified to reach the theoretically safe level of platelet counts of $20,000/mm^3$. Further, though the amount of bleeding (from the gums and by way of epistaxis) in such a patient may not be clinically significant, it is distressing to the patient and parents. Therefore, it needs to be controlled.

Since the sudden onset of a petechial rash in a well child, with the rest of the clinical examination being absolutely normal, leaves almost no differential diagnosis, a bone marrow examination is not considered mandatory prior to initiating steroid therapy. If one finds large platelets on the peripheral smear, it denotes a good response on the part of megakaryocytes and rules out bone marrow abnormality. It is rare for megakaryocytopenia to precede reduction of other cell lines in leukemia. However, if the clinical features of ITP are not unequivocal, or the peripheral smear does not support the diagnosis, it may be safe to perform a bone marrow examination prior to starting steroids, as it would otherwise jeopardize the outcome in acute lymphatic leukemia.

Acceptable Option—Hospitalize and Give IVIG

Since the use of steroids is fraught with an inherent danger of side effects and could also adversely affect the outcome in the event of a leukemia being missed, IVIG may be a good alternative. IVIG, administered in the dose of 0.8 to 1 g/kg/day for two days, rapidly raises the platelet count above 20,000/mm^3. However, it is expensive and needs intravenous therapy and therefore, hospitalization. There is also a risk of aseptic meningitis due to the treatment. However, the invasive procedure of bone marrow examination can be avoided, since steroids are not being used.

Ethically Unacceptable Option—No Treatment

There are no convincing data to suggest that treatment affects either the short term or long-term outcome of ITP in pediatric patients. Though counts of less than 10,000/mm^3 are considered 'unsafe', intracranial hemorrhage may not occur even with counts as low as 5000/mm^3 or less. On the other hand, there is no guarantee that intracranial hemorrhage will not occur at a platelet count of 20,000/mm^3 or more. Intracranial hemorrhage is rare, and considering the rarity of the event, it is not clear whether treatment of ITP cases has really reduced the incidence of intracranial hemorrhage. Further, treatment or the lack of it, does not seem to influence the incidence of chronic ITP. Therefore, barring the need to raise the platelet count to a theoretically safe level of 20,000/mm^3, there may be no advantage in treating ITP patients with either modality. Therefore, one could opt for no treatment. 70 to 80 percent of the cases would spontaneously resolve and get 'cured' within a maximum of six months. However, as per the standard guidelines, with such a low platelet count, one should still opt for treatment.

Unacceptable Option—Platelet Transfusion

It is futile to try and raise the platelet counts by transfusing platelets. The transfused platelets are destroyed by the antiplatelet antibodies, thereby not allowing a sustained rise in the counts. This treatment should only be attempted in the event of an intracranial hemorrhage. In this situation, one hopes to buy time, while organizing other treatment options like emergency splenectomy.

Case Progression

This child was treated with steroids after a bone marrow aspiration was normal. The platelet count improved over three days to 55000/mm^3, but thereafter there was no further significant sustained rise. The counts ranged from 55000/mm^3 to 70,000/mm^3 even after two weeks of steroid therapy, at which time the drugs were stopped. The child continued to manifest a petechial rash from time to time and would off and on develop mucosal bleeds; but was otherwise asymptomatic. Even after six months, there was no change in the clinical picture.

What are the options for further management?

Ideal Option—Observe Closely without Drug Treatment

As this child is reasonably asymptomatic, one may observe closely for any significant bleed that may necessitate treatment. If the bleeding is minor and gets controlled quickly, it is better to just observe the further progress.

Unacceptable Option—Restart Steroids and Continue Long-term
Long-term steroids carry the risk of attendant toxicity and should be prescribed only if there are significant clinical symptoms; they should not be used in a child whose counts are lower than normal but who is not significantly symptomatic clinically.

Unacceptable Option—Splenectomy
While splenectomy is curative, one has to weigh the lifelong risk of overwhelming post splenectomy infections (OPSIs) against the current disability and against the alternate option of long-term steroids. Though the risk of OPSI can be partially minimized by advising pneumococcal vaccine and penicillin prophylaxis, splenectomy should be advised only if the symptoms of chronic ITP are sufficiently severe to affect the quality of life. It may also be considered, if steroid therapy is mandatory and yet is leading to unacceptable toxicity.

Experience gained...

> If the patient presents a week or more after the onset of symptoms, it should be safe not to opt for any treatment. However, when the patient presents early in the course of the disease, the treatment options are debatable.

Treatment of ITP
Immune thrombocytopenic purpura presents either as a newly diagnosed disease (it is no longer referred to as acute ITP because it may not present acutely), or persistent ITP (lasting for 3–12 months) or chronic ITP (>12 months) or recurrent ITP (presenting 3 months after complete remission) or refractory ITP (failure to respond).

ITP is a diagnosis of exclusion, and an antibody test is not required for diagnosis. It is rare below 2 years of age.

Treatment is not based on platelet count alone but also on the presence of significant bleeding and presence of risk factors (early in the course of presentation). IVIG 1 g/kg in a single dose is the drug of choice but prednisolone or methylprednisolone for 7 days may be alternatives. Anti-D (50–75 µg/kg in a single dose IV) is considered only in Rh+ve and Coombs -ve children having Hb >10%. It acts within 12 hours, IVIG takes 24 hours while steroids take 3 days to show a response. Platelet transfusion is ineffective as the transfused platelets would be destroyed by antibodies. Immature platelet function >10% denotes a recovering platelet count.

ITP must be differentiated from other causes of thrombocytopenia that include inherited disorders such as Wiskott–Aldrich or Chédiak-Higashi syndrome (immunodeficiency), Bernard–Soulier or Von Willebrand disease and also bone marrow disorders or hypersplenism.

CASE 41

■ Reactive Arthritis Secondary to Mediastinal Malignancy

Events...

A 12-year-old child was seen for complaints that had started four years ago. At that time, he had developed an acute onset of pain and swelling in the right ankle joint that lasted for two days. He got relieved with Ibuprofen and was never investigated. He had a similar episode six months later, at which time the right ankle arthritis was treated as reactive arthritis and he did get better after a week of Ibuprofen. Routine investigations done at that time were non-contributory. A few months later, he suffered another relapse and thereafter, such recurrences became more and more frequent and would also last longer than the previous episodes. At no time did physical examination reveal any other abnormality except the right ankle arthritis. Repeated investigations did not yield any particular diagnosis. Each time, he was treated with non-steroidal anti-inflammatory drugs but never steroids. X-rays done on a few of these occasions had not shown any significant radiological changes.

What are the options for further management?

It is important to consider a provisional diagnosis before embarking on decision-making about further management.

Analysis

This child has had recurrent arthritis of the right ankle joint for last four years, without involvement of any other joints or any other system. This is obviously a local problem in the right ankle joint. **Recurrent monoarthritis** could be either an allergic manifestation (**reactive** arthritis) or due to a **local** malformation which is aggravated by unnoticed trauma. It is unlikely to be due to an **infection** as it has gone on for very long. **Collagen vascular disease** is also not possible for the same reason. **Sickle cell disease** may develop recurrent bone or joint involvement but often at multiple sites, and there would have been some evidence of such a disease clinically. **Leukemia** may present with a joint involvement but would not remain silent for a long time.

Ideal Option—Investigate Further

As the disease has been localized to the right ankle joint alone, it is rational to order a MRI of that joint. It is likely to pick up a lesion that may have been missed earlier on the X-ray. Though a congenital malformation would be obvious on MRI, demonstration of any other lesion would not offer any clue to the etiology of the disease. In fact, it is more important to rule out the spread of the disease beyond the only joint that is clinically visibly involved. Thus, demonstration of polyarticular disease or other bony involvement would bring in different etiologies other than diseases restricted to a single joint. Thus, MRI should evaluate the entire skeleton. Another alternative could be a radionuclide bone scan that would pick up any hot spot in other parts of the skeleton.

Routine hematological tests may not reveal any additional information and at best, would rule out some of the disorders mentioned above. Whatever the etiology, ESR is likely to be high and would not offer any additional information.

If a radiological lesion is found in the right ankle joint, one may consider an open biopsy for histopathological diagnosis. Since the provisional diagnosis is reactive arthritis, the biopsy report is likely to be nonspecific; however, it would rule out the rare possibility of a slowly growing local malignancy.

Unacceptable Option—Empirical Trial with Steroids

Using steroids in this child is irrational as it may mask the underlying disease. Moreover, if this is considered to be an allergic reactive arthritis, it may settle down by itself and there is no advantage of using drugs other than symptomatic anti-inflammatory agents.

Case Progression

A month before he presented to us, he had started developing mild breathlessness that went on increasing gradually, for which he was eventually hospitalized.

On admission, a physical examination showed a sick pale child with respiratory distress. Examination of the respiratory system revealed dullness over the right side of the chest with diminished breath sounds, without any foreign sounds. These physical signs did not correlate with the surface anatomy of a lobar or pleural distribution. The right ankle joint was swollen and tender with restriction of movements in all directions. All other joints were normal. Other systems were normal.

Final Outcome

Since this child had developed a gradually increasing breathlessness with chest signs that suggested a mediastinal mass, a chest X-ray was ordered that showed a large mediastinal tumor. A biopsy suggested that it was an undifferentiated malignancy.

Analysis

Therefore, one is now forced to conclude that the recurrent reactive arthritis was in response to a malignancy that had initially remained silent, and has now surfaced, four years after the initial manifestation. In retrospect, if one had planned a skeletal survey of the entire body as an aid to evaluate the subclinical involvement of other joints or bones, one may have come across a small silent mediastinal mass that could have given us the diagnosis much earlier. But of course, this is hindsight.

Reactive Arthritis

The classic triad of arthritis, urethritis and conjunctivitis—Reiter syndrome is uncommon in children. Typically, reactive arthritis presents in isolation as arthritis following gastrointestinal or urogenital infections commonly *Campylobacter, Chlamydia, Yersinia,*

Mycoplasma, *Salmonella*, or *Shigella*—a result of an aberrant immune response that may occur weeks to months after an infection. The disease presents typically as acute onset asymmetrical oligoarthritis mainly affecting lower limb joints including the sacroiliac joint and spine. It is often accompanied by tendonitis and enthesitis. Nocturnal pain and morning stiffness are common. Extra-articular manifestations are also known including urethritis and conjunctivitis.

The diagnosis of reactive arthritis is based on the exclusion of other causes of arthritis with circumstantial evidence of a triggering infection. Many other conditions such as psoriatic arthritis, inflammatory bowel disease with arthritis and ankylosing spondylitis closely mimic reactive arthritis.

There are no specific tests for confirmation and the treatment is symptomatic. While the disease is often self-limiting, it is also known to run a chronic course and even recurrence is also seen.

Experience gained...

> In an undiagnosed condition, one may have to consider imaging to assess various anatomical sites that could be involved in the disease process, so that a particular site may become accessible to biopsy. Reactive arthritis may be secondary to infections or malignancy, and from that point of view one may have to plan extensive investigations.

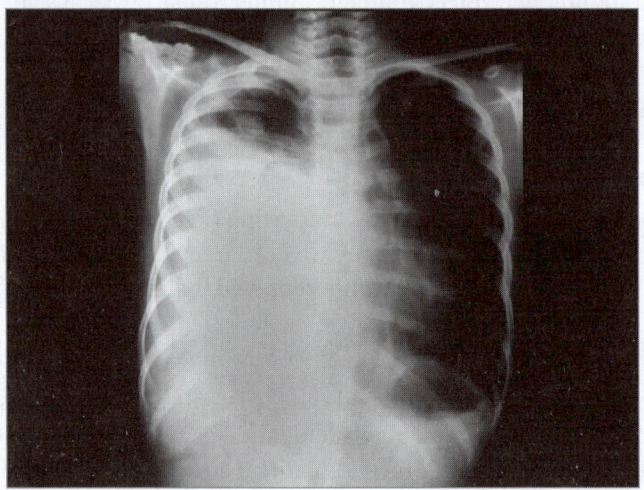

Large mass in the mediastinum.

Management Dilemmas in Office Practice 85

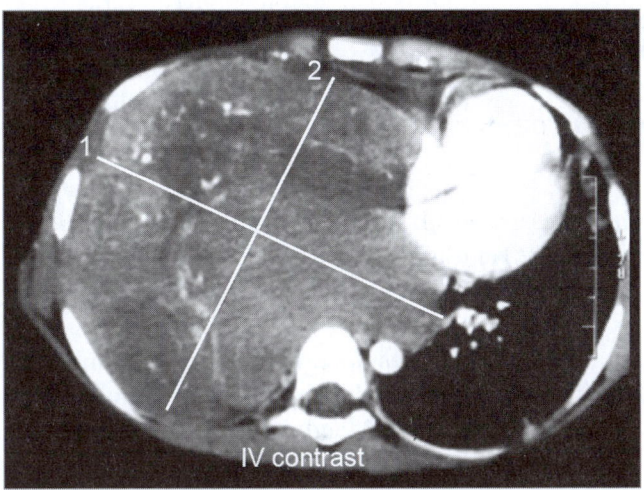

CT scan showing large mediastinal mass.

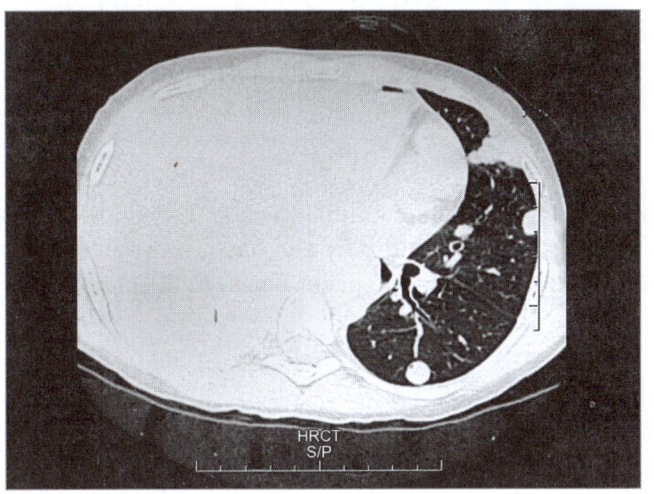

CT scan showing large mass.

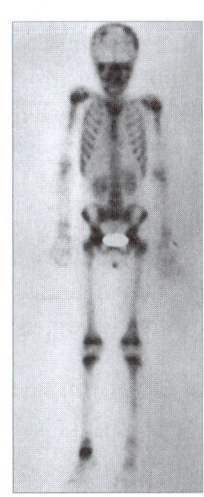

Bone scan.

CASE 42

■ Mismanaged Gastroenteritis

Events...

An 18-month-old child presented with vomiting for a day followed by loose stools. There was no fever or abdominal pain. He was seen by a pediatrician and prescribed a combination of ofloxacin and metronidazole. In spite of this therapy being continued for the next four days, there was no improvement as the loose stools continued and the frequency of vomiting had, in fact, increased. The vomiting was never bile stained. Routine stool examination had shown a few pus cells and presence of reducing substances. The child was advised a soya milk formula and was asked to avoid solid food. However, since there was no improvement whatsoever, he was advised hospitalization for parenteral therapy. At that stage, the parents opted for another opinion.

What are the options for further management?

In order to be able to take the right decision and choose the correct action, one must have a probable clinical diagnosis, for which, many more details in the history need to be known. This should be followed by a thorough clinical examination.

Additional History

On detailed enquiry, he had lost one kilogram over this week and was now anorexic and irritable. Apparently, he had been a healthy child so far and had grown well. He was never bottle-fed and consumed family food. There was no major illness in the past and the family was educated and hygienic.

Physical Examination

It revealed a well-nourished child without dehydration, who was irritable but not very sick. The abdomen was soft and not distended. The systemic examination was normal.

Analysis

This child has been a healthy child all along, without any risk factors for gastrointestinal infections since he was not bottle-fed and the family was reasonably hygienic. Hence, the present episode of gastrointestinal infection may at best, be a viral infection that he must have contracted accidentally. Even, if one considers it to be a bacterial infection, there should have been no hurry to start an antibiotic, because not all bacterial infections need an antibiotic to get cured. Further, the combination of an antibiotic with metronidazole is irrational, as dual infections are extremely rare and much more, so at this age, in such a healthy child. An ideal action in the initial stages of any such illness is to maintain hydration and nutrition as much as possible. Vomiting in acute gastroenteritis is usually a short lasting and self-limiting symptom and does not require any drug treatment. At the most, an occasional dose of metoclopramide or domperidone may be justified. Routinely, one would have expected this child's loose stools to get better within 3 to 4 days, while the vomiting should have come under control within a day. As the progress in this child was quite different, one will have to logically explain the possible reasons behind such an unanticipated course.

Prolongation of vomiting and loose stools may be due to a drug resistant infection or due to complications of the disease itself. A drug resistant infection would have led to worsening of his condition and not just a prolongation of his symptoms. Complications, such as dehydration and electrolyte disturbances, sepsis, intussusception, or hemolytic uremic syndrome are ruled out as there are no symptoms and clinical signs to suggest the same. Thus, in this child, prolongation of symptoms is likely to be related to iatrogenic factors such as side effects of drugs or the dietary changes that were introduced.

Persistent vomiting is possibly attributed to the drug, especially metronidazole, or it could be the result of the soya formula which is often not palatable. Loose stools may be a manifestation of malabsorption following acute gastroenteritis and may have been aggravated by an unnecessary restriction of food and use of antibiotics.

Ideal Option—Withdraw all Drugs, Start Normal Diet

As discussed above, persistent infection is not the cause for this child's prolongation of symptoms. The cause is quite likely to be iatrogenic and therefore, the ideal option is to withdraw all medications and put the child on a normal diet and wait for a spontaneous recovery.

Unacceptable Option 1—Hospitalize and Start an IV Antibiotic

As this child does not look sick and is not dehydrated, there is no need for hospitalization. Though this child has been treated with antibiotics right from the first day of his illness, he has not responded. Nor has he deteriorated. Hence, parenteral antibiotics are ruled out.

Unacceptable Option 2—Change Antibiotic and/or Use Prebiotic/Probiotic/Racecadotril

A change of antibiotic is not justified because the progress of the illness does not suggest a drug resistant infection. In the first place, there is no reason to suspect drug resistance in community-acquired infections. In fact, in such a healthy child from a hygienic family, a bacterial GI infection itself is not common.

Drugs like prebiotics and probiotics are not indicated in such a situation. They may be reserved for a few specific conditions, such as antibiotic associated diarrhea due to *Clostridium difficile*. One may argue that this is exactly the situation in this child, since the diarrhea has persisted after the use of an antibiotic. However, one needs to differentiate between antibiotic induced diarrhea and antibiotic associated diarrhea. The former condition is a side effect of antibiotics, and the child is not sick. On the other hand, antibiotic associated diarrhea is a superimposed secondary infection due to *C. difficile*, in which the child may pass blood and mucus in stools and appears quite sick. Racecadotril is an antisecretory drug and is not useful in diarrhea caused by other mechanisms. Moreover, even in infections causing secretory diarrhea, its benefits are marginal. Thus this option is no good.

Unacceptable Option 3—Investigate for Resistant Infections, Immunodeficiency and Malabsorption

As mentioned above, this is not likely to be a drug resistant infection. In fact, stool culture has very few indications in clinical practice and should be reserved for cases of protracted diarrhea in a malnourished infant. Even in such cases, the mere growth of *E. coli* does not guide us to any specific action, as further sub-typing of *E. coli* alone can label the organisms grown to be pathogenic or otherwise. Collecting a stool sample for a culture is also not an easy proposition.

This child is obviously immunocompetent as is evident by the status of his health and the fact that he has had no major illness in the past. He has been immunized up to date and has not shown any adverse reaction.

Similarly, this is not a primary malabsorption; that would have presented much earlier in life. If this is a secondary malabsorption following acute gastroenteritis, this should settle down by itself and in fact, continuation of drugs may interfere with its recovery.

Case Progression

It was decided to withdraw all the drugs and allow normal food that the child used to consume. There was no improvement over the next 24 hours and the parents were worried, more so because no drugs had been prescribed in spite of the child not getting better over the last eight days. They were reassured again, and they agreed to continue following the same advice.

Final Outcome

By the next day, the vomiting had stopped, and the stools gradually came back to normal. The parents were grateful to us for their child's recovery, and we were grateful to them for their patience.

Experience gained…

> Acute diarrhea in a healthy child does not need any specific treatment other than ORS and continuation of the normal feeding pattern. There is neither a need for soya formula nor any justification to use drugs like antibiotic combinations, prebiotics, probiotics and racecadotril. In fact, using drugs in such patients, leads to prolongation of the illness and confuses the doctor, as it happened in this case.

Acute Gastroenteritis

Exclusive breastfeeding prevents diarrheal diseases though loose stools are common in breastfed infants. In spite of several loose stools in a day, the infant remains happy and playful. However, if a breastfed infant with loose stools appears sick, a serious underlying disease must be evaluated. Infants on bottle-feeding and toddlers are susceptible to frequent episodes of infective diarrhea.

A typical viral infection starts with vomiting along with mild or no fever followed by loose stools within the next 24 hours; often by then, vomiting stops on its own. Fever also abates within a day or two but loose stools may continue, at times even for a week or more. Persistence of loose stools by itself, does not suggest active disease in the presence of an otherwise active and normal child. This persistence is due to transient malabsorption of carbohydrates in particular and settles down by itself without any change in the diet. Such a viral illness is more common in infants and toddlers.

Whenever the presentation of acute gastroenteritis differs from a typical viral illness, one must look for other etiologies. High fever, abdominal pain, and stools with mucus and/or blood indicate acute bacillary dysentery. However, at times, stools may be watery during the initial day or two in bacillary dysentery, but mucus and blood appear thereafter. In such cases, high fever and the sick look of the child denotes the possibility of a bacterial infection.

The sequence of appearance of symptoms is also important to note. If the illness starts with loose stools with or without fever, followed by vomiting in the next day or two and by then, loose stools stop, it is not gastroenteritis. It may be due to parenteral diarrhea as a result of extra-intestinal infections (UTI or pneumonia), especially in infants or toddlers. Other causes of acute gastroenteritis include food poisoning, food intolerance (without fever) and inflammatory bowel disease. Parasitic infections rarely present acutely.

Treatment naturally depends on etiology. Viral gastroenteritis is treated with ORS and zinc—10 mg/day for a week. Zinc is supposed to help in the healing of mucosal injury thereby improving absorption of nutrients. Acute bacillary dysentery is treated with antibiotics covering gram-ve bacteria such as cotrimoxazole or cefixime.

CASE 43

■ Inadequate Feeding Investigated for Failure to Thrive

Events...

A 6-month-old infant presented with a history of vomiting off and on for the last three months and occasional loose stools. He was apparently well till he was three months old, after which his vomiting started insidiously. It usually occurred during or immediately after feeds, though it was not always related to feeds and was never bile stained. There were occasional episodes of loose stools that were treated with different drugs. After trying some home remedies and medicines from general practitioners, he was referred to a pediatrician at the age of five months because he had hardly gained weight over the last three months. At that time, the pediatrician noted delayed gross motor milestones and failure to thrive. In view of recurrent vomiting and loose stools (though occasional), recurrent infections and/or metabolic disorders were considered. Several tests were done but all of them were within normal limits. In view of growth faltering and delayed milestones, he was investigated for primary or secondary hypothyroidism, but it was ruled out. Since the metabolic screen and immune functions were normal, he underwent MRI of the brain and tests for congenital infections that were also normal. The only abnormal laboratory parameters were hypoproteinemia with both albumin and globulin fractions being below normal, microcytic hypochromic anemia and the presence of lactose in the stools. His mother was advised to stop breast feeds and try soya formula. As he persistently vomited the soya formula, he was prescribed some protein powder to be taken with water. As there was still no improvement, he was referred for further management.

What are the options for further management?

In order to be able to take the right decision and choose the correct action, one must have a probable clinical diagnosis, for which, many more details in the history need to be known.

Additional History

He was born of a full-term normal delivery, with a birth weight of 2.9 kg. He was exclusively breast fed till three months of age. However, on direct questioning, it was realized that he had gained just 1.2 kg over the first three months, in spite of being apparently normal.

Analysis

It is clear that this infant has failed to thrive right from the beginning, even when he did not have vomiting or any other symptoms. Though he continued to grow poorly, he had not developed any other symptoms. If he was suffering from an occult infection or a metabolic disorder, he would have presented with a few more symptoms depending upon the nature of the disease. Congenital infections would have presented with a low birth weight and would have progressed to manifest other symptoms in addition to failure to thrive. Though his gross motor milestones are delayed, he does not have cognitive defects and hence, this may merely represent malnutrition and not a primary brain disorder. It is not surprising that several laboratory and imaging tests were normal. The only abnormal test results reported in this child, such as hypoproteinemia, anemia and lactose in stools denote malnutrition. At this age, malnutrition without any other symptoms suggests a primary error in feeding, rather than secondary malnutrition.

Physical Examination

Poorly built and nourished
Weight 4.6 kg
TPR normal
Loss of subcutaneous fat from all over
Liver just palpable
Other systems normal
Gross motor age three months
Vision and hearing apparently normal

Alert, not sick
Length 61 cm
Moderate pallor
No other abnormality
Spleen not palpable

Head circumference 42 cm
Mild edema of feet

Fine motor, cognitive development normal

Analysis

This child has severe protein energy malnutrition. At this age, a liver that is just palpable in such a child denotes predominant calorie deficiency rather than protein deficiency. Since there are no clinical findings to suggest any other disease, this is primary malnutrition due to lactation failure, which has been further compounded by faulty advice on feeding. Vomiting and occasional loose stools in this child can also be explained by faulty feeding that would disturb gastrointestinal functions. There could have been episodes of intercurrent infection but that is unlikely to be the primary problem.

Comment

Several management errors are evident in this case. It is a well-known fact that there are hardly any contraindications to breastfeeding and therefore, stopping breastfeeding for nonspecific trivial reasons is just not acceptable. This infant had gained only 1.2 kg in the first three months; it is too inadequate for an exclusively breastfed baby. Whenever there is inadequate weight gain in an infant, it is not always easy to assess the adequacy of breast milk. There are some clues that need to be evaluated with caution. Baby's comfort level and happiness, frequency of urination, mother's impression about engorgement of her breasts and dripping of milk from the other breast while feeding, are some of the points that may help to define adequacy of milk or otherwise. One needs to confirm the proper technique of breastfeeding and especially, proper latching at the breast. Prior to consideration of supplementary feeds, mothers' needs to be supported and properly guided in an attempt to achieve successful breastfeeding. It is only when all such measures fail, and the inadequacy of breast milk is confirmed, that supplements must be advised. So the first error in this child's management was to stop breastfeeding and no due consideration was given to inadequacy of breast milk and need for supplementation.

Soya milk formula is rarely required in routine practice. Primary lactose intolerance is extremely rare and infants with secondary lactose intolerance do not need soya milk formula, except in cases of malnourishing protracted diarrhea of infancy which has a multifactorial pathogenesis. Therefore, in routine clinical practice, stool examination for lactose is not called for and if reported, should be ignored. As such, soya has an obnoxious taste; no wonder, the vomiting worsened in this infant.

Since it was deduced that this infant neither tolerated breast milk nor soya milk formula, he was advised protein supplements in water. This infant was calorie deficient and required calorie replacement rather than protein supplements. In fact, malnourished children in general need more calories that are supplied mainly by carbohydrates and partly by fats. Their protein intake should be, such that it supplies 8 to 10 percent of the total calories. High protein diet may even be harmful as the proteins need to be broken down to supply calories; as a result, the metabolic load increases and leads to stress on the kidneys, which in turn leads to nausea and vomiting with failure to thrive. So, in this infant protein supplements may further worsen his health.

While such a malnourished infant needs more calories, the process of nutritional rehabilitation should proceed slowly as per the infant's response and tolerance to the feeding program. It is important to encourage breastfeeding irrespective of milk production, as frequent sucking by the baby is the stimulus for milk production. Supplementary feeds at this age could be cereals, pulses, vegetables, and fruits besides animal milk. The volume per feed, frequency of feeding and consistency of feeds need frequent adjustments besides the composition of feeds. Minor intolerance to supplementary feeds is likely but should not be a reason to abandon feeding as minor relevant modifications usually suffice to settle the problem. Improvement takes time to show, often up to several months, and till then minor problems need to be attended too. However, interruption to feeding is rarely required. It is important to realize that early intervention is the key to success and periodic growth assessment is the best parameter of adequate nutrition in infancy.

Experience gained…

> In the absence of a proper feeding history, vomiting and failure to thrive was considered to be a pathological problem and it resulted in various laboratory and imaging tests.

CASE 44

■ Infant with Atypical Kawasaki Disease

History

A 4-month-old infant presented with a low-grade fever for three days followed by a high spike of fever two weeks ago. There were no other symptoms; the infant was feeding well during the first three days of low-grade fever. He was observed at home on the advice of the pediatrician and was hospitalized on the day he spiked high fever.

Analysis

A young infant with high fever demands urgent investigations to rule out an acute bacterial infection. As there are no symptoms other than fever, it is difficult to localize the disease merely on history. In fact, physical examination may also fail to localize the disease at this age. Common bacterial infections at this age include UTI, pneumonia, and meningitis, and they must be ruled out by proper investigations. The odd point in this infant's history is the *low-grade* fever for three days at the onset of the illness, during which his feeding was not disturbed. In acute bacterial infections at this age, refusal to feed and irritability or drowsiness are often the main presenting features. Other causes of fever at this age include malaria and environmental (heat) fever.

Physical Examination

Febrile and sick looking infant
Weight 5.8 kg   Length 63 cm   Head circumference 40 cm
General examination and systemic examination normal

Analysis

As expected, physical examination has not helped to pinpoint the disease and hence, urgent investigations are mandatory. An infant with heat fever is not likely to 'look sick'. Therefore, this is unlikely to be heat fever.

Investigations

Hb 8 g%   WBC 10,500/mm^3 P 62   L 35   E 3
Platelets 2.3 lacs/mm^3 Peripheral smear—normal
Chest X-ray normal   CSF normal
Routine urinalysis—20 to 25 pus cells/hpf   Urine culture—no growth

Analysis

The only suspicious test result is that of routine urine examination, though by itself, it is not diagnostic.

Case Progression

As there was no other clue to the probable diagnosis, it was decided to treat this infant with antibiotics for UTI and observe the progress. He did not respond to this therapy and fever continued, though he did not develop any other symptoms.

Plan for Further Management

Since the infant has neither improved with the antibiotic therapy nor deteriorated, and since there is no localization of the disease even after some more time has elapsed, it is unlikely to be an infection. Therefore, it is necessary to investigate further for rare diseases. One would repeat CBC and urinalysis/urine culture before proceeding to other tests.

Repeat Tests

Hb 6.5 g% WBC 13,000/mm^3 P 72 L 26 E 1 M 1
Platelets 3.8 lacs/mm^3 Urine normal

Analysis

Fall in hemoglobin and increase in platelet count may suggest active infection or inflammation. As mentioned above, infection seems unlikely at this juncture. Therefore, one may look for a noninfective inflammatory disorder, such as autoimmune disease or malignancy. A malignancy that can present as fever alone at this age and in which routine laboratory tests may not be abnormal, is neuroblastoma. A hematological malignancy would have presented with abnormalities in the hemogram; other malignant disorders present with a localized lump, as in the case of hepatoblastoma or Wilms' tumor. Autoimmune disease is rare at this age. In an attempt to pursue these diagnoses, one may plan urinary catecholamines, CT abdomen and chest. Other tests done for pyrexia of unknown origin include a bone marrow examination for any infiltrative disorder and an echocardiogram for bacterial endocarditis.

Case Progression

These tests were carried out and except for the echocardiogram, they were all normal. Echocardiogram showed coronary aneurysms and a diagnosis of **Kawasaki** syndrome was made. He was treated with IVIG; since the first dose did not control the fever, another dose was administered. There was no response to the second dose either. At this stage, echocardiogram was repeated, and it revealed an increase in the size of aneurysms involving all the coronary arteries. Methyl Prednisolone was administered; however, even this did not prove to be beneficial. At this point in time, he was seen to have developed a swelling in the neck that had increased in just over 12 hours and was pulsatile. Diagnosis of aneurysm was made and was confirmed to be arising from the subclavian artery. This meant that he was suffering from generalized vasculitis. Such a manifestation of Kawasaki disease is known and carries a high mortality. This child was administered infliximab antibody. He was to be posted for cardiac bypass, but succumbed before surgery.

Comment

Atypical Kawasaki

Typical Kawasaki disease is diagnosed by standard criteria which evolve over the first few days. They include fever >5 days with four out of 5 features—strawberry tongue and cracked lips, a purulent conjunctivitis, skin rash, and edema over hands and feet with periungual desquamation single cervical lymph node enlargement >1.5 cm during subacute phase. Irritability is a constant feature though not included in the diagnostic criteria, it is extreme in infants and young children. Reactivation of BCG scar is often noticed. The first week may show thrombocytopenia but by the second week, thrombocytosis and leukocytosis are evident.

- Incomplete Kawasaki—fever <4 days, 3 or less out of 5 features but with echo abnormality.
- Atypical Kawasaki—additionally involving lungs and kidneys.
- Other features are also seen and they include aseptic meningitis, arthritis either at the onset or delayed, gastroenteritis, jaundice, sterile pyuria, uveitis, perianal desquamation, and gallbladder hydrops.
- Complications include myocarditis, pericarditis, CCF, coronary aneurysm, shock, and macrophage activation syndrome.
- Treatment consists of IVIG 2 g/kg single dose and aspirin 30-50 mg/kg/day till fever subsides. If fever continues >48 hours, repeat IVIG or consider steroids or infliximab. Alternatively, cyclosporine 5 mg/kg in two divided doses for 5 days. Continue aspirin 3-5 mg/kg/day for 4-6 weeks or till ESR comes down to normal.

An autoimmune disorder that can present so early in life is Kawasaki disease. As discussed above, Kawasaki disease may present in many atypical ways and the full-blown picture may evolve only after sometime. To consider IVIG therapy in time, one may have to suspect the disease early enough. However, this has also resulted in Kawasaki disease being overdiagnosed. This should be avoided, because it not only entails huge expenses but also unnecessarily increases the parental anxiety.

CASE 45

■ Fungal Pneumonia

Events...

An 8-year-old child presented with fever and severe cough for last three weeks. He was apparently alright when he started getting a moderate fever that was followed by a severe cough over the next two days. He received oral Amoxicillin, but there was no response at the end of five days of antibiotic therapy.

What are the options for further management?

In order to be able to take the right decision and choose the correct action, one must have a probable clinical diagnosis.

Analysis

Fever and cough suggest an acute respiratory infection. Severe cough denotes an airway disease. It is not common for acute bacterial respiratory infection to present with severe cough, except intracellular infections such as mycoplasma or pertussis. Therefore, it could also be a viral infection.

Ideal Option—Offer Symptomatic Therapy and Carefully Observe

Since the child is obviously stable at this stage, one could consider observation with symptomatic therapy. Thus, while one would use paracetamol for fever, use of a cough syrup would depend upon the type of cough—either a cough suppressant or an expectorant. In the absence of any previous history of cough suggestive of hyperreactive airway disease, bronchodilators may not be necessary.

Acceptable Option—Treat with a Macrolide

In view of probable Mycoplasma infection, one may consider treating with a macrolide. Laboratory tests at this stage may not be productive since Mycoplasma antibodies (IgM) may not appear within the first few days of illness. At this stage, a chest X-ray is also unlikely to offer any clue to the diagnosis, as the clinical manifestations are mainly due to airway involvement.

Unacceptable Option—Treat with Amoxicillin

In this child, amoxicillin has been started on the second day of the illness, without any specific probable etiological diagnosis. Since significant cough is a prominent presenting symptom in this case, it suggests airway disease, which is either viral or due to mycoplasma/pertussis. Therefore, though amoxicillin is a good antibiotic for many respiratory infections, it is not the ideal choice in this case.

Case Progression

He continued to run the same degree of fever and was still coughing, though there were no new symptoms. Clinical examination did not reveal any significant respiratory findings. A CBC was asked for that was unremarkable.

What are the options for further management?
Analysis

This child's general condition has remained nearly the same over the last eight days. Clinically, there is no worsening in terms of higher (than before) spiky fever or breathlessness, thereby suggesting absence of any complications. This goes against a bacterial pneumonia that is unresponsive/partially responsive to oral amoxicillin. Further, even after so many days, there are no localizing signs of a lobar pneumonia. The CBC at this stage is also unremarkable. Therefore, this is unlikely to be a typical acute bacterial lobar pneumonia caused by *Streptococcus pneumoniae* or *H. influenzae*. Thus, it may be an atypical infection like Mycoplasma, pertussis or even a viral infection.

Case Progression

Finally, a chest X-ray was asked for that showed bilateral pneumonia.

Analysis

The chest X-ray showed bilateral pneumonia. Acute bacterial pneumonia is usually unilateral, localized to a single lobe though *Mycoplasma pneumoniae* may be bilateral. Bilateral radiological lesions can be seen in disseminated or miliary tuberculosis, in which case cough is not a dominant symptom. However, bronchogenic spread of tuberculosis following a primary complex may result in severe cough.

Though the significant cough may suggest a foreign body, the age is unusual, and the involvement is bilateral. Also, it is only after the foreign body gets infected that such a child will manifest with fever, not at the onset. Bronchiectasis, another illness characterized by significant cough, is a chronic condition and hence ruled out.

What are the options for further management?
Ideal Option—Investigate for Etiology

As amoxicillin was used initially but did not help, it would be necessary to change therapy. Bilateral pneumonia may suggest either Mycoplasma infection or any other organism but not acute bacterial disease. So, trial with macrolide at this stage may be justified and laboratory tests for IgM antibody against Mycoplasma be ordered. Irrespective of antibody test result, if child does not show clinical improvement, search for other infections would be mandatory. However, if a macrolide had already been used as a drug of first choice at the first visit and if it had failed, a search for another infection would be necessary at this stage. Further investigations would include bronchoalveolar lavage and CT scan. BAL would demonstrate the etiological agent and CT scan may help to delineate a pathology that is not depicted on the chest X-ray, such as mediastinal lymphadenopathy, small pleural effusion, or interstitial lesions. It will also help to confirm the presence of pneumonia, that may have been inferred wrongly on the chest X-ray. As the lesion is bilateral, it is most unlikely to be either congenital malformation or inhaled foreign body.

Acceptable Option—Try Broad-spectrum Antibiotics

If for some reason, the above-mentioned investigations are not immediately feasible, it may be acceptable to give a short trial with a parenteral broad spectrum antibiotic at this stage. Since this patient has neither improved, nor deteriorated, while on treatment with amoxicillin, it may be argued that the organisms are partially sensitive, or there are issues about bioavailability. Therefore, a parenteral broad-spectrum antibiotic with a wider coverage may work. However, as discussed above, it is quite likely that the etiological agent is atypical. In which case, this strategy won't work, and one will have to fall back on trying to establish an etiological diagnosis.

Case Progression

A broad-spectrum antibiotic was tried. As expected, the trial failed. However, though he still did not show any response, he did not deteriorate either. By the end of two weeks, he developed mild breathlessness. Chest X-ray and CBC was repeated. While CBC did not reveal any significant abnormality, chest X-ray showed some worsening of the bilateral lesions. At this stage, he was getting hypoxic and was hence referred for further management.

What are the options for further management?

Physical Examination at Referral Center

Fairly built and nourished	Looks sick
Weight 25 kg	Height 122 cm
Pulse 110/min	Temp 100°F
RR 35/min	No respiratory distress
No cyanosis	No clubbing
No lymphadenopathy	Bone and joints normal

Systemic Examination

Respiratory system – Percussion note normal, Vesicular breath sounds
– Scattered crepitations both sides
No hepatosplenomegaly
Other systems normal

Analysis

This patient is obviously deteriorating at this stage. As breathlessness did not develop suddenly, it is unlikely to be pneumothorax. Pleural effusion may be an accompaniment of pneumonia but is unlikely to develop at the end of two weeks. If pleural effusion develops over time slowly, it may not result in breathlessness. The onset of breathlessness suggests a worsening of lung function. Therefore, what originally started as an airway disease has now progressed to affect the lung function. In the absence of signs of parenchymal involvement, it is logical that the airway disease has now involved the interstitium. Infectious diseases involving the interstitium could be **viral,** tuberculous, or fungal. Since the disease has gone on for two weeks and has now deteriorated, it is less likely to be viral. **Tuberculosis** is also unlikely, because it is miliary tuberculosis that can lead to breathlessness, and miliary TB is not a common presentation in a healthy child at this age. Further, absence of hepatosplenomegaly is against the diagnosis of miliary tuberculosis. **Fungal** infection at this age is rare but may be seen in an immunocompromised patient. However, the history does not suggest that this child is immunocompromised.

At this stage, one may also consider **non-infective** conditions. While histiocytosis and sarcoidosis are possible, fever and cough are unusual presenting symptoms of **histiocytosis.** Further, this child also does not have any skin lesions or polyuria, which are the other features that often make one suspect histiocytosis. **Sarcoidosis** though rare, is a possibility in this child. It may be suggested by the detection of mediastinal lymphadenopathy on CT scan. Systemic vasculitis such as **Wegener's** granulomatosis may present with other system involvement and child would have been much sicker with neutrophilic leukocytosis and thrombocytosis. **Malignancy** is most unlikely. Thus, at this stage further tests are mandatory.

Thus, this child seems to have developed respiratory dysfunction due to worsening of pneumonia. As this pneumonia has taken more than two weeks to deteriorate, it may have been caused by either tuberculosis or fungal infection. Bilateral pneumonia in both these conditions is interstitial.

Ideal Action at this Stage

It is most urgent to investigate this child further, to find out the exact etiology as he is already hypoxic, and if not diagnosed quickly and correctly, may deteriorate further. BAL or/and CT scan should be ordered. Blood tests are unlikely to help in etiological diagnosis. Simultaneously, he also needs proper oxygenation and further support in terms of mechanical ventilation if necessary. Antibiotics may be discontinued at this stage. Hypothetical anti-TB treatment is not justified; one should attempt a quick diagnosis and only if tuberculosis is confirmed, anti-TB therapy should be initiated.

Case Progression

BAL did not yield any organism in this child, while the CT scan did demonstrate interstitial lung lesions scattered all over. There was no mediastinal lymphadenopathy.

Analysis

In TB, cough is a symptom of endobronchial involvement, which would basically be a spread from a primary complex. Therefore, one expects to find a mediastinal lymph node in such a case. On the other hand, though interstitial lung lesions are consistent with miliary TB, one expects hepatosplenomegaly which this child does not have; further, children with miliary TB do not cough so badly. Therefore, TB seems to be ruled out. Absence of mediastinal lymphadenopathy also rules out sarcoidosis.

Case Progression

At this stage, the option was to choose between lung biopsy or lung aspiration. As noninfective causes seemed less likely, lung aspiration was considered the intervention of choice, and it did grow **Aspergillus**.

Final Outcome

He was treated with an antifungal agent and improved over the next two weeks.
(If one would have drawn a blank even on lung aspiration, one may have considered empirical anti TB treatment at this stage).

It was necessary at this stage to find out why this child developed a fungal infection. His immune profile was ordered that turned out to be normal.

Experience gained...

> In retrospect, it is a conjecture that tis child must have been exposed to a fungal infection, when he was nebulized during his initial treatment. Nebulization is commonly offered as a treatment modality in cases of severe cough in children, and often no proper hygienic care is instituted. Disposable masks are rarely used, and care of the tubing is mostly ignored. Thus, the oxygen mask, tubing or the nebulizing chamber may infect a child, if such equipment is not handled properly.

Fungal Pneumonia

Pneumonia refers to inflammation of lung parenchyma and may result commonly from infection, but also at times from other noninfective causes such as immunological disorders, malignancy or aspiration syndromes. Inhalation of foreign body or oil instilled into the nostrils that trickles down the airways may also cause pneumonia. Infective pneumonia may often be caused by bacteria but also by viruses, fungi and parasites. Etiology of pneumonia needs to be suspected clinically and on the basis of local epidemiology.

Fungal pneumonia is generally seen in immunocompromised individuals (congenital immune deficiency, HIV infection, steroid or chemotherapy and severe malnutrition). It may also be seen in individuals who have exposure to contaminated soil or bird droppings. Fungal pneumonia is generally a chronic process—though it may start as fever accompanied with cough, wheezing, and breathlessness, these symptoms persist and deteriorate over time and there maybe hemoptysis. Diagnosis is suspected, based on risk factors. Imaging of the chest may reveal localized mass (fungal ball) and diagnosis is confirmed by a tissue biopsy and culture of a specimen collected through bronchoalveolar lavage.

Treatment depends on the type of pathogen. In general, the drug of choice is Amphotericin B that is administered parenterally though oral voriconazole is preferred for aspergillosis and Caspofungin for Candida infection. Treatment has to be continued for a long time—few weeks to months though in a healthy individual, 2-3 weeks may be adequate. The cost of Amphotericin is high, and the drug has considerable side effects when given for a long time. Lipid-based formulations are also available, though much more costly. Oral drugs are comparatively cheaper.

CASE 46

■ Palatopharyngeal Incompetence

Events...

A 2-year-old child presented with cough and wheeze since birth. He was born of a full term normal delivery and had cried well at birth. 12 hours after birth, he was noticed to be mildly breathless and cyanotic for which he was shifted to NICU. Physical examination revealed tachypnea, central cyanosis, and hypoxia on pulse oximeter. He was investigated for a probable heart defect, but it was ruled out by a 2D echocardiogram. The chest X-ray and ECG were also normal. He was given oxygen by hood, which maintained the oxygen saturation within normal limits. As soon as he was started on breastfeeds, he developed a cough and had to be fed through a nasogastric tube for sometime. Because of severe cough especially on feeding, gastroesophageal anomalies including GER and tracheoesophageal fistula were ruled out by appropriate investigations. Over the next four weeks, his tachypnea and hypoxia had improved considerably, and he could maintain normal oxygen saturation on room air. He could also feed on the breast, though at times he would get choked and end up with coughing. He had shown a modest gain in weight and had no abnormal physical findings. So, he was discharged and advised empirical treatment for GER.

At 3 months of age, he was fairly comfortable, except for the severe bouts of cough that would occur maximally on waking up from sleep. This kind of cough continued, and in addition, he used to get fever off and on, for which he received many courses of antibiotics over the next two years, without any long-lasting benefit. In view of this persistent cough, and having ruled out relevant underlying causes, it was decided to treat this child as asthma, though there was no family history of atopy. In spite of compliant inhaled steroid therapy for the next six months, there was no response in the bouts of cough. As a result, the parents tried alternative systems of medicine only to find that they also did not work. That is the time they came for a second opinion.

What are the options for further management?

To plan further action, it is necessary to formulate a working diagnosis, based on which further investigations or management may be undertaken.

Analysis

The chief complaint of this child has been violent bouts of cough that started almost at birth and has continued till two years of age, though probably with diminishing severity. This is obviously an airway disease. It has not affected the growth of the child significantly. So this is not a progressive illness, and is hence, not infective in origin, but is most likely to be mechanical. Fever in this child has never been a prominent symptom as compared to the cough, and hence it may not signify episodes of infection. Moreover, if this was an infective condition, it would signify a serious underlying cause, which would have resulted in failure to thrive. Fever can result from any inflammation, including an aspiration syndrome leading to chemical pneumonitis that is often mistaken for an infection. This child was treated as asthma with inhaled steroids since all the investigations were negative. However, asthma never starts right at birth, and therefore, it is no surprise that he did not respond. Cardiac defects have been already ruled out, shortly after birth. Therefore, though this child has been thoroughly investigated for aspiration syndrome, the provisional diagnosis on this analysis still remains an aspiration syndrome. It is not easy to confidently rule out all the causes of aspiration syndrome.

Ideal option—Re 'view', have a Fresh Look

Though this child has always been under the care of many pediatricians, it is rational to have a fresh unbiased look at the problem. One must begin with a detailed history and thorough physical examination.

When asked leading questions, the parents revealed that most of his severe bouts of cough occurred after getting up in the morning after a long duration of sleep. He would become comfortable after an hour or so, and subsequently he was reasonably free from severe cough throughout the day. Another fact that came to light was that he did better with solid food, so that the parents attributed his improvement over time, to a reduced consumption of milk. During history taking, it was noticed that the child had a nasal twang to his voice; when questioned about it, the parents said that this was since birth, and therefore, they did not consider it abnormal.

Physical examination revealed an averagely grown comfortable child, who was not tachypneic or cyanosed. There was generalized hypotonia with normal deep tendon reflexes, delayed gross motor milestones and a mild delay in cognitive functions. As mentioned earlier, there was a definite nasal twang to the voice. There was no other abnormality of the nervous system, or any other system. On careful examination of the oral cavity, it was noticed that the palate was not moving well on crying. These findings gave a clue to the cause of aspiration syndrome. He had a swallowing dysfunction due to palatopharyngeal incoordination as a result of palatal weakness. The mild delay in milestones is consistent with such a possibility.

The parents were counseled and advised to make him sleep in the prone position to prevent pooling of secretions. They were also advised to feed him carefully, particularly solid food, to avoid aspiration. It was likely that he was improving naturally over time, as his development had also improved over time.

Less Acceptable Option

Clinical analysis suggests that the diagnosis in this child is almost certainly aspiration syndrome, probably due to palatopharyngeal incoordination. Nevertheless, one may wish to reinvestigate and confirm the same. Therefore, one may consider a radionuclide milk scan that will positively document aspiration into the lungs. Once the aspiration has been proved, one may try to define the cause. H type of fistula can be ruled out by bronchoscopy, with methylene blue instilled into the esophagus. If this is ruled out, one would think of a swallowing dysfunction that may be secondary to a central nervous system disorder, involvement of the cranial nerves, or a myopathy. In that event, a CT scan or MRI of brain may delineate the central abnormality, if any. However, as mentioned earlier, none of these tests may be able to define the cause clearly. In such an event, the management largely rests on prevention of aspiration by positioning and feeding techniques. Since history suggests that this child is naturally but gradually, improving over time, this kind of management may further help the recovery.

Experience gained...

> When one is confronted with a chronic problem that has defied all tests, it may be ideal to start afresh with an unbiased detailed history and thorough physical examination before embarking on further laboratory tests. This case illustrates how a relook helps to diagnose the condition.

Aspiration Syndromes

A typical aspiration event presents with sudden choking and vomiting while feeding followed by cough and/or breathlessness. It may lead to respiratory infection. Rarely, the event may be serious enough to endanger life due to sudden cessation of breathing. Transient mild self-limiting occasional episode may occur even in a healthy infant, especially during bottle-feeding—this is due to gastroesophageal reflux (physiological). When infants present with other symptoms such as cough, breathlessness or failure to thrive, along with symptoms suggestive of aspiration described above, one suspects gastroesophageal reflux disease (GERD). In such cases, the underlying cause must be evaluated. Confirmation of GERD is not easy and ideally may need esophagoscopy and 24-hour esophageal pH monitoring, as mere imaging (barium swallow or radioisotope milk scan) may not be adequate. This is the reason why diagnosis of GERD is often based on strong clinical judgment. Tracheoesophageal fistula usually presents early in life though H-type fistula may present later in life. TOF with esophageal atresia is suspected if severe gastric distension is also present in a neonate presenting with choking while feeding; these infants may present with breathlessness following aspiration. Achalasia cardia or chalasia may also be present with aspiration. Severe cough (pertussis) or a large vomit can also result in aspiration. GERD may also be due to bronchodilator drugs used for bronchial asthma. Swallowing incoordination is common in a developmentally delayed child due to palatopharyngeal incoordination or as a result of lower cranial nerve palsies. Nasogastric tube feeding in a comatose child may also be a risk factor for aspiration and so also morbid obesity.

Management is symptomatic with the use of antacids and H_2 blockers/PPI (Proton-pump inhibitor) for a few weeks. Supportive measures include a head-up reclining position and thickened small and frequent feeds. Surgical intervention in the form of fundal plication may be necessary in infants with life-threatening GER, achalasia or TOF.

CASE 47

Hemophagocytic Syndrome

History

A 10-year-old male child presented with a history of generalized abdominal pain a month ago, without any other symptoms. After a few days of failed trial with antacids, abdominal USG reported probable appendicitis, for which he was operated, though he did not have any localized pain in the right iliac fossa and his CBC and routine urinalysis was normal. On the second postoperative day, he started running fever which did not get controlled with antibiotics. Repeat abdominal USG showed a localized collection of pus at the site of operation, which was immediately drained. Subsequently, antibiotics were changed, but the fever continued. CBC was repeated which revealed pancytopenia. Considering a diagnosis of sepsis and DIC, antibiotics were further changed but without any response. At this point, he started developing mild breathlessness and cough, which is when he was transferred for further management.

Analysis

Abdominal pain without any localization even after a few days from its onset, and a normal WBC count are not compatible with the diagnosis of appendicitis. Unless there is definite tenderness and guarding/rigidity localized to the right iliac fossa, it is difficult to consider a diagnosis of appendicitis. Fever on the second postoperative day could be due to local complications such as pus collection, which was rightly suspected, proved and appropriately managed. However, since the fever did not subside in spite of this, it is clear that the cause of fever was something different. Irrespective of the cause of the original abdominal pain and the subsequent development of pus in the abdominal cavity, if the continuation of fever is believed to represent sepsis (and breathlessness to denote ARDS), there are some odd points. Typically in sepsis, one may expect leukocytosis with thrombocytopenia and not necessarily pancytopenia, which may suggest bone marrow suppression that may have resulted from either drug toxicity or infection. At this juncture, it is difficult to consider what the primary pathology could be, though he is now admitted for secondary bone marrow disease that would need further investigations.

Physical Examination

Well-built and nourished	Looking sick	
Weight 32 kg	Height 138 cm	
Temp 102°F	Pulse 140/min	RR 40/min
No chest retraction	No cyanosis	Mild edema feet
Mild icterus	Significant pallor	Purpuric spots
Subconjunctival bleed	No lymphadenopathy	Bones and joints normal
No engorged neck veins	Hepatojugular reflux absent	

Systemic Examination

Liver 4 cm +, firm, mildly tender; Liver span 10 cm
Spleen not palpable
RS—occasional crepitations, no other localizing signs
Other systems normal

Analysis

Significant pallor with bleeding suggests either bone marrow aplasia or leukemia. The presence of hepatomegaly may favor leukemia. Tender hepatomegaly could be due to incipient cardiac failure, though there are no other signs such as cardiomegaly, engorged neck veins or positive hepatojugular reflux. Mild icterus may be a rare accompaniment of cardiac failure, though it may also denote hepatitis. Leukemia may also involve the liver and lead to icterus (by way of leukemic hepatitis or enlarged lymph nodes at the porta hepatis pressing over bile duct). Mild edema of the feet may indicate hypoproteinemia either due to liver disease or nutritional deficiency. Tachypnea with occasional crepitations suggest involvement of lung parenchyma that is not a feature of leukemia. Thus, at this stage, the exact diagnosis is elusive and further investigations such as bone marrow aspiration or biopsy would be needed.

Investigations

Hb 6 g%   WBC 1800/mm^3 P 54 L 40 E 2 M 4   Platelets 20,000/mm^3
Serum bilirubin 2.2 mg%   direct 1.6 mg%
ALT 95 units   AST 82 units
Serum proteins 5.5 g%   Albumin 2.5 g%   Globulin 3 g%
Serum electrolytes normal   Blood urea and serum
                                                                                          creatinine normal
Chest X-ray apparently normal   SpO$_2$ 85% in room air
Blood culture normal
Bone marrow aspiration showed hemophagocytosis—no evidence of leukemia

Analysis

This child has hemophagocytosis, though the primary cause does not seem to be clear as yet. It may result from infections, autoimmune disorders, or malignancy. In view of biochemical hepatitis, it may be a primary viral infection such as CMV. Such an infection can even explain the lung lesion; in CMV infections such lesions are known to be interstitial with minimal clinical and radiological evidence. Leukemia is ruled out. Autoimmune disorder may be a possibility though further investigations may be necessary.

Management

Hemophagocytosis needs urgent management as it may be a fatal disorder. The child was given supportive therapy in the form of blood/platelet transfusions, oxygen and IV fluids. Antibiotics were discontinued. IVIG and/or steroids have been tried in this condition.

However, in this case since the primary cause is not known yet, IVIG may be a better option. Simultaneously, further investigations for viral infections and autoimmune diseases were ordered and they were all negative.

After all the above-mentioned supportive management, this child stabilized as far as his hematological problems were concerned, though his fever continued. At this point, some tests were repeated again and the results were as follows:

Hb 9.5 g%   WBC 6,500/mm^3 P 60 L 35 E 3 M 2   Platelets 2.3 lac/mm^3
ESR 105 mm
Liver function tests returned to normal

Case Progression

This child managed to scrape through his hematological complications, but the primary disease was still elusive. With an enlarged liver and pneumonia, options were to pursue CT scan of the chest, BAL, or liver biopsy. A CT scan was done, that showed a small pneumonia in the right middle lobe without any mediastinal lymphadenopathy. Since it was inconclusive, a liver biopsy was performed which revealed miliary tuberculosis. This child did well on ATT with steroids.

Final Diagnosis

Miliary TB with hemophagocytosis.

Hemophagocytic Lymphohistiocytosis

Hemophagocytic lymphohistiocytosis (HLH) occurs secondary to infections or other inflammatory diseases and drugs and is seen in all age groups. But primary HLH due to perforin deficiency is rare and is seen in young infants. HLH should be suspected when there occurs an unexpected sudden deterioration in the course of a disease. Standard diagnostic criteria include fever, splenomegaly, bicytopenia, increased triglycerides and ferritin, low fibrinogen, high CD25, low NK cells and bone marrow showing hemophagocytosis. Presence of 5 out of 8 criteria confirms the diagnosis of HLH. HLH and macrophage activation syndrome are similar with small subtle differences. While HLH presents with hematological abnormalities (bicytopenia or pancytopenia and hemophagocytosis in the marrow), MAS presents without it. Thus, rheumatologists call it as MAS while hematologists call it as HLH. Pathogenesis is the same in both though treatment differs a bit. HLH is treated with dexamethasone, etoposide and stem cell transplant while MAS is treated with steroids and cyclosporine, though refractory MAS is treated the way HLH is treated.

Management Dilemmas in Office Practice

CASE 48

■ Leukemia Presenting as Scurvy
History
A 5-year-old female child presented with a painful inability to walk over last one month. There was a mild progression of symptoms in the sense that she was now finding it difficult to even stand or squat. There was no pain at rest. The pain was aggravated by movements or weight bearing. She also complained of a backache for the last 15 days.
  No history of any trauma
  No history of fever or any swelling of bones or joints
  No history of bladder or bowel disturbances
  No history of sensory disturbances
  She was treated with analgesics with temporary relief.

Analysis
In view of a painful inability to walk without any symptoms of inflammation such as fever or reported swelling, it is likely to be neurogenic pain and or weakness, probably arising from a spinal cord lesion. Being slowly progressive over a month, it may suggest a slowly developing compressive lesion. Backache may point to the local lesion in the spine.

Physical Examination
Fairly built and nourished
Weight 18 kg   Height 105 cm
TPR normal   BP 85/55 mm of Hg
Vague tenderness over the legs
Bones and joints normal
No restriction of movements at any joints
Spine normal–no tenderness/no swelling
No other relevant abnormality on general examination

Systemic Examination
CNS—normal   No sensori—motor deficit
DTR ++ all over   Plantar flexors   No clonus
Other systems normal
Stands with support with difficulty, walks few steps with difficulty.

Analysis
Except vague tenderness over the legs, there are no other physical signs. Therefore, there is no clue to the probable diagnosis. Though there is no neurological localization on physical

examination, an evolving spinal cord compression must be ruled out in such a patient; the physical signs may become apparent as the lesion progresses. However, the disparity between the symptoms (inability to walk/stand) and the lack of neurological signs is striking. This makes us consider the differential diagnosis of muscle or bony pain. **Myalgia** is generally acute as in case of leptospirosis or viral infection, such as influenza, dengue fever or chikungunya. Hence one may consider **bony pain** that may be due to scurvy, leukemia, sickle cell disease, rickets or fluorosis. **Scurvy** is usually seen in children with severe malnutrition. **Sickle cell disease** would affect the growth of the child so that she would be stunted, and the pain would be usually acute, localized and accompanied with swelling. **Leukemia** usually presents acutely, so that by now since a month has passed, there should have been other symptoms and signs. Though hypocalcemic **rickets** is associated with limb pains, the history would not be so acute, this is not the age for it to manifest for the first time, it would lead to difficulty in walking as against inability to walk, and there would be physical signs to go by. Therefore, since there is nothing to suggest any of these diseases, the child needs to be investigated further.

Investigations

Hb 10 g%
Dimorphic anemia
X-ray lower limbs

TLC 8000/mm^3
Platelets adequate
– penciling of the cortex, signet ring appearance
– reported as scurvy

P 14 L 80 M 3 E 3
ESR 50 mm

MRI spine normal

Analysis

At this point, on direct questioning, it transpired that this child consumed only milk, chicken and eggs. For the last 6 weeks, the family had stopped consuming chicken and eggs due to the fear of 'bird flu', so that the child was consuming only milk.

The anemia could be explained on the predominant milk diet, of late. Though the X-rays were reported as scurvy, clinically it was difficult to accept the diagnosis in the absence of malnutrition and gum bleeds, in spite of the milk diet. Further, all the classical radiological signs of scurvy were not there. However, in the absence of any other diagnosis, it was decided to administer a large dose of vitamin C and the patient was asked to follow-up.

Two Weeks Later

This child directly came for a follow-up after two weeks when she sustained a fracture of the ulna following a trivial fall from the bed (a height of 18 inches). Meanwhile there had been a negligible improvement following the dose of vitamin C. A few days back, this child had also developed a transient right ankle joint swelling and pain that lasted for 4 days and was completely relieved by Ibuprofen. At this point the child was markedly pale on physical examination though there were no other abnormal findings, other than the fracture and the vague tenderness in the lower limbs (which had been there all along).

Analysis

A fracture sustained after a trivial fall suggests a pathological fracture. In conjunction with marked pallor (which had suddenly progressed over the last two weeks) and the vague tenderness over the legs, leukemia was a strong possibility and the child was hospitalized for investigations.

Investigations

Hb 5.6 g% WBC 8,000/c.mm P 12 L 84 M 2 E 2 No abnormal cells on peripheral smear examination
    Bone marrow examination confirmed the diagnosis of acute lymphatic leukemia.

Lessons Learnt

1. Acute lymphatic leukemia may have a varied presentation over a few weeks and the diagnosis may evolve gradually.
2. Full blown clinical manifestations of scurvy are seen in severely malnourished children. Occasionally, bony pain may be the only manifestation. Such a child demands radiological confirmation, as biochemical tests are not routinely available. In absence of pathognomonic radiological features, the findings may be simulated by rickets, calorie malnutrition or leukemia, as seen in this case.

CASE 49

■ Poststreptococcal Reactive Arthritis

A 7-year-old child presented with low grade fever along with joint pain and swelling for last 15 days. He was apparently alright three weeks ago, when he had moderate to high fever and throat pain, for which he received symptomatic treatment. He recovered, and remained well for a few days, but thereafter started running low-grade fever again, this time with involvement of the joints. He developed pain and swelling in both knees, right ankle, left shoulder and also a few proximal interphalangeal joints. Movements of the involved joints were restricted and painful. It was persistent nonmigratory arthritis. He also complained of morning stiffness. He had no cardiac involvement and other systems were normal. He was put on aspirin in the dose of 75 mg/kg body weight per day in divided doses. However, there was no relief even after a week of therapy and arthritis persisted.

In view of an acute onset of polyarthritis following acute pharyngitis, rheumatic fever with arthritis was a strong possibility, though there were many atypical manifestations.

Investigations

Hb 10 g% WBC 12,800/mm^3 P 69 L 25 E 4 M 2
ESR 56 mm at one hour ASLO 600 todd units
2 D echocardiogram normal

Analysis

This child has had a recent streptococcal infection as is evident by the high ASLO titer. This is also corroborated by the history of acute pharyngitis just a week prior to the development of arthritis. So there is no doubt that this is poststreptococcal arthritis, but it does not fulfill the standard criteria of rheumatic fever with arthritis.

This child developed arthritis within a week of acute pharyngitis. It has involved both large and small joints, it has been an asymmetric involvement with shoulder joint affection, it has not been migratory, and it has been persistent in spite of aspirin therapy for two weeks. There is no cardiac involvement in this child.

Obviously, this presentation and progression nearly rules out rheumatic fever. Therefore, this child's diagnosis is **poststreptococcal reactive arthritis.**

Relevant Information

It differs from rheumatic fever in that cardiac involvement though known is rare. Joint swelling and pain last for some weeks and responds poorly to aspirin. However, ultimately after a few weeks, there is complete improvement without residual affection, contrary to juvenile chronic arthritis. Thus, though the pattern of joint involvement may partly simulate juvenile chronic arthritis, its progression is different.

Poststreptococcal reactive arthritis and rheumatic fever are both immunological complications of acute streptococcal infection, but do not share similar HLA alleles. This genetic difference is responsible for varying manifestations and prognosis.

There is no unanimity in the management of this condition. The general view is to advise penicillin prophylaxis at least for a year, for those who do not have cardiac involvement, and follow a regimen similar to that of rheumatic fever for those who develop cardiac disease.

CASE 50

Suspected Kawasaki Disease Presenting in 2nd Week

History

A 6-year-old child presented with fever for last 10 days and skin rash for last six days. Fever was high and spiky and was not associated with any other symptoms for the first four days. On day five, he developed a macular rash mainly over the extremities that was not itchy. According to the records, he was toxic and had a skin rash, congested eyes and glossitis, but there were no other abnormal physical findings. Antimalarial therapy was tried without benefit. At this stage, he was investigated.

Hb 9 g%   WBC 18000/mm^3 P 73 L 24 E 3
Platelets 2.6 lac/mm^3 ESR 70 mm
Peripheral smear did not show any abnormality
Widal test –ve   Blood culture—no growth

He was put on ceftriaxone as a trial for probable typhoid fever but had shown no response to therapy after 5 days.

At this stage he was referred for further management.

Physical Examination

Fairly built and nourished   Sick looking   Not irritable
Weight 19 kg   Height 106 cm
Temp 103°F   Pulse 120/min   Respiratory rate 32/min
Macular skin rash mainly over the extremities   No peeling of skin
Eyes not congested   Mouth normal   Palms and soles normal
No lymphadenopathy   No mucosal involvement of urethra or anus
Bones and joints normal   No limb or bony tenderness
Systemic examination normal

Analysis

There is no evidence of any infection as even at the end of 10 days, there is no localization nor deterioration in this child's condition, even when he has not improved. Infections that can go on for a long duration such as a **deep-seated abscess, EB viral infection, leptospirosis** or **rickettsial** infections would have offered some clues by the end of 10 days, with localizing signs related to some system involvement. **Bacterial endocarditis** is one infection that can present with no apparent localizing signs. However, it is rare in the absence of a cardiac defect and further investigations would rule it out. Fever and rash could be due to systemic inflammatory disease. Typically, **systemic vasculitis** presents with an evanescent skin rash that coincides with the spikes of fever that usually come up twice a day; in between, the child remains fairly well. A child with systemic vasculitis should also manifest some other soft clinical features such as arthralgia or arthritis, pleuritis or pericarditis and hepatosplenomegaly. However, these may take some time to show up. Since his previous records mentioned the presence of congested eyes and glossitis, it may suggest the possibility of **Kawasaki disease.** Details of congested eyes and glossitis would have helped a great deal. Nonpurulent conjunctivitis with sparing of limbus, and a strawberry red tongue and mouth without mucosal ulcers would be expected in Kawasaki syndrome. While trying to arrive at a reasonably correct diagnosis, absence of such detailed information is a handicap. These physical signs may have disappeared as the disease progressed and are hence not seen at this stage. Few other physical findings such as lymphadenopathy and evolving changes in skin rash such as periungual peeling would have made the diagnosis of Kawasaki syndrome more certain.

Case Progression

It was decided to repeat his blood counts and order a 2 D echocardiogram that would rule out bacterial endocarditis and pick up coronary artery involvement, if any.

Repeat blood count showed increasing neutrophilic leukocytosis and thrombocytosis.

2D echocardiogram was normal.

However, in view of the risk of this being Kawasaki syndrome and already in its second week of presentation, it was decided to treat this child with IVIG empirically.

He improved within the next three days and was asked to continue low dose aspirin for the next three months at which time 2D echocardiogram was repeated and found to be normal.

Experience gained...

This case illustrates the difficulties in diagnosing cases that suggest Kawasaki syndrome but lacks few of its classical features. In such conditions, one may have to take into account a calculated risk of further action. IVIG may be considered in case of doubt, but it is safe to wait for the first 8 to 10 days of the illness, to observe further progress of the clinical profile that may unfold a definitive diagnosis one way or another. In the early stages of the disease, hasty decisions regarding further management should be avoided.

Extra...

The clinical course of Kawasaki disease can be divided into three stages:

Phase	Duration	Characteristics
1. Acute phase	10 to 14 days	• Fever, exanthema, enanthema • lymphadenopathy, peripheral edema carditis
2. Subacute phase	2 to 4 weeks	• Peeling of skin • End of this phase is marked by return of ESR • and platelet count to normal
3. Convalescent phase	Months or years	Affected vessels undergo remodeling

Criteria for the Diagnosis of Kawasaki Disease

Fever more than five days (four days, if treatment with intravenous immunoglobulin eradicates fever) plus, at least four of the following clinical signs not explained by another disease process:

1. Bilateral conjunctival infection.
2. Changes in the oropharyngeal mucous membranes, including one or more of injected and/or fissured lips, strawberry tongue, injected pharynx.
3. Changes in the peripheral extremities, including erythema and/or edema of the hands and feet (acute phase) or periungual desquamation (convalescent phase).
4. Polymorphous rash, primarily truncal; nonvesicular.
5. Cervical lymphadenopathy with at least one node >1.5 cm.

Differentiating Kawasaki Disease from Mimics

A character which is common to other illnesses	Differentiating features
Fever	Abrupt onset, no preceding respiratory symptoms high, often up to 38.5 to 40:C° not responding to antipyretics at least for five days
Conjunctivitis	• Mainly bulbar conjunctiva involved • Perilimbal sparing • Nonpurulent • Anterior uveitis on slit lamp examination
Buccal mucosa and lips	Vesicles, ulcers of mucosa and exudates over the tonsils are uncommon
Skin rash	Perineal confluence is especially common, though rash maybe all over
Lymphadenopathy	• Unilateral, anterior cervical, usually single node but USG reveals grapelike clusters of enlarged nodes • Diffuse lymphadenopathy and splenomegaly are NOT typical
Extremities Peeling of skin	• Rash is edematous and indurated • Typically begins at the tips of fingers (less commonly of toes) just below the distal edge of the nails beginning after the first week • Desquamation of perineal skin at the end of first week

CASE 51

■ Galactosemia

History

A 10-month-old infant born of a nonconsanguineous marriage presented with progressive abdominal distention and failure to thrive over the last two months. There were no other symptoms at the time of the presentation. The history dates back to three months of age when he was first noticed to have jaundice that lasted for the next three months. There was no history of clay-colored stools, but he did pass high colored urine. He had not gained much weight since infancy, but the parents claimed that after some homeopathy treatment, the infant recovered, the jaundice regressed and he started putting on weight, so that he looked fairly normal by the age of 6 months. He remained well for two months and then started developing progressive abdominal distention and loss of weight.

On direct questioning, the developmental milestones were normal. The child was breastfed and weaned at 5 to 6 months of age.

Analysis

This child's illness seems to have first manifested at around three months of age with jaundice. Jaundice presenting for the first time at three months of age is rare. Occasionally, a slowly progressive jaundice that did start in the neonatal period, may not be reported by the parents for the first few weeks, till it becomes noticeably deep. Since there is a history of passing high colored urine, it appears to be a **direct hyperbilirubinemia.** Even without this history, one would have guessed it to be direct hyperbilirubinemia, because infants with indirect hyperbilirubinemia, usually do not present with weight loss; also, they are otherwise not so sick (the first week of life being an exception). Direct hyperbilirubinemia could be due to **extrahepatic biliary atresia,** neonatal hepatitis syndrome or inborn errors of metabolism. Generally, all these conditions should have be presented much earlier, within a few weeks of birth; however, occasionally, it may be possible that some of these conditions are very slowly progressive, and hence manifest late. This infant has failure to thrive, which could be consistent with most of the afore-mentioned conditions. In view of the absence of clay-colored stools, it is unlikely to be primary biliary obstruction; however, such a history cannot be completely relied upon and operative cholangiography remains the gold standard of diagnosis. **Neonatal hepatitis** may be due to congenital or acquired infections or other causes. Hepatitis due to an acquired infection could be consistent with the presentation at three months of age, but it is rare in early infancy. In the absence of any developmental delay, convulsions or vomiting, **metabolic** disorders also seem less likely. Thus, it is quite likely that this must have been neonatal hepatitis noticed rather late in the course of illness and hence presented only at three months of age. Apparently, the jaundice progressed for the first few months and then regressed. Such a regression may be either natural or induced by drugs like steroids in certain cases. We do not know the relevance of homeopathy drugs to this infant's improvement. However, as he was reported to be better and gained weight over next two months, it may be concluded that the condition was in remission, whatever the cause of its remission. Amongst the causes considered earlier, extrahepatic biliary atresia does not go into remission like this, whereas neonatal hepatitis may, though if it does go into remission, it is quite likely that it subsequently resolves and does not relapse. Metabolic disorders may be progressive, though they are also known to have a waxing and waning course. Thereafter, this infant developed progressive abdominal distention and failure to thrive without jaundice. This may suggest progressive hepatomegaly with or without ascites; in this setting, failure to thrive denotes liver cell dysfunction. Therefore, this infant could have now developed cirrhosis of liver, as a complication of the initial insult in infancy. If so, it could either be a metabolic disorder or a rare case of an acquired neonatal hepatitis.

Physical Examination

Poorly built and nourished Chronically sick looking
Weight 7.2 kg Length 67 cm Head circumference 43 cm
Pulse 115/min RR 30/min BP 80/45 mm
Mild edema feet Moderate pallor No icterus

Systemic Examination

Liver 5 cm, firm to hard, not tender Liver span 10 cm
Spleen 2 cm, firm Free fluid +
Engorged abdominal veins with flow away from umbilicus
Other systems normal

Analysis

Physical signs suggest cirrhosis with portal hypertension and liver cell failure as denoted by the presence of ascites. However, the clinical examination has not given any additional clues to the etiology of the same.

Investigations

Hb 8 g%   WBC 8,000/mm^3 P 52 L 44 E 3 M 1   Platelets normal
Serum bilirubin 1.4 mg%; Direct 0.9 mg%
ALT 90 units   AST 65 units
Alkaline phosphatase 120 KU   PT 18 sec; Control 12 sec
Serum proteins 6.2 g%   Albumin 2.6 g%   Globulin 3.6 g%
SAAG 1.4   CMV IgG and IgM—strongly positive
Mother's CMV IgG—positive; IgM—negative
Urine—reducing sugar present
Galactosemia confirmed by enzyme studies

Analysis

Laboratory tests seem to suggest chronic liver cell failure due to CMV hepatitis as well as galactosemia. However, the diagnosis of both congenital or perinatally acquired CMV infection, is best confirmed by viral studies. Interpretation of IgG and IgM antibodies can be tricky. Many babies acquire CMV infections postnatally, which may not be causally related at all to the infant's liver disease. On the other hand, enzymatic studies confirming galactosemia are definitive.

Final Diagnosis

Galactosemia.

CASE 52

■ Mismanaged UTI Presenting as Breathlessness

History

An 8-year-old child presented with acute onset of breathlessness over 24 hours for which he was admitted to a hospital for a week. He is reported to have settled quickly, within 24 hours of admission, though he was kept in the hospital for a week and was treated with some drugs, details of which were not available. Thereafter, he was apparently well for a week at home and then developed breathlessness again and was also reported to be drowsy. At this stage he was referred for further management. There was no past history of recurrent cough, nor a family history of atopic diseases. However, he used to have recurrent fever since early childhood, and was treated with antibiotics off and on with temporary benefit. There were no other accompanying symptoms during these episodes of fever.

He also gave a history of poor appetite and generalized weakness and was not growing well over last few years.

Analysis

This child has presented with an acute onset of breathlessness that got better quickly but recurred within a few days again. Therefore, essentially we are dealing with recurrent breathlessness of short duration. The most common cause of recurrent breathlessness is **bronchial asthma.** However, this child did not have recurrent cough or wheezing in the past, nor is there any family history of atopy. However, even in the absence of such a history, one should be cautious in ruling out asthma, as it remains the most common cause of such recurrent breathlessness. It also happens to be a condition that gets relieved in a short time. **Acute allergic** laryngitis is another condition that would recur but would have presented with stridor. **Cardiac asthma** is rare in children and should not have got better within a short time, only to recur again.

If we ignore the recurrence of breathlessness, we may consider conditions that present acutely with breathlessness. **Inhaled foreign body** is unlikely at this age without a history of cough. Further, for it to present as breathlessness, the foreign body would have to be placed at the carina, which would lead to a hyperacute presentation. Finally, it would have required bronchoscopic removal; there is no such history. Other conditions such as **tension pneumothorax** and **pulmonary embolism** are also hyperacute in their presentation and are therefore ruled out. Infective diseases such as **pneumonia** would not present with a sudden onset of breathlessness and that too without preceding fever. Obviously, it cannot be an **empyema** as it would have followed a poorly treated acute bacterial pneumonia. Pneumothorax and pleural effusion are other causes of an acute onset of breathlessness. In a **tuberculous pleural effusion,** fever is an accompanying symptom. Though **pneumothorax** can develop suddenly in a case of histiocytosis or due to bursting of an emphysematous bulla in asthma, such a child would have been relieved only by intercostal drainage and no such procedure was performed in this child.

This could have been **metabolic acidosis** that was wrongly considered to be breathlessness. It may have been temporarily treated unknowingly (with soda-bicarb having been given unjustifiably for acute respiratory failure), and therefore, it recurred again. Considering that this child is also reported to have had poor growth and generalized weakness over the last few years, this is a likely possibility. The most common cause of such a condition is **chronic renal disease.** Correlating the recurrent fevers that this child suffered from since early childhood, he may have had undiagnosed urinary tract infections that may have led to chronic renal disease. If he does have a chronic renal disease, such children are known to suffer from hypertension that could lead to cardiac failure and present as acute breathlessness. **Diabetic ketoacidosis** may also similarly present with tachypnea, which is wrongly interpreted as breathlessness, but it is unlikely to have got better without proper diagnosis and insulin administration. The only reason why such a condition should recur once treatment has been instituted, is noncompliance. Drowsiness during the current episode may represent encephalopathy, either due to hypertension or uremia.

Physical Examination

Poorly built and poorly nourished	Weight 15 kg	Height 102 cm
Moderate pallor	No clubbing	Temp normal
Pulse 115/min	RR 35/min	BP 165/100 mm
Deep and rapid respiration	No respiratory distress	
No lymphadenopathy	Bones and joints normal	
Systemic examination		
Respiratory system—normal breath sounds	No foreign sounds	
CVS—mild cardiomegaly	No signs of cardiac failure	
Other systems normal		

Analysis

Hypertension and metabolic acidosis as depicted by deep and rapid respiration, with failure to thrive suggests chronic renal failure. Recurrent fever may represent recurrent UTI due to either an anatomical malformation or VUR. Mild cardiomegaly denotes left ventricular enlargement due to long standing hypertension. Absence of cardiac failure also suggests chronic long-standing hypertension.

Investigations

Hb 7 g%	Normocytic normochromic anemia
WBC 15,000/mm^3	P 75 L 23 E 1 M 1
Urinalysis—20 to 25 pus cells	proteins + +
Urine culture—no growth	Serum creatinine 3.8 mg%
Abdominal USG—bilateral hydronephrosis	
VCUG—Grade 4 VUR	

Analysis

As expected this, child has end stage renal failure due to neglected and poorly managed UTI.

Final Diagnosis

End stage renal failure secondary to UTI.

CASE 53

Gaucher Disease

History

A 3-year-old child presented with fever and cough off and on for last one year and stiff neck for last three months. He was apparently well for the first two years of life, though he had delayed development since early infancy. For the last one year, he had been sick off and on. He was investigated for recurrent cough, but no diagnosis was reached. He used to be treated with antibiotics and cough syrups with variable benefit. He also had blood transfusions on two occasions in the past one year.

Three months ago, he started complaining of neck pain that gradually worsened and movements of the neck became quite painful. He was suspected to be suffering from TB spine, though the X-ray did not show classical changes. He was prescribed anti-TB therapy but in spite of compliant treatment for two months, there was no improvement. At that stage he was referred for further management.

Physical examination revealed a stunted and wasted child with a developmental quotient of about 60%, who also had significant splenohepatomegaly and moderate anemia. His neck was stiff, and offered a resistance to movements in all directions, though there was no apparent swelling or tenderness at the local site. He was alert, had no evidence of raised intracranial tension and there was no neurodeficit. Other systems were normal.

Analysis

This child's most unusual complaint is neck pain for the last three months. In isolation, such neck retraction may suggest a local inflammatory or infective disease or an intracranial pathology especially in the posterior fossa. However, this child has a multiorgan disease, since he has an involvement of the brain as suggested by delayed development, respiratory system affection as denoted by recurrent cough, reticuloendothelial system disease represented by splenohepatomegaly, moderate pallor with past history of blood transfusion twice suggesting bone marrow involvement and involvement of the skeletal system as evident by neck stiffness. The disease has been going on almost since early life and has never had any acute symptomatology. Hence, infection or malignancy is ruled out. Therefore, it favors the possibility of a storage disorder. Though bony defects are known in storage disorders, symptoms of bony involvement are rare. However, all other manifestations do strongly denote a storage disorder, such as Gaucher disease, especially in view of the large spleen. On reviewing the literature, cervical spine involvement leading to neck stiffness which presents as marked neck retraction, is well-recognized in Gaucher disease.

Final Diagnosis

Gaucher disease.

CASE 54

Autoimmune Disorder

History

A 8-year-old female child presented with high fever for last two weeks and a macular skin rash at the peak of fever that would disappear temporarily with control of fever. On day 10 of persistent fever, she developed difficulty in breathing and pain in the right side of chest, for which she was admitted. She had been admitted in the past for undiagnosed fever on two occasions, and in one of those episodes, she had complained of joint pains, for which she was investigated for possible rheumatic fever. However, records showed that she was not advised any long-term penicillin prophylaxis.

Analysis

The fact that she had not developed any other localizing symptom till day 10 of fever may go against acute bacterial infection. The difficulty in breathing and pain in chest on right side suggests pleural involvement in the form of pleural effusion or pleuropneumonia. Acute bacterial pleuropneumonia would not develop so late in the course of the illness. However, breathlessness may denote pleural effusion.

Fever with macular rash appearing each time at the peak of fever suggests probable immune mediated condition. Such immune-mediated condition may be either autoimmune or infection induced immune disorder. Such evanescent skin rash coming at the peak of fever rules out a viral infection. However, Hodgkin's disease may cause an allergic skin rash and may be possible in this child. Thus, at this stage one may consider either autoimmune disorder or lymphoma. In autoimmune disorder, pleural effusion is likely to develop. If it is lymphoma, pleural involvement is unlikely though difficulty in breathing may result from large mediastinal lymphadenopathy. Thus, this child mostly suffers from systemic vasculitis, the exact syndrome may evolve over time.

Physical Examination

Poorly built and nourished Febrile, toxic, sick looking

Weight 19 kg	Height 110 cm	BP 90/40 mm
Temp 102°F	Pulse 150/min	RR 35/min.
Moderate pallor	Mild edema feet	No lymphadenopathy
Bones and joints normal	Macular skin rash all over	

Systemic Examination

Respiratory system—impaired note and diminished breath sounds all over right side of chest below 5th intercostal space, no foreign sounds

Liver 4 cm, firm, not tender Liver span 9 cm
Spleen 3 cm, firm No free fluid
Other systems normal

Analysis

This child has evidence of pleural effusion with hepatosplenomegaly and moderate anemia. It is a multisystem disorder. Combination of pleural effusion and hepatosplenomegaly is against tuberculosis as pleural effusion is a manifestation of immune host with strong hypersensitivity response while hepatosplenomegaly is indicative of dissemination of infection in a child with poor immune function. Hepatosplenomegaly with moderate anemia suggests either hemolytic anemia or infiltrative disorder. Infiltrative disorders are not likely to result in pleural effusion. If it is hemolytic anemia, it is likely to be acquired rather than congenital in view its presentation at this age for the first time. If it is acquired hemolytic anemia, it may be autoimmune disorder that may also explain pleural effusion. Mild edema feet may signify either cardiac failure due to anemia or it may be nutritional hypoproteinemia.

Investigations

Hb 6.5 g% Retic count 8.5%
Peripheral smear—microcytic hypochromic anemia with normoblasts seen
Hemoglobin electrophoresis normal
WBC 18,000/mm^3 P 78 L 18 E 3 M 1
ESR 110 mm at the end of one hour
Chest X-ray—pleural effusion
Serum proteins 6.4 g% Albumin 2.8 g% Globulin 3.6 g%
ALT 85 units AST 70 units Alkaline phosphatase—normal
BUN 80 mg% Serum creatinine 1.9 mg%
Routine urine—Albumin ++
ANA –ve Coombs' –ve APLA + ve

Analysis

Besides evidence of hemolytic anemia and pleural effusion, there is also involvement of kidney and liver as seen biochemically. This proves multisystem involvement disorder. High ESR and positive APLA test denotes autoimmune disorder though one cannot label the disease at this stage.

Final Diagnosis

Autoimmune disorder.

CASE 55

Idiopathic Thrombocytopenic Purpura

History

A 9-year-old female child presented with bluish patches over the skin noticed for last three weeks. Her illness started insidiously with the spontaneous appearance of bluish patches on the skin which would change color over the next few days and then gradually fade, by which time other similar lesions would appear elsewhere on the skin. They were scattered all over with no specific predilection to any area. She had no other symptoms—no fever, no bleeding from any other site, no abdominal or joint pain. She remained active and playful throughout this period. She had not been on any drug nor was she administered any drug for these complaints. She had grown normally and had no significant illness in the past. There has been no past or family history of a bleeding disorder.

Analysis

Spontaneously appearing bluish patches, which change color and fade over time, suggest **ecchymosis**. A **fixed drug eruption** may look similar; however, this child has been absolutely healthy prior to this complaint and was not on any drugs. Though there is no family history, a **mild congenital deficiency** of one of the coagulation factors may present as ecchymosis for the first time at 9 years of age. However, being a mild deficiency, the symptoms should come up after minimal trauma and not spontaneously. Though this child has been regularly developing ecchymotic patches over the last three weeks, she has otherwise remained well without developing any other symptoms. Hence, it is unlikely to be a progressive disease such as leukemia or **bone marrow aplasia**. Conditions like **chronic liver disease** or **systemic vasculitis** are also unlikely, because except for the ecchymotic patches, this child has no other symptoms. **ITP** is the most common condition presenting this way at this age, but generally it would remit within a short time. Since, new lesions keep appearing in this child over last three weeks, it seems less likely. On the other hand, **functional disorders of platelets** could present in this fashion. The only other distant possibility is that of **child abuse** or self-inflicted injuries by the child herself.

Physical Examination

 Comfortable, not sick looking
 Ecchymotic patches scattered all over, with a few purpuric lesions
 No pallor, organomegaly or bony tenderness
 No other abnormality detected on general or systemic examination

Analysis

In view of the physical findings, chronic liver disease is ruled out, while conditions, such as leukemia and systemic vasculitis are less likely, though this needs to be confirmed by investigations.

Investigations

Hb—10 g%,   WBC count—8600/mm^3 P 54 L 38 E 6 M 2
Platelet count—1.7 lac/mm^3
PT and APTT—normal

Analysis

As most of the above-mentioned diseases are ruled out clinically as well as by laboratory tests, it is likely that this is a case of thrombasthenia or platelet function defects. To confirm the same, specialized tests need to be ordered.

Case Progression

The platelet function tests turned out to be normal. In view of this, child abuse was strongly suspected. However, there were no psychosocial problems with either the child or the family members. Since no definite diagnosis was reached, it was decided to repeat the tests. While the results were similar, this time it was reported that the platelets were reduced on the peripheral smear, though the count reported was 1.6 lacs/mm^3. This was surprising; in fact, there were only 4 or 5 platelets visualized per oil immersion field, which correlated with a rough platelet count of 40,000 to 50,000/mm^3. Only then it was realized that the platelet count that was reported was wrong; due to the microcytic anemia that this child had, the small RBCs were being counted as platelets by the counter. A bone marrow examination subsequently confirmed the presence of megakaryocytes and therefore, the diagnosis of ITP.

Final Diagnosis

Idiopathic thrombocytopenic purpura.

Experience gained...

> It is mandatory to correlate every platelet count with the adequacy of platelets on peripheral smear.

CASE 56

Sudden Falls in a 12-year-old

Case

A 12-year-old female child presented with two episodes of suddenly falling down, over the last two months. It happened for the first time during morning prayers in school when she suddenly collapsed. She regained consciousness in a minute or two and was normal thereafter. She had another similar episode when walking with her mother in the market. At that time, she did not fall down but apparently was supported by her mother; she looked blank for a few seconds and had one or two jerky movements of her limbs before she regained consciousness. No family history of syncope/sudden death of unknown cause.
Physical examination was normal.

Should you investigate this child? If so, which tests?

Before considering tests, we need to analyze history and guess what may have actually happened. This sudden transient loss of consciousness and postural tone without preceding symptoms and quick recovery may suggest vasovagal syncope. Neurocardiogenic syncope (vasovagal) is preceded by a prodrome—a feeling that the child is going to fall in the form of light headedness, dizziness, or such similar symptoms. This is also the typical age for such an occurrence. This is a benign condition and does not warrant any tests or treatment. However, other possibilities must be carefully ruled out. If the event occurs suddenly without any prodrome, or during physical exertion, or there is a history of sudden death in the family, or there are symptoms, such as palpitations or breathlessness suggestive of cardiac disease, then one should strongly suspect a cardiogenic syncope, which needs proper evaluation. Long QT syndrome often has a family history. These episodes did not suggest vertigo as there would have been other symptoms, such as a rotational feeling before or after the attack, and it would not cause momentary loss of sensorium. Vertigo is not so transient; further, two isolated episodes are unlikely—once it occurs it continues for a few days till it resolves. Seizures would have presented with abnormal movements or stiffness before loss of consciousness. During a seizure, the eyes of the patient are open, as against in a syncopal attack when they are closed (in this girl's second episode, the mother noticed the eyes to be closed). Further, the child is confused or drowsy before recovering fully. While atonic seizures may not have any abnormal movements or stiffness, they are extremely rare.

Even though there is no suggestion of a cardiac event in this child, an ECG should always be done, because in combination with a good history and clinical examination, it is highly sensitive for picking up cardiac syncope. If one is strongly suspecting a cardiac event on history, and the ECG turns out to be normal, one may have to resort to ECG during exercise or Holter monitoring. 2D echocardiogram can only pick up structural abnormality.

EEG or neuroimaging is not indicated in this child as clinically, a neurological event has been ruled out. A 'Tilt-table' test may be carried out to confirm neurocardiogenic syncope. However, one opts for it only when one is considering medications for frequent episodes;

it is not required in this case. Once the ECG is normal, it is best to reassure parents that these episodes are most likely to be benign syncope and therefore, it is safe to wait and watch.

Further Progress in this Child

Treating physician carried out all tests including "tilt-table" test, ECG, echocardiogram and EEG. All tests were normal. Parents were reassured about the benign nature of the symptoms.

Lessons Learnt

> A 'sudden collapse' is not easy to analyze unless one gets a first-hand account from a person who observed the episode. More often than not, people around the victim are busy doing some or other action, rather than observing exactly what happened. Thus, many a times, the physician may have to consider all possibilities to rule out serious illness and hence may need to investigate.

CASE 57

■ Dengue Shock Syndrome

History

A 5-year-old child presented with a history of fever for four days followed by vomiting for two days. Fever was moderately high and continuous, responding temporarily to acetaminophen. There were no other symptoms during the first-four days. He did not receive any other medication. On day five, the fever subsided but he started vomiting frequently, which continued over the next day. It did not get controlled with domperidone, and soon he became dehydrated for which he was hospitalized. The vomiting was not bile stained. There was no history of diarrhea, abdominal pain, high colored urine, yellow discoloration of eyes, or headache. He had apparently been a healthy child so far without any major illness in the past.

Analysis

This child had a self-limiting fever for four days that got better without any antibiotics. So this must have been a viral infection. However, there is no clue to a specific viral disease as there were no other localizing symptoms. Anyway, most viral infections share a common symptomatology. He started vomiting on day five, which coincided with the recovery of fever. This is unusual. As he did not receive any drug other than paracetamol, **drug-induced** vomiting can be definitely ruled out. Common febrile illnesses that are associated with significant vomiting are gastroenteritis, hepatitis or meningitis. It is an early symptom, occurring right at the onset of disease in **gastroenteritis** and **hepatitis.** Besides, absence of diarrhea or high-colored urine following vomiting nearly rule them out. In **meningitis,** vomiting would be accompanied by headache and the fever would have continued. So meningitis is also ruled out. Undiagnosed vomiting is often labeled as **gastritis,** though dyspepsia and epigastric pain would be the classical accompanying symptoms. **Metabolic** disorders may be triggered by viral infections, though it is uncommon for them to manifest for the first time at this age in a healthy child. Vomiting may be a non-specific feature of adrenal failure, myocarditis, or pancreatitis but such conditions would have presented with many other symptoms besides vomiting.

We must try to connect the preceding fever for four days to the subsequent occurrence of vomiting thereafter. In this child, the fever was mostly due to a viral infection. Anatomically, stomach, liver, or brain, are the common organs that lead to vomiting when diseased. If this virus was to infect one of these organs, vomiting would have started early, right at the onset of the disease. So this viral infection could have led to complications in a manner that one of these organs got involved. In other words, this may be either a gastropathy, hepatopathy or encephalopathy resulting from immunological or metabolic complications of a viral infection. Such complications do not involve the stomach, though the liver or brain can be involved. If the brain had been affected by such a complication, altered mental status would have been a prominent symptom. Thus, this is likely to be a hepatopathy due to immunological or metabolic complications induced by a viral infection. At this juncture, there is no further clue to pinpoint the probable etiology.

Physical Examination

Fairly built and nourished Lethargic
Weight 18 kg Height 104 cm
Temp normal Pulse 128/min Respiratory rate 32/min
BP 90/60 mm of Hg Grade II dehydration CRT prolonged
Peripheral pulses weak Peripheries cool
No pallor No icterus
No other findings on general examination.

Systemic Examination

Liver 3 cm +, firm, not tender Liver span 6 cm Spleen not palpable
Respiratory system—diminished breath sounds at the right base, no foreign sounds
Other systems normal

Analysis

This child is in compensated shock as evident by tachycardia, cool peripheries, prolonged capillary refill time, weak peripheral pulses and moderate dehydration. Diminished breath sounds without foreign sounds at the right base suggest a pleural effusion. In conjunction with signs of shock, this denotes capillary leak syndrome. In such a case, hepatomegaly may suggest hepatopathy due to hypoperfusion. As these complications followed a viral infection, it indicates a possibility of dengue shock syndrome.

Investigations

Hb 15 g% WBC 4,700/mm^3 N 60 L 32 M 6 E 2 Platelets 1.2 lacs/mm^3
Urine normal ALT 50 units AST 45 units
Other liver functions normal
Abdominal USG showed hepatomegaly with enlarged congested gallbladder.
Dengue IgG and IgM +ve

Final Diagnosis

Dengue shock syndrome.

Lessons Learnt

> Any single organ may bear the brunt of hypoperfusion or shock ahead of other organ involvement, in the early stages. Thus, the patient may present with symptoms related to a particular organ dysfunction, which may mimic a primary disease of that organ. This is what happened in this case, wherein the vomiting was a symptom of liver involvement, but it was not primary hepatitis. The clue to such an indirect involvement of the liver was the onset of vomiting late in the course of illness.

CASE 58

■ Capillaria Hepatica

History

An 8-month-old infant presented with fever for last two months. He was irritable, had a poor appetite and had lost 500 g of weight over last two months. There were no other significant symptoms. His weight gain over the first-six months had been normal and he had been a healthy infant prior to this illness.

There were no detailed records of the progress of his illness. Several antibiotics were empirically tried without any benefit. Routine investigations had shown eosinophilia in peripheral blood but no other abnormality.

Analysis

Fever in an infant would invariably suggest infection. As fever has been going on for two months, it is likely to be a chronic infection. History does not indicate any localization. Antibiotics have failed to control this disease. However, there has been no worsening. This may suggest either a nonbacterial infection or tuberculosis. At this age, tuberculosis, if left untreated, would have disseminated and led to TBM. Hence, it is unlikely in this child. Nonbacterial infections may be viral, fungal, or parasitic. Chronic viral infection may be HIV. Fungal infections are generally the result of underlying immune deficiency and may be an accompaniment of HIV infection. Parasitic infection is likely in view of eosinophilia though such infections rarely cause fever, except malaria.

Physical Examination

Averagely built and nourished
Weight 6.8 kg
No pallor
Length 70 cm
No icterus
Not acutely sick though irritable
Head circumference 43 cm

Systemic Examination

Liver 3 F+, firm, not tender
Spleen not palpable
No other abnormality
Liver span 8 cm
No ascites

Analysis

Hepatomegaly is the only positive finding on physical examination. Fever with hepatomegaly may indicate a chronic infection as discussed above. It is unlikely to be hepatoblastoma as the liver would have been hard in consistency and larger in size. Further, the clinical presentation would have been in the form of distention of abdomen rather than persistent fever. Any other malignancy, such as leukemia is also unlikely.

Investigations

Hb 10 g% WBC 18500/mm^3 P 52 L 21 E 24 M 3 ESR 45 mm at the end of 1 hour
LFT normal
Chest X-ray normal Mt test –ve
Abdominal USG-hepatomegaly, otherwise normal
Liver biopsy—*Capillaria hepatica*—parasitic infection

Treatment

Child was treated with albendazole for two weeks and recovered well.

Lessons Learnt

1. Fever with hepatomegaly but without liver dysfunction suggests infection other than viral hepatitis.
2. Persistent eosinophilia denotes parasitic infection, though it may also be due to leukemoid reaction as in tuberculosis or due to eosinophilic leukemia.
3. Most parasitic infections do not cause fever though this has been a rare parasite.

■ Fever with Skin Rash

Preamble

Fever accompanied with skin rash often poses a diagnostic challenge, especially when it is the only presenting feature. It may be the *presenting manifestation* of many **infections** (viral, bacterial, fungal, parasitic) besides **hypersensitivity reactions** or **collagen vascular disorders**. However, there are many other disorders where fever and rash coexist, but the rash is not the presenting or a prominent manifestation. In such conditions, the diagnosis does not depend only on the assessment of the skin rash. Such examples include malignancies like lymphoma, opportunistic infections in HIV infected persons, typhoid and malaria.

Diagnostic Approach

While attempting a clinical diagnosis, there may be many aspects of the rash which may need to be taken into consideration. These include the morphologic type of the rash, its distribution, the sequence of its appearance/disappearance, phenomena following the rash like desquamation, and of course the temporal relationship of the rash with fever. Amongst these, the morphology may or may not be helpful, since its specificity is often low. In other words, a given morphologic type of rash can exist in various disorders and in a given disorder, different morphological types of rashes have been described.

Morphological Types

Classification of the type of lesion helps to a small extent as far as specific diagnosis is concerned. *Target lesions* may help to narrow down the diagnostic probabilities as in case of erythema multiforme, which is of two types—the first one is benign and self-limiting while the other is the more severe form, such as Stevens-Johnson syndrome or toxic epidermal necrolysis (may be caused by *Mycoplasma*).

Maculopapular rash is seen in viral infections, drug reactions and immune complex mediated diseases.

Vesicular rash may be seen in coxsackie, echovirus, varicella, herpes simplex, Stevens-Johnson syndrome.

Purpuric rash may be seen in viral (hemorrhagic viral fevers), bacterial (meningococcemia, rickettsia, rat bite fever, relapsing fever) and parasitic (malaria) infections. A purpuric rash may begin as a blanching macular rash which then evolves into a typical purpuric rash after a few days making the initial diagnosis difficult. The rash may be petechial even in uncomplicated dengue fever.

Nodular lesions are seen in fungal infections, tuberculosis, rickettsial diseases and malignancy. Erythema nodosum represents an immune mediated lesion due to many infections.

Diffuse erythema is seen in scarlet fever, Kawasaki disease as well as Stevens-Johnson syndrome, staphylococcal scalded skin syndrome and toxic epidermal necrolysis.

Distribution of Rash

A rash that starts on the legs peripherally and spreads to the chest and abdomen (centripetal) suggests meningococcemia or rickettsial disease. A rash that starts centrally and spreads peripherally is characteristic of a drug rash and most viral infections, except echo and coxsackie. Streaky facial involvement is likely to be due to parvovirus B19 (fifth disease or erythema infectiosum).

Desquamation

Desquamation occurs during the crescendo phase of staphylococcal exfoliative toxin syndrome (as maximal disease manifestations evolve); during the decrescendo phase of Kawasaki disease (typically days 10 to 20 after onset, beginning in the periungual region); and only during the convalescent phases of streptococcal scarlet fever and of staphylococcal and streptococcal toxic shock syndrome. Desquamation of palms and soles is likely to be a full-thickness loss (as if molted) after Kawasaki disease, streptococcal scarlet fever, and toxic shock syndrome. In Kawasaki disease, unlike streptococcal scarlet fever, toxic shock syndrome, and staphylococcal exfoliative toxin syndrome, total body desquamation does not occur or is fine and superficial, occurring in only about 10% of patients, particularly in the groin and perineal area.

It is clear that evaluation of skin rash alone may not lead to the specific diagnosis. Even in the absence of a definite diagnosis, the first step should be to rule out serious and/or potentially troublesome diseases. Once they are ruled out, evolution of skin rash and the disease profile itself usually offers a clue to the diagnosis. Therefore, it is practical to divide diseases that present with fever and skin rash into the following four categories:

i. Those which may be **life-threatening** and require urgent attention—meningococcemia, sepsis with DIC, staphylococcal toxic shock syndrome. These are usually diagnosed within the first few days of the onset of the illness. The characteristics of life-threatening skin rashes are—it affects the entire body, the rash involves skin and mucous membranes and may form blisters. In general**,** purpuric rashes and bullous rashes could be life- threatening and require urgent attention.

ii. Those which require **careful follow-up**, because though the diagnosis is not definite at a given point in time, these may evolve into conditions that require timely intervention: Stevens-Johnson syndrome, toxic epidermal necrolysis, staphylococcal scalded skin syndrome, scarlet fever, rheumatic fever, Kawasaki disease, leptospirosis and dengue fever, drug rash other than Stevens-Johnson syndrome.

   While many of these conditions can be life-threatening, timely diagnosis has definite therapeutic implications in all of them.

iii. Those that **unfold** themselves **slowly**—collagen vascular diseases, systemic onset juvenile rheumatoid arthritis, SLE, dermatomyositis.

   In this group, the rash may appear quite sometime after the onset of fever. The final diagnostic label may take weeks to months. While the diagnosis evolves, usually there is no immediate danger to life.

iv. Those that are **short-lasting** and **self-limiting**—conditions that do not have much therapeutic implications—measles, rubella, rosella, adeno- and enteroviral infections, infectious mononucleosis.

CASE 59

Systemic Inflammatory Disorder

History

A 12-year-old female child presented with fever for last four weeks and a skin rash for last three weeks. She was apparently alright one month ago, when she started getting high-grade, continuous fever. Initially, it was not accompanied with any other symptoms, but after a week she reported a skin rash that was most prominent at the peak of the fever and would often subside by itself once the fever was relatively less. There was a mild itching when the rash was most prominent. On direct questioning, she gave a history of transient pain and swelling in the left ankle joint that lasted for just 12 hours and subsided on its own. Thereafter, she had felt a similar pain in the small joints of one hand, without swelling, which had also lasted just for a day.

The physical examination as reported had not revealed any significant abnormality. The investigations done included a CBC with peripheral smear, ESR, urinalysis, chest X-ray, blood culture, urine culture, Widal test and antibody tests against the EB virus, leptospirosis, and rickettsia. All the tests were negative except for a mild neutrophilic leukocytosis and a high ESR by the end of the first week of fever. Repeat tests had shown an increasing neutrophilic leukocytosis with thrombocytosis and the ESR had increased.

This prompted the physician to try a broad-spectrum antibiotic, considering the probability of acute bacterial infection but there was no response.

At this juncture, some more tests were ordered that included an abdominal ultrasound, a CT scan of the chest and abdomen, ANA and RA factor. The ANA was weakly positive and RA factor was negative.

She was then referred for further management.

Physical Examination

Fairly built and nourished	Sick looking	
Weight 30 kg	Height 142 cm	
Temp.103°F	Pulse rate 112/min	RR 30/min
Bones and joints normal	No lymphadenopathy	Mild pallor
Skin rash—macular, discrete, all over the body		Nails normal
No mouth ulcers	No conjunctivitis	No alopecia
Systemic examination normal	No hepatosplenomegaly	

Analysis

This child has a prolonged fever with a skin rash as the only diagnostic lead. If this fever represents an infection, there is no localization of the infection so far, since there are no other positive findings on physical examination. The character, time frame and the evolution of the rash do not fit into the pattern of any **exanthematous** illness, which is therefore ruled out. It is unlikely to be a **drug-induced** rash since these are not evanescent. **Infectious mononucleosis** can present with prolonged fever and can manifest with a rash following administration of amoxicillin. However, there are no other physical findings to suggest the same, and again, once such a rash develops, it would persist and not be evanescent. Malignancies like lymphoma may present with prolonged fever and a skin rash; since the rash is usually allergic in nature, it may itch, and may also be evanescent. However, the rash would not necessarily come up at the height of fever, and the imaging studies done so far should have picked up lymphoma. The investigations had revealed an increasing neutrophilic leukocytosis with thrombocytosis and a high ESR. These suggest an acute inflammatory disease which could be either infective or noninfective. The evanescent skin rash that is most prominent at the peak of fever and disappears by itself, suggests a **noninfective inflammatory** disorder. Moreover, there has been no clue to any infection so far nor was there any therapeutic response to antibiotics. Thus, it is quite likely to be a systemic inflammatory disease that possibly cannot be labeled at this stage, and will evolve over time. It could be a systemic onset of juvenile chronic arthritis. Though **systemic lupus erythematosus** is an important consideration in a 12-year-old girl, it is less likely in this child since she does not have leukopenia (which is often characteristic of SLE) and there are no other clinical features of SLE as of now.

Management

This child was looking quite sick due to her prolonged fever and loss of weight and appetite. Since she was not responding to anti-inflammatory drugs, it was decided to consider oral steroids. However, as the diagnosis at this stage was merely presumptive, it was decided to perform a bone marrow examination to confidently rule out any leukemic process (though, of course, the hematological tests done on peripheral blood earlier, were normal). Once the bone marrow was reported to be normal, she was put on oral steroids, and she recovered within the next few days. The fever came under control within four days, and she regained her appetite and weight over the next few days. Steroids need to be continued for long periods in such children with a systemic onset of juvenile chronic arthritis. Further management depends upon the evaluation of joint disease at a later stage in which case, she would need disease modifying drugs such as methotrexate besides anti-inflammatory drugs.

Lessons Learnt

When a macular rash develops almost a week after the onset of high fever, and then both fever and rash persist, common exanthematous illnesses are ruled out. A rash that is evanescent, becoming obvious at the peak of fever only to subside when the spike of fever reduces, suggests vasculitis as a part of a systemic inflammatory disorder. Such a diagnosis is supported by the absence of localization of any infection. In such conditions, it is always safe to rule out acute leukemia by a bone marrow examination, because if missed by chance, prognosis would change drastically with use of steroids.

CASE 60

■ Meningococcemia

Events...

A 2-year-old child presented with mild fever and vomiting for a day. The fever was moderate, and he had vomited 3 or 4 times. The next morning, the mother noticed a few scattered macular lesions over the body, for which she sought advice from a physician. He diagnosed these skin lesions to be 'purpura' but found no other abnormal physical findings. There was no hepatosplenomegaly or pallor, and the child did not look sick. He ordered a CBC with platelet count. Except for mild neutrophilic leukocytosis, there was no other abnormality; the hemoglobin and the platelet count were normal. So, an antibiotic was prescribed and the parents were asked to follow-up the next day. However, the child deteriorated over the next eight hours and was rushed to the hospital in a state of shock. A diagnosis of meningococcemia (without meningitis) was made, and he was treated with Penicillin, steroids and appropriate intravenous fluids, but he succumbed to his illness within the next two hours.

Explanation...

In the presence of fever, a purpuric rash is an emergency, and its cause must be found at the earliest. The first step is to differentiate thrombocytopenic purpura from nonthrombocytopenic purpura. The latter could be vascular purpura, or it may be due to thrombasthenia. However, fever is not a feature of platelet function defects. Therefore, if investigations suggest a non-thrombocytopenic purpura in a febrile child, one should carefully look out for vascular causes of purpura. This child did not have any other symptoms suggestive of Henoch–Schönlein purpura. So, the sudden development of vascular purpura in the presence of fever suggests that it is secondary to an evolving serious infection. This child deteriorated rapidly thereafter and went on to develop circulatory shock. Though sepsis with disseminated intravascular coagulation can present similarly, such a child would have progressed over 3 or 4 days and then developed DIC and purpura. On the other hand, the rapid deterioration seen in this child is typical of **meningococcemia**. Purpura fulminans may also present similarly; while in such cases the purpura is obvious, in meningococcemia it may have to be fished out.

While it is difficult to anticipate further progress in a child who presents with purpura, it is enough to warrant hospitalization and close observation. In fact, though the other physical findings were reported to be normal when this child was first seen for the purpuric rash, early signs of compensated shock (which may often be subtle) should be carefully looked for in such cases. These include disproportionate tachycardia and tachypnea, delayed capillary refill time and evidence of hypoperfusion as suggested by a change in behavior and reduced urine output.

This child also had significant vomiting. In this setting, it could have been attributed to either gastrointestinal, hepatic or central nervous system affection. Gastrointestinal infections can lead to a complication like hemolytic uremic syndrome over a few days, which then presents with purpura. Hepatic diseases may present with bleeding due to coagulation defects but are unlikely to develop purpura. Retrospectively, one does not know whether this vomiting suggested a subtle affection of the central nervous system secondary to hypoperfusion.

Thus, in an acute illness, often it may not be easy to interpret the significance of vomiting.

Experience gained...

Purpuric rash in presence of fever is an emergency; both thrombocytopenic and a non-thrombocytopenic purpura have an equally grave significance in this setting.

An early diagnosis of meningococcemia is mandatory to ensure success of therapy. It needs a high index of suspicion. The purpuric rash may have to be fished out, so also the subtle signs of compensated shock.

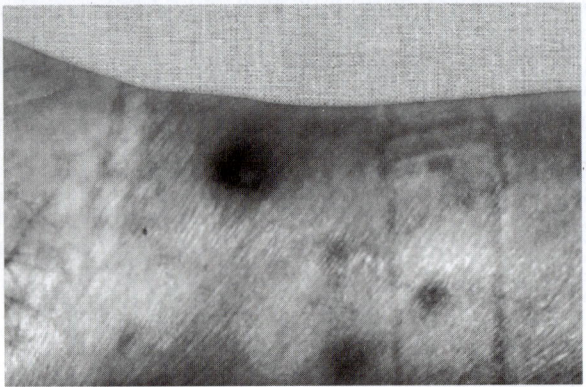

Gangrenous lesion with purpura.

CASE 61

■ Stevens–Johnson Syndrome

Events...

A 4-year-old child presented with fever for five days followed by a bullous skin rash for which an opinion was sought. He complained of burning while micturition and defecation, and also had a difficulty in eating. He had received some medications for his fever, the details of which were not known. Physical examination revealed a sick child with vesiculobullous lesions all over the body, severe mucosal ulcers in the mouth and a nonpurulent conjunctivitis.

Explanation...

Like purpura, every vesiculobullous skin rash should be considered potentially life-threatening, especially in a sick child and such a child should be hospitalized, carefully observed and properly treated. This child may have developed **Stevens-Johnson syndrome**—an extreme form of a skin reaction to a drug. This condition has to be treated like a case of severe burns, with isolation and prevention of infection, proper hydration and at times, antibiotics. A close differential diagnosis in such a case could be a staphylococcal scalded skin syndrome.

Experience gained...

> Vesiculobullous skin rashes in a sick child usually represent potentially life-threatening illnesses that need urgent diagnosis and management. Varicella presents with a vesicular rash and the disease is usually benign. However, if such a child is sick looking or the rash is hemorrhagic, it could be a potentially serious disease.

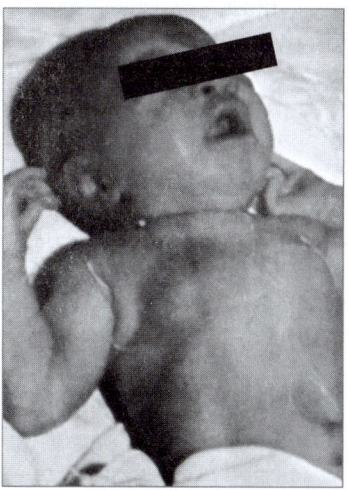

Bullous lesions.

CASE 62

Dengue Shock Syndrome

Events...

A 6-month-old infant presented with moderate fever for four days and a macular skin rash, mainly over the trunk, for a day. There were no other symptoms. It was considered to be a viral infection and was treated symptomatically. The fever subsided over the next two days and so also the skin rash. After remaining afebrile for a day, the parents reported excessive lethargy that was initially considered to be a post-viral generalized weakness. Therefore, their physician just reassured them. However, over the next 12 hours, he started vomiting and was rushed to the family physician. A physical examination revealed that the infant was drowsy though the family doctor did not find any other significant abnormalities. He surprisingly noted that the baby had gained one kilogram in just 24 hours, though he could not explain this. The infant was referred for further management.

Explanation...

Two events in this child were unusual and hence, not anticipated. The first one was that he became lethargic and started vomiting *after* an apparent recovery from an illness that was presumed to be a viral infection. Considering that he had recovered without any antibiotic, the presumption that it was a viral infection was probably correct. Many viral infections *end* with a skin rash; this is what seemed to happen in this infant also. Therefore, the subsequent unusual progress that was seen in this child, was not expected. The second unusual event in this child was the sudden gain in weight. On direct questioning, he was not passing an adequate amount of urine. On careful physical examination, the pediatrician noted tachycardia with puffiness of the face, abdominal distension without organomegaly and diminished breath sounds at both bases. It was clear that he had developed capillary leak syndrome with a resultant extravascular collection of fluid and intravascular dehydration. This was **dengue shock syndrome.** He was luckily revived with intravenous fluids.

Experience gained...

> While most viral infections are benign, a few of them may result in complications that may be dangerous. It is important to recognize such infections for timely action. However, the diagnosis of viral infections is mostly a clinical conjecture and often, it is not possible to diagnose *a specific* viral infection. Many viral infections share the same symptoms and signs that may also be common to a few noninfective illnesses such as Kawasaki syndrome. Thus, there may be no clinically discernable difference between dengue and any other viral infection. Hence, every illness, including a seemingly benign viral infection, should be considered to have fully recovered only after the recovery has been sustained for a certain period. In an acute illness, such a period of observation may extend just for a few days. But in chronic diseases, it may be necessary to monitor the child for a few weeks to months, as in tuberculosis where a relapse may occur as late as a year after completion of treatment.

CASE 63

■ Rickettsial Disease

Events...

A 3-year-old child presented with fever for four days and a skin rash for last two days. The fever was moderate to high. The rash increased over two days and led to black patches over one ear lobe and one toe. Physical examination revealed a sick child with high fever, who had a maculonodular rash scattered all over, with two gangrenous patches over the ear lobe and one toe. This suggested vasculitis that may be secondary to infection or autoimmune disease. As there were similar cases reported at around the same time in the community, it was thought to be an infection. It was confirmed to be *rickettsial disease.* When suspected, the diagnosis of rickettsial infections can be confirmed by the Weil Felix test.

Experience gained...

> This case illustrates a point that in the evaluation of any skin rash, there are times when the morphology is important (gangrenous lesions), though at other times, a greater emphasis must be laid on the accompanying symptoms and physical signs (as illustrated in the child with meningococcemia). Such treatable conditions should not be missed.

CASE 64

■ Severe Combined Immunodeficiency

Events...
A 3-month-old infant presented with fever for last six weeks, cough and diarrhea off and on during this period, and a skin rash for last two weeks. He did not feed well and had failed to gain weight. He was treated with antibiotics with no significant change in his illness. BCG vaccine was administered at birth and had led to a nonhealing ulcer.

Physical examination revealed a sick malnourished infant with a nodular rash over the trunk, hepatosplenomegaly, scattered crepitations in the lungs on both sides and an ulcer at the site of BCG vaccine.

Explanation...
Disseminated infection at multiple sites in an infant who has failed to thrive suggests an underlying immune deficiency. A nonhealing ulcer at the site of BCG vaccination denotes a T cell defect or combined immune deficiency. Isolated B cell defects present well beyond the first 3 or 4 months of age, only after the maternally transferred antibodies have disappeared. In view of the nonhealing BCG ulcer, this may be an infection resulting from the BCG strain of tubercle bacillus that has spread to distant parts of the body due to immune deficiency. It could also be some other opportunistic infection as well.

Immunological tests revealed **severe combined immunodeficiency.** Skin biopsy from a nodule confirmed tuberculosis, and PCR demonstrated it to be the BCG strain of tubercle bacillus. This infant succumbed to the disease in spite of appropriate drug therapy.

Experience gained...

> Occasionally, a rash may help reach the diagnosis not by its morphology, but by providing a histopathological tissue diagnosis. Vasculitis is another lesion that can be proved by skin biopsy, which helps in the diagnosis of an immune disorder.

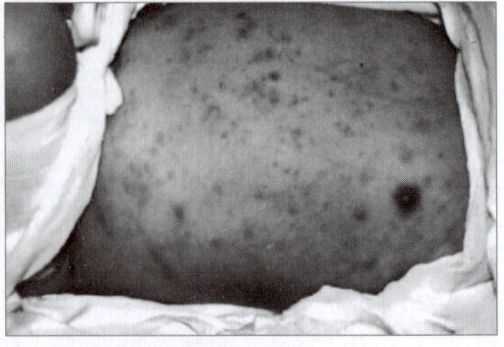

Nodular lesions.

Management Dilemmas in Office Practice

CASE 65

■ Streptococcal Infection

Events...

A 6-year-old child presented with high fever for two days followed by a skin rash. Physical examination showed a severely congested throat with enlarged, tender, jugulodigastric lymph nodes and an erythematous blanching skin rash over large areas of the body. This suggested a *streptococcal infection* that needs prompt treatment, so as to avoid postinfective immune complications, such as rheumatic fever.

Experience gained...

> This is an example of a treatable infection, which presents with fever and a rash. If not properly recognized and managed, it may result in secondary complications with risk of permanent sequelae.

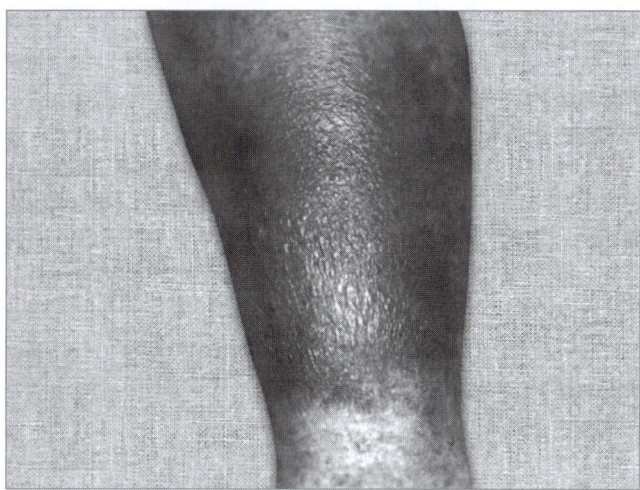

Diffuse erythema of streptococcal infection.

CASE 66

■ Hodgkin's Lymphoma

Events...

An 8-year-old child presented with severe cough for last two months, skin rash for last one month and fever for last three weeks. He was apparently alright two months ago when he developed a severe cough that was considered to be pertussis. The CBC was non-contributory and chest X-ray was normal. He was treated with erythromycin and a cough suppressant, but the cough worsened over time. At the end of a month of persistent cough, he developed a macular skin rash that was itchy and was diagnosed to be a drug rash. He was prescribed antihistamines that did not relieve his itching. In fact, he was getting irritable, and by then, had lost 4 kg of weight. A week later, he started running fever that added to his sickness. At that stage, since repeat investigations did not offer any clue to the diagnosis, he was referred for further evaluation.

Explanation...

The initial diagnosis of pertussis seems to be rational. One would expect the cough in pertussis to worsen over the first 2 to 3 weeks and then gradually subside over another few weeks. It is also not unusual that the CBC and chest X-ray were normal. When he developed a skin rash, it was not easy to connect the rash to a disease that was believed to be pertussis and so an easy way out was to label it as a drug rash. What was missed was the fact that he had lost considerable weight and that needed to be accounted for. Thereafter, he started running fever. A fever that comes up five weeks after the onset of cough may suggest a chronic infection like tuberculosis. However, tuberculosis rarely causes severe cough and normally it would have started with fever. Thus, a non-infective condition was thought of. In view of the severe cough, it was decided to repeat the chest X-ray that showed widening of superior mediastinum; CT scan of chest confirmed it to be a large lymph node. Now it was possible to connect the allergic skin rash to the primary disease, as an urticarial rash is known in Hodgkin's lymphoma. It could also explain the deteriorating health in this child. The diagnosis of Hodgkin's lymphoma was later confirmed.

Experience gained...

> Generally speaking, all the symptoms and physical signs in a patient must be correlated to a single diagnosis. Thus, in this child, an itchy skin rash had to be connected to a disease that started as cough and went on to cause a significant deterioration in the general health over the next two months. This case illustrates that while the skin rash would not have led to a diagnosis in this child, accompanying symptoms and the temporal profile should have helped to arrive at the correct diagnosis.

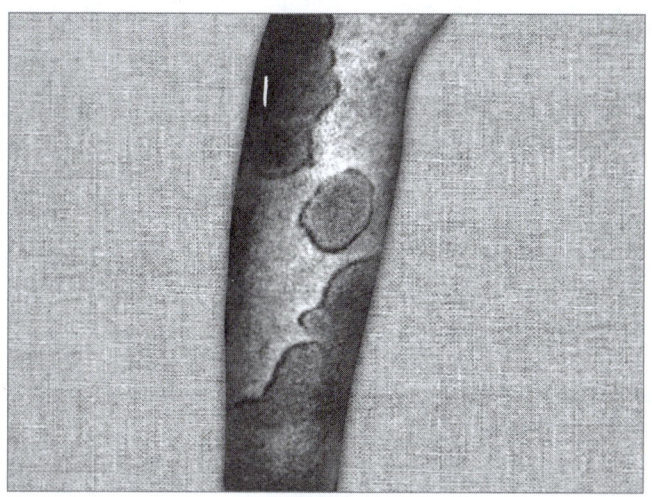
Urticarial lesion.

■ Inborn Errors of Metabolism

Preamble
There is an inborn fear of such disorders in the minds of pediatricians. Most of these diseases involve complex metabolic processes that seem to be difficult to study. There are more than 300 such disorders that are known to science so far. Clinical presentations of many of these disorders not only overlap with one another, but they also simulate many infective diseases. Some of them manifest acutely as life-threatening emergencies that need urgent action. Others present as recurrent episodes of similar complaints that may defy correct diagnosis. This poses a challenge to pediatricians.

Core Knowledge
Broadly there are three types of metabolic disorders. The first group consists of disorders that result from accumulation of small toxic molecules, and they include organic acidemia, aminoacidopathies and carbohydrate metabolism defects. Most of them present in neonates, though some of them do present later in life, in spite of the fact that the accumulation of toxic molecules occurs right from early in life. Such examples are phenylketonuria and galactosemia. The second group refers to energy deficiency diseases and mitochondrial disorders are a classical example of this group. Unlike the first group of disorders in which the fetus is protected through maternal circulation, these disorders often start in fetal life. They may present with birth defects or intrauterine growth retardation and affect the brain, liver, heart and skeletal muscles. The third group is lysosomal storage disorders, and depending on the tissue that is primarily affected, the manifestations vary. Connective tissue storage leads to coarse facies, contractures, cataract, and cardiac valve involvement. Developmental delay due to involvement of the brain, hepatosplenomegaly and skeletal dysplasia may be other manifestations. The first two groups of disorders present acutely and must be recognized early to avoid permanent sequelae, while the third group of disorders present with chronic progressive manifestations.

The clinical profile of metabolic disorders often simulates many common diseases met with in office practice. However, the course of events may differ in many ways and often, there are subtle clues that must be picked up in order to suspect these disorders. It is enough, if we suspect inborn error of metabolism and refer the patients in time for further management. Though, it is ideal that the initial workup be done by the primary pediatrician who happens to see the patient first, because some of these disorders may demonstrate laboratory abnormalities only during the crisis and not thereafter. Many children who are actually suffering from one of these disorders but who present as an acute emergency, improve on withdrawal of oral feeds and administration of intravenous fluids (including dextrose). Though this treatment is unintentionally instituted as a part of the general management of that emergency, it sometimes happens to be the specific treatment of acute episodes of these disorders.

When to suspect a metabolic disorder?

One should suspect a metabolic disorder whenever there is an unexpected clinical presentation and/or progress that does not fit into the pattern of any common classical disease. One should also suspect a metabolic disorder when clinical manifestations develop suddenly and may also recover quickly only to recur again. History of consanguinity and sibling deaths should add to the suspicion of such disorders as most of these diseases have an autosomal recessive transmission.

The following **unexplained situations** demand a search for metabolic disorders:
1. Acute onset of vomiting, coma or acidosis, especially, if it is intermittent.
2. Sepsis
3. Motor deficits, developmental delay or regression
4. Acute liver cell failure, hepatosplenomegaly
5. Cardiomyopathy and skeletal muscle weakness
6. Urolithiasis.

The initial laboratory workup should include serum electrolytes, ammonia, lactate, pyruvate, glucose, arterial blood gas and urinary ketones. In an acute emergency situation, whenever there is no definite diagnosis possible, the priority is to resuscitate the child before attempting to diagnose. However, it is ideal to collect and freeze samples of plasma and urine for subsequent analysis, in case an inborn error of metabolism is suspected. As mentioned above, the laboratory abnormalities may not persist once the crisis is over and one may miss the diagnosis till the patient presents with another episode. Blood samples should not be frozen.

The ensuing case scenarios represent some of these problems and demonstrate how subtle clues help in suspecting these disorders.

CASE 67

■ Metabolic Disorder Presenting as Complication of Diarrhea

Events...

A one-year-old child presented with loose stools for two days. He was treated symptomatically, following which the diarrhea improved partially. But on the third day of his illness, he started vomiting which persisted for a day. At that stage, he was not dehydrated, his abdomen was not distended and there were no other positive findings. A day later, this was followed by a sudden onset of convulsions and coma. Physical examination did not offer any clue. He was hospitalized in a critical care unit and received IV fluids and anticonvulsants. He was put on mechanical ventilation and empirical antibiotics. He recovered completely within the next two days. All routine investigations including CSF were normal, except that he had metabolic acidosis with a high anion gap.

Explanation...

Acute gastroenteritis usually starts with vomiting followed by loose stools. This child started vomiting on the third day—that was unusual. If vomiting develops late in the course of such an illness, it is likely to be a side effect of drugs used or a complication, such as paralytic ileus, intestinal obstruction or intussusception. Since this child did not receive any drugs and had no positive findings on physical examination to suggest these complications, the vomiting remains unexplained. This could have prompted one to anticipate an unusual course of events. Subsequently, this child developed convulsions and coma. This could have been considered to be a neurological complication of intestinal infections, in the form of toxic encephalopathy, or as a result of dehydration related problems, such as electrolyte disturbances or venous sinus thrombosis. Certain viral infections that cause diarrhea can also cause encephalitis. However, toxic encephalopathy is usually seen in shigellosis which is characterized by high fever which this child did not have; further, children with toxic encephalopathy recover quickly from their convulsion and altered sensorium. Similarly, this child was not dehydrated on examination; therefore, electrolyte abnormalities like hyponatremia or venous sinus thrombosis are unlikely to be the cause of his convulsion and coma. Finally, the CSF was normal and his recovery quite quick (and unanticipated), which rules out encephalitis. In other words, these neurological events are also difficult to explain on the basis of a gastrointestinal infection.

In fact, a sudden development of neurological manifestations and also, an equally quick recovery, rules out infection. Vascular complications may develop suddenly but they are unlikely to recover so quickly. Such a clinical profile is seen in a metabolic disorder. Though metabolic disorders typically present at an earlier age, there is always a spectrum to their severity. The milder variety can present later in life and are typically triggered by intercurrent illnesses/infections. The metabolic acidosis with a high anion gap was inconsistent with the lack of dehydration in this child and thereby, also suggested the possibility of a metabolic disorder such as organic acidemia or aminoacidopathy. In fact, intravenous fluids and the withholding of oral feeds (since the child was unconscious) may have unintentionally helped the child to recover, as the offending food agents were automatically withdrawn. Further tests would be necessary to pin down the exact defect.

Experience gained...

An unexpected course of events must arouse the suspicion of a metabolic disorder. These disorders may simulate an infection but subtle clues serve as a guide to the correct diagnosis. In this child, unanticipated recovery and metabolic acidosis with a high anion gap offered a clue to the right diagnosis.

CASE 68

■ Metabolic Disorder Presenting as Unexplained Encephalopathy

Events...

A 6-month-old infant presented with mild fever and occasional vomiting for two days, followed by the sudden development of altered sensorium. He was doing well till the onset of fever and had no major illness in the past. Physical examination showed that he was comatose but did not offer any clue to the diagnosis. He was investigated and all routine tests were normal including CBC, CRP, CSF, blood sugar and electrolytes. He was put on intravenous fluids and observed for further progress. He recovered after three days and looked quite normal thereafter.

Explanation...

This infant had trivial symptoms that suddenly led to the development of coma. He also improved unexpectedly without any diagnosis. While one could have considered it to be viral encephalitis to begin with, he would not have recovered so quickly. Further, ideally the CSF should have been abnormal in viral encephalitis. Therefore, this is not an infective illness, but is likely to be a metabolic disorder. In such cases where the diagnosis is elusive in an acutely serious condition, it is best to collect blood for a metabolic workup. That should include blood ammonia, lactate, pyruvate, blood gas and urine for ketones. This infant had raised blood ammonia levels that paved the way for further tests to define the exact metabolic disorder.

Experience gained...

> In an acute serious manifestation, especially when the diagnosis is not possible on clinical grounds and laboratory tests, it should be a routine to freeze plasma (not blood) and urine samples for further evaluation, if required. This is most vital as many metabolic disorders demonstrate laboratory abnormalities only in an acute crisis and those abnormalities may not persist once the child recovers. Thus, the diagnosis can be missed, and one may wrongly rule out a metabolic disorder.

CASE 69

Urea Cycle Defect

Events…

A 2-year-old child presented with mild fever and breathlessness for two days and was suspected to have pneumonia. There was no past or family history of asthma or atopy. His chest X-ray was reported as pneumonitis. He was treated with IV antibiotics, IV fluids and oxygenation, and recovered as expected within the next couple of days and was discharged. He suffered from another similar episode after a few months. The CBC showed mild neutrophilic leukocytosis and the chest X-ray was again reported as pneumonitis. So, he was treated again on the same lines and recovered. Considering it to be the second episode of pneumonia, he was investigated in detail, specifically for immunodeficiency and cystic fibrosis. When these conditions were ruled out, a CT scan of chest was done to rule out any congenital malformation that could have led to the recurrent pneumonia. The CT scan was normal. GER was also ruled out and so also H type of tracheoesophageal fistula. Since all these tests were negative, finally, the parents were reassured that this recurrence of pneumonia was merely an accident. Unfortunately, he had a similar episode for the third time, which is when he was referred as a case of recurrent pneumonia.

Explanation…

This child had a *mild* fever and was reported to have 'breathlessness'. Nowhere in his clinical notes was it mentioned whether he had respiratory distress. Therefore, he could well have had 'tachypnea' but not respiratory distress. This tachypnea was out of proportion to the extent of abnormality reported on the X-ray (usually, the word 'pneumonitis' is used to describe a small ill-defined abnormality on the X-ray which if reported as pneumonia, would sound outrageous). Further, his improvement was also too quick, thereby suggesting that it may not be related to antibiotic therapy. Hence, it was most unlikely that this child had pneumonia. At this stage itself, one would have given a thought to an alternate diagnosis. If this child was tachypneic due to pneumonia and required oxygenation, one would have confirmed the hypoxia by at least a pulse oximeter if not an arterial blood gas.

During the current admission, there was no evidence of any respiratory signs at all, and as suspected, he was not in respiratory distress but only had tachypnea. Therefore, the diagnosis of pneumonia was definitely amiss and there was no need to toe the line of recurrent pneumonia any further. This raised the possibility of it being metabolic acidosis and hence blood gas analysis was asked for. It confirmed metabolic acidosis and also showed respiratory alkalosis which explains the hyperventilation. Subsequently, further tests were ordered that proved the diagnosis of urea cycle defect.

Experience gained...

Hyperventilation of unknown origin may be a manifestation of a metabolic disorder. In fact, what looks like a respiratory disease superficially may turn out to be metabolic acidosis due to diabetes, renal tubular acidosis, or acidosis secondary to inborn errors of metabolism. The mild fever does not go against a metabolic disorder; it is known to trigger their clinical manifestations.

CASE 70

Galactosemia

Events...

A 4-month-old infant presented with jaundice noticed by the parents for last three days. He was apparently well till then and was exclusively breastfed. He had high colored urine and yellow stools. He was investigated and found to have direct hyperbilirubinemia, with mildly raised ALT and AST. The torch titers were noncontributory and abdominal sonogram was normal. Considering it to be a case of hepatitis, a liver biopsy was performed that did not help to pinpoint the diagnosis, as it showed mild inflammatory changes of a non-specific nature. By then, he developed a change in sensorium without any other symptoms and was considered to be in liver cell failure. He recovered on supportive treatment, but the jaundice had worsened in spite of an apparent 'recovery from liver cell failure'.

Explanation...

This infant presented with direct hyperbilirubinemia at four months of age. The common age of onset of direct jaundice is either early in the neonatal period as is seen in neonatal hepatitis— biliary atresia syndrome or often later in childhood. Though a choledochal cyst could be present at any age, the USG in this infant was normal. Thus, presentation at four months of age itself should have alerted us to the possibility of an uncommon etiology. Further, the development of the 'so called' acute liver cell failure did not follow the usual sequence of deepening jaundice, edema, ascites, and bleeding diathesis. When he recovered after supportive treatment, the jaundice had, in fact, deepened contrary to expectations. So, there were many unusual points that would have suggested a search for another diagnosis. This child on investigations turned out to be galactosemia.

Experience gained...

> An unusual age of presentation of direct hyperbilirubinemia and unanticipated progress of the disease should alert the physician about a probable metabolic disorder. Many such diseases will evolve into a full blown classical clinical picture only over time, and till then, it is a high index of suspicion based on atypical features of onset, duration and progress of the disease that should make one search for an alternative diagnosis. This is particularly true, if the provisional diagnosis has been made on flimsy grounds.

CASE 71

■ Phenylketonuria

Events...

A 5-month-old infant presented with fever for a day followed by convulsions and coma. He was exclusively breastfed and had no major illness till the onset of the present complaints. He was diagnosed as viral encephalitis and treated accordingly. He recovered after two days. Investigations could not prove the diagnosis. Meanwhile, there was a history of first-degree consanguinity and the infant was noticed to be of a fair complexion (when both parents were not). Add to this, the diagnosis of viral encephalitis was uncertain. So it was decided to investigate this infant for probable phenylketonuria and this diagnosis was proved.

Experience gained...

> Many metabolic disorders may offer subtle clues as happened in this child. The provisional diagnosis of viral encephalitis was never a satisfactory one and the pediatrician correctly looked for signs that would have been easily overlooked. History of consanguinity led to a strong suspicion. Such a history would not come forth unless asked for, and one may not ask for it unless one suspects a genetically transmitted disorder.

Management Dilemmas in Office Practice | 153

CASE 72

■ Mitochondrial Encephalopathy with Lactic Acidosis

Events...

A 1-year-old child presented with a history of fever for two days followed by generalized convulsions. There was no past history of a similar illness or any major disease in the past. Physical examination revealed left upper motor neuron hemiparesis without any other neurological abnormalities. In particular he had no meningeal signs, change in sensorium or signs of raised intracranial tension. Other systems were normal. On investigation, the Mantoux test was 8 mm positive, chest X-ray was normal and so also the CSF. CT scan showed no evidence of basal meningitis or hydrocephalus. Since this patient had presented as an acute infantile hemiplegia, and since one of its common causes was tuberculosis, this diagnosis was entertained. Since the CSF is occasionally known to be normal in very early cases of TB meningitis (this child had indeed presented quite early), he was diagnosed as a case of TBM, with the intention of repeating the CSF after a few days to confirm the diagnosis. He was treated accordingly, and he quickly recovered within a few days. In view of the speedy recovery, the CSF was not repeated, and he was sent home on anti-TB treatment. He completed therapy as planned and remained very well without any sequelae. A few months later, he had a similar episode again and was reinvestigated. Considering that relapse of TBM is quite unusual, he was investigated in detail and found to have metabolic acidosis. This was confirmed to be mitochondrial encephalopathy with lactic acidosis (MELA).

Experience gained...

> The diagnosis of TBM was on uncertain grounds with most of the typical features missing. While not all features are evident in every case, absence of most of the features should have warned against the diagnosis. Relapse of TBM being rare, and that too after compliant treatment, gave the clue to an alternate diagnosis.

CASE 73

Metabolic Disorder with Cardiomyopathy

Events...

A 3-month-old infant presented with cardiac failure that was ascribed to viral myocarditis for want of any better diagnosis. He was treated with anti-failure line of treatment but there was no improvement. In fact, over the next few weeks he started deteriorating and eventually died of refractory cardiac failure. There was no satisfactory explanation to these events. Two years later, parents brought their two months old second child with similar complaints and they reminded us of the previous sibling's death due to a similar illness. It was at this time that a history of first-degree consanguinity was elicited. This gave the clue to a probable metabolic disorder like a fatty chain abnormality. He was put on carnitine and relevant investigations were sent, but the exact diagnosis could not be proved. This infant also died after a few weeks.

Experience gained...

> It was the death of the previous sibling that gave a clue to a probable metabolic disorder in this infant. Not all metabolic disorders can be proved, either due to unavailability of laboratory tests or due to limitations of science itself. There are more than 300 metabolic diseases known to science and the list is ever increasing. Even then, every attempt must be made to come to a diagnosis in the hope of helping every child, and also for genetic counseling.

CASE 74

■ Ataxia Presenting as Metabolic Disorder

Events…

A 4-year-old child presented with fever followed by an acute onset of ataxia. He was diagnosed to have post-infectious cerebellitis, which recovered naturally without any intervention. The diagnosis was totally clinical and was never confirmed as the child made a quick recovery. He came back again after a few months with ataxia, but this time he worsened with neuroregression. At that time, it was realized that this was a metabolic disorder.

Experience gained…

> The first episode of unexplained ataxia should alert one to the possibility of an evolving disease that may not be obvious to begin with. However, the parents could at least be sounded on the need for further evaluation.

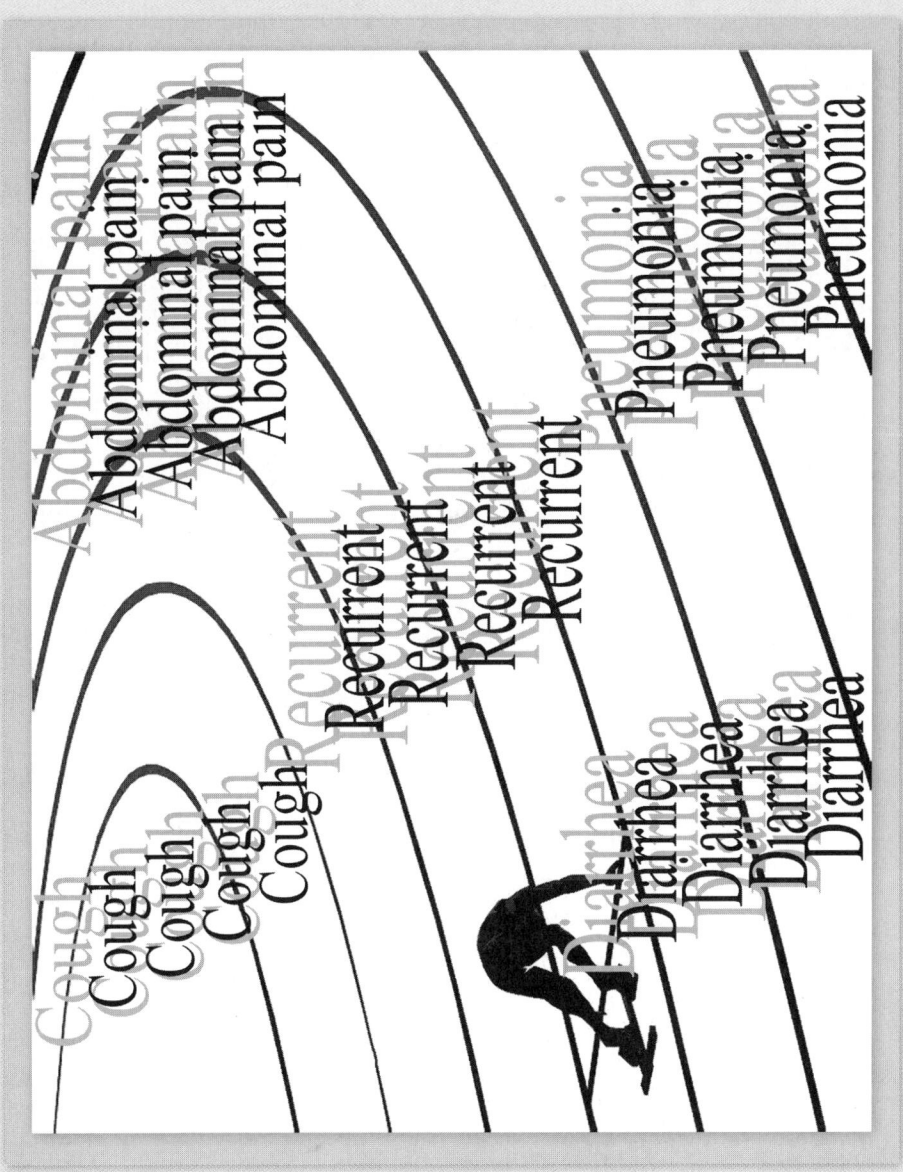

SECTION 3

Recurrent Problems

■ Introduction

Recurrent symptoms are common in clinical practice. The first step is to differentiate between persistent and recurrent symptoms. There may be an apparent overlap as presented by the patient, but a detailed history can easily separate the two. After all, a persistent cough (as in whooping cough) also has small cough-free intervals but not long enough to call it a recurrent symptom while cough in asthma is typically recurrent and episodic. A symptom is described as episodic if it occurs at the same time in the same way while a recurrent symptom may occur at any varying time.

Another important concept is to differentiate whether the recurrent symptoms represent a persistent disease or they are actually due to recurrent disease. For example, tuberculosis presents as fever and/or cough off and on but the disease is "on" all the time. A specific question "is the patient completely well or not in between recurrent symptoms?" would easily differentiate between the two. A patient with recurrent fever/cough in tuberculosis is unwell in between episodes of symptoms while in a recurrent viral infection, the patient is normal in between two episodes. Further, there is often a long interval (weeks) between recurrent symptoms in recurrent viral infection while there is a small interval (days) between recurrent symptoms in a persistent disease.

This section illustrates the analysis of actual cases that we encountered.

An Approach to Recurrent/Persistent Pneumonia

Both these terms—"recurrent/persistent" and "pneumonia"—must be clearly defined before we understand the approach to such a problem. In other words, the evaluation of recurrent/persistent pneumonia entails a definite diagnosis of pneumonia in the first instance. Subsequently, one needs to be sure whether it is recurrent or persistent. However, there may be limitations to the clinical and radiological diagnosis of pneumonia which need to be appreciated. Similarly, it may not be easy to differentiate between 'recurrent' and 'persistent', at least on clinical grounds.

Clinical Diagnosis of Pneumonia—Limitations

Pneumonia is a pathological term. On physical examination of the chest, its clinical signs could be an impaired note on percussion, diminished breath sounds, bronchial breathing and crepitations—distributed over a *localized* area. However, other pathologies, such as atelectasis, cavity or pleural effusion may mimic pneumonia by giving rise to similar findings. Atelectasis with a patent bronchus would present with bronchial breathing, and accumulated secretions may lead to crepitations. A cavity may present exactly like pneumonia, the only difference being high pitched bronchial breath sounds in pneumonia versus low-pitched bronchial breath sounds in a cavity. Of course, it is difficult for most clinicians to differentiate between high- and low-pitched sounds. Further, such subtle differences depend upon many variables, and hence, are not reliable. A pleural effusion may also simulate pneumonia. In a large pleural effusion, if the underlying lung has collapsed but the bronchus is patent, it could result in bronchial breath sounds, since fluid is a good conductor of sound. Though there would be no foreign sounds in a pleural effusion, occasionally, a pleural rub may mimic other foreign sounds.

Finally, even a 'genuine' pneumonia may not present with all its typical physical signs, because these depend upon the stage of development of the pneumonia, the extent of involvement and the patency of the bronchus leading to the involved area of the lung. Therefore, at times, pneumonia may present with localized crepitations only, and may be mistaken for other pathological lesions. When accompanied with a collapse, pneumonia may present with diminished breath sounds without bronchial breath sounds, as is seen in cases of tuberculous pneumonia.

Radiological Diagnosis of Pneumonia—Limitations

The classic radiological sign of pneumonia is a dense opacity with an air bronchogram, though absence of an air bronchogram may not rule out pneumonia. At times, the air bronchogram may not be visualized, either due to technical issues like exposure or due to coexisting pathology. However, often, a mere infiltration or haziness may be reported as pneumonia, though it may or may not be truly so. In a child with asthma, atelectatic segments may be mistaken for pneumonia.

On the other hand, densely opaque radiological shadows may actually represent other pathologies such as a congenital malformation, and even extraparenchymal mediastinal lesions such as duplication of esophagus or encysted pleural effusion. While interpreting an opacity/haziness on the chest X-ray, it is important to localize the lesion anatomically.

In pneumonia, the opacity is restricted to a lobar or segmental pattern. Such a demarcation is facilitated by a lateral film.

In other words, each time the radiologist reports a pneumonia, it may or may not be so. The term 'pneumonitis' is a loose term and conveys nothing in particular.

Differentiation between Recurrent/Persistent—Not Easy

Clinically, the terms 'recurrent' and 'persistent' are not easy to differentiate. Ideally, there has to be a clear period of normalcy between two episodes, to call it a recurrent problem. However, a persistent problem may not have persistent symptoms and hence, may be erroneously considered to be a recurrent problem. For example, tuberculosis presents as fever 'off and on'—the disease is persistent, though the symptoms seem to suggest recurrent illnesses. On the other hand, if radiological clearance is not documented after apparent clinical recovery, it may be construed to be a recurrent problem when it surfaces again, though actually, it has been persistent all along. Thus, though one needs to clearly differentiate between these two situations that may look similar, it may not always be possible. In such an event, one should consider both the probabilities during the course of evaluation. However, pneumonia recurring in the same anatomical area demands a search for a local abnormality, irrespective of whether it is construed as recurrent or persistent pneumonia.

Correctly Diagnosed Pneumonia—Issues regarding Etiology and Progress

Though pneumonia may be correctly diagnosed, its etiology may not necessarily be an infection. Noninfective causes of pneumoma include collagen vascular diseases (e.g., Wagener's granulomatosis), lipoid pneumonia, kerosene aspiration, etc. Even when it is an infection, it may be bacterial, viral, fungal or parasitic. If bacterial, apart from the usual gram +ve and gram -ve organisms that typically cause community acquired pneumonia, one need to consider tuberculosis and atypical intracellular pathogens (*Mycoplasma, Chlamydia*). The etiology of pneumonia is almost always guessed clinically, based on epidemiology, onset/duration/progress, accompanying symptoms and physical signs, and is supported by relevant laboratory tests.

Once an infective pneumonia is diagnosed, it is important to select the correct antibiotic and cover the most probable organism based on epidemiological grounds. If the infective organism is resistant to a chosen antibiotic, there may not be any change in the patient's condition. But if the organism is partially resistant to a chosen antibiotic, then it may result in a partial or temporary improvement, only to relapse again within a short time. Such a relapse may be wrongly considered to be a recurrent pneumonia.

At times, a child with tuberculosis is wrongly being treated with antibiotics and a transient remission in fever is interpreted as a response. The failure of the radiological lesion to improve simultaneously is attributed to the fact that radiological clearance takes a long time, and is therefore, not considered to be inconsistent with a 'cure'. Such a patient is bound to have a recurrence of fever, at which time he may be erroneously considered to be a case of persistent pneumonia. On the other hand, a radiological lesion, especially in the upper zone in an infant, may persist for 1-2 months with the patient having clinically recovered within a short time. This is a situation where there is a clinical cure but radiological persistence. Obviously, in this case, it is not persistent pneumonia and continuation of therapy is not required.

The most common cause of what seems to be a persistent pneumonia in spite of compliant correct antibiotic therapy is the development of a complication, such as empyema. In fact, it must be a rule that if a patient suffering from pneumonia shows no improvement in fever within 3-4 days of antibiotic therapy, it is mandatory to search for a collection of fluid in the pleural cavity through imaging techniques. In fact, as infants suffering from acute bacterial pneumonia are at risk of developing empyema early in the course of disease, it is ideal to rule out such a complication even at the initiation of treatment. Depending upon the nature, the degree, and the timing of accumulation of fluid, one may have to resort to different modalities of drainage. However, there is no need to change the antibiotic, because this does not represent drug resistance. In such a patient, as soon as the fluid is drained, the fever abates. This should not be considered as persistent pneumonia. Other complications include a lung abscess that usually settles with a longer duration of therapy.

Significance of 'True' Recurrence

Recurrence of pneumonia may either be at the same site or at a different site. This would make a difference when it comes to evaluation. In case of a recurrent pneumonia at the **same site**, one need to evaluate for a local structural defect, while if the pneumonia recurs at **different sites**, one may have to look at generalized disorders. Further, if recurrent pneumonia is an **isolated** manifestation without an involvement of any other systems, then it is quite likely to be a local functional abnormality as is seen in ciliary dyskinesia, IgA deficiency or cystic fibrosis in infancy. On the other hand, if recurrent pneumonia is **associated with widespread infections** in other parts of the body, it is likely to be a generalized immunodeficiency, such as HIV or congenital immune deficiency syndrome.

Although such problems are rare in routine office practice, functional (ciliary dyskinesia or cystic fibrosis) or immunological defects (IgA deficiency or HIV) may result in persistent or recurrent pneumonia. Therefore, in selected situations, they need to be considered. A child with ciliary dyskinesia presents with sinusitis and bronchitis and may be easy to diagnose in the presence of dextrocardia (Kartagener's syndrome). Cystic fibrosis presents in infancy with failure to thrive, pneumonia and respiratory failure. Subsequently, intestinal malabsorption is the hallmark of its clinical profile. IgA deficiency is often picked up when a child with recurrent respiratory infections in early childhood develops ataxia-telangiectasia after a few years. Till then, it is usually difficult to diagnose IgA deficiency unless it is clinically suspected and then confirmed by laboratory tests. HIV related pneumonia may be caused by stubborn bacterial infections, fungi, or *Pneumocystis carinii*, besides tuberculosis. Most of these infections are difficult to control due to a state of immune suppression (and not as a result of drug resistance, as is often misbelieved). These 'uncontrolled' infections may present as persistent pneumonias.

Drug Resistance

Finally, some pneumonias may be *truly drug resistant*, though this is rare in routine office practice. Often, drug sensitive pneumonias are wrongly labeled drug resistant for various reasons. A wrongly chosen antibiotic is the common scenario where pneumonia is labeled as drug resistant. Atypical bacterial pneumonia (often referred to as afebrile pneumonia) is caused by intracellular organisms such as *Mycoplasma* or *Chlamydia* and these organisms are susceptible to macrolides or quinolones. It is difficult to diagnose these infections on clinical grounds alone, though there may be subtle clues. Pneumonia caused by such organisms involves both the airway and lung parenchyma. As a result, these patients present with severe cough, which is not a predominant symptom in pneumonias caused by the usual community acquired bacteria. Such atypical pneumonias may not respond to commonly used synthetic penicillins or cephalosporins and masquerade as drug resistant pneumonias. At times, the organisms may be drug sensitive but there may not be a clinical response. This may be due to an incorrect dose or route of administration; one may get the desired response simply by increasing the dose of the antibiotic or administering the antibiotic parenterally.

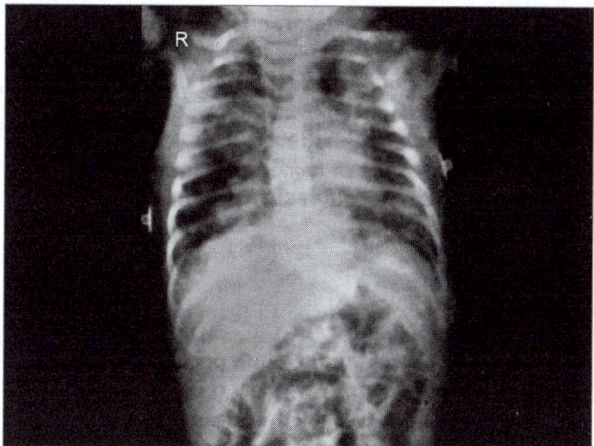

Lipoid (oil) pneumonia.

Lastly, one must attempt to correlate the clinical profile with radiology and other laboratory tests. Most of the problems are created when the clinician depends heavily on investigatory modalities and ignores the clinical profile. The following section depicts case scenarios that illustrate the various issues discussed above.

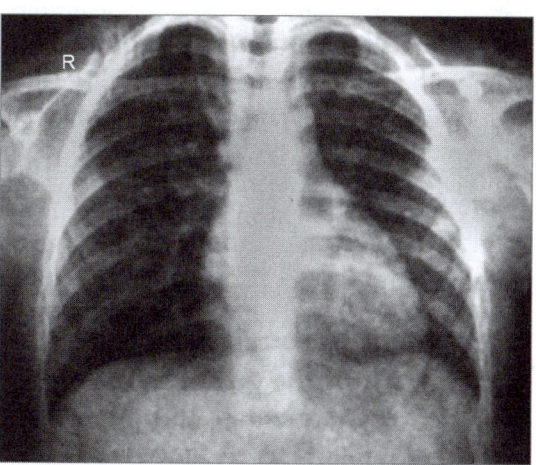

Recovery from lipoid pneumonia.

CASE 75

Clinical Recovery, Radiological Persistence

Events...

A 2-year-old child presented to a pediatrician with fever and cough for last two days. Physical examination did not reveal any positive findings, so he was treated symptomatically. Since he did not improve over next 3 days, he was investigated. The CBC was normal, and the chest X-ray showed a patch of dense haziness in the right paracardiac region. Considering it to be acute bacterial pneumonia, he was treated with an antibiotic. He became asymptomatic within a day and the antibiotic was continued for a week. A repeat chest X-ray done thereafter did not show any improvement in the radiological lesion. Hence, the antibiotic was changed, but it again failed to clear the radiological lesion. This time, it was decided that since radiological clearance is known to take a few weeks even after complete clinical resolution, the chest X-ray would be repeated only after a month. However, at the end of another month, the shadow still persisted.

Explanation...

It is always necessary to correlate the clinical and radiological findings in any given case. Generally, pneumonia is localized to the lobe and hence classically, the clinical findings are restricted to a 'lobar' pattern, as depicted by the surface anatomy of the lobes of the lungs. They may vary according to the size and stage of the pneumonia, such that there may not always be an impaired note or bronchial breathing; sometimes, there may be only crepitations. All the same, these findings are always distributed in a 'lobar' pattern. It is incorrect to interpret radiological shadows without a clinical correlation. Since, this child did not demonstrate any physical findings to suggest pneumonia, it could have meant that the radiological shadow was unrelated to the clinical symptoms.

Even if the diagnosis of pneumonia were to be justified on the basis of the chest X-ray alone, this child could not have got better within a day of starting the antibiotic if it was bacterial pneumonia. At the most, it could have been a spontaneous recovery of viral pneumonia. However, such a localized viral pneumonia is rare, they are usually interstitial. Therefore, it is quite likely that this was not a pneumonia at all. Further, in this child, the antibiotic was changed at a point when the child had already 'responded' in terms of fever, because the radiological lesion had not cleared. This was unjustified, because the original antibiotic had already 'worked' and secondly, repeating the chest X-ray within a short time was not warranted, since radiological clearance may take longer. In fact, in this child the chest' X-ray did not clear even at the end of a month.

Therefore, in other words, at the end of a month, there is a persistent radiological shadow, though clinically, the child had completely recovered long back. This, therefore, may not be pneumonia at all. This persistent shadow may represent either a congenital malformation of the lung or it may be an extraparenchymal lesion arising from any other mediastinal structure. In such a case, a lateral chest X-ray would correctly delineate the anatomy. In case there is still some doubt, one could resort to a CT scan of the chest.

This child was suspected to have an extraparenchymal shadow, which was confirmed to be a **duplication of the esophagus**. Thus, this was not pneumonia at all, though it was wrongly considered to be persistent pneumonia.

Experience gained...

> This case drives home to the point that often, a radiological impression tends to override the clinical setting; one must remain cautious to prevent such a mishap.
>
> It also illustrates the point that a preexisting silent condition can come to light accidentally, because of a X-ray that is done for some other reason.

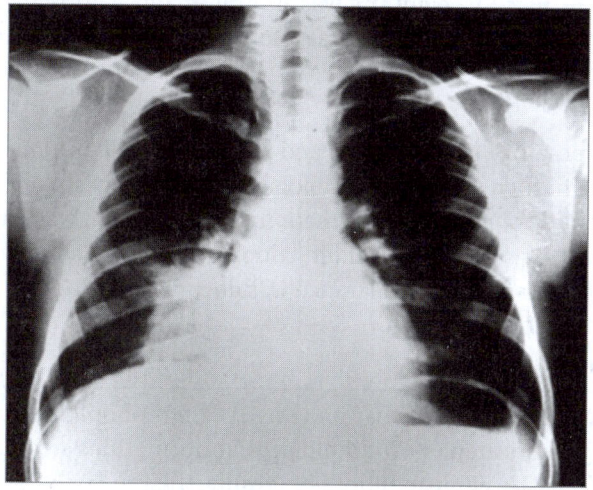

Lower lobe pneumonia.

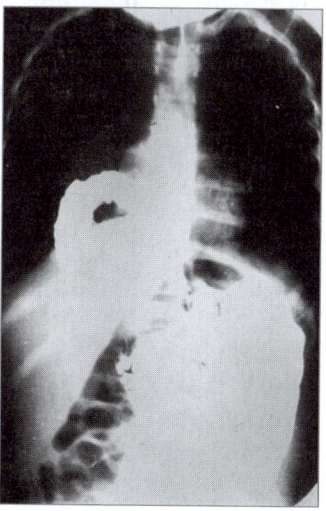

Barium study to demonstrate duplication of esophagus.

CASE 76

Clinical Recovery, Radiological Persistence

Events...

A 6-month-old infant presented with fever and cough for the last 4 days. He had signs of pneumonia in the right upper zone. He also had neutrophilic leukocytosis and the chest X-ray confirmed the diagnosis with the apical segment of the right upper lobe being involved. He was treated with IV amoxicillin with clavulanic acid and recovered clinically within the next few days. A repeat chest X-ray after a month showed a persistence of the apical shadow, though the infant had gained weight and was asymptomatic. A CT scan of the chest confirmed that there was no other abnormality. He was referred for persistent pneumonia.

Explanation...

As this infant had remained symptom free and had grown well, obviously his pneumonia had been well treated. If in such a case, the radiological shadow persists, one needs to confirm that it does not represent a congenital malformation. In this child, it was confirmed by a CT scan of the chest. He was advised no active intervention and was asked to follow-up after another 4 weeks, at which time radiological clearance was documented.

Experience gained...

> This case emphasizes the point that imaging findings should not override the clinical condition, though persistence of radiological abnormalities need an explanation and should subsequently be confirmed to have resolved completely. It is worth noting that apical segment pneumonia in an infant may often take several weeks to clear radiologically though the infant remains otherwise well. It does not call for any specific action and the shadow does disappear over time.

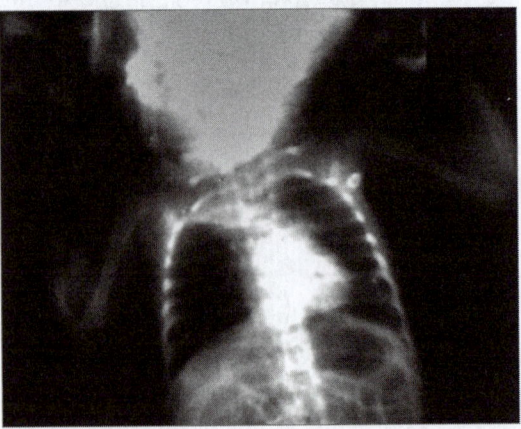

Persistent upper lobe lesion.

CASE 77

■ Clinical Recovery, Radiological Persistence

Events...

A 5-year-old child presented with high fever and cough for last 10 days. She was initially treated with oral Cephalexin by the family physician for 4 days, but as the fever did not subside, she was referred to a pediatrician. A CBC and chest X-ray was asked for and the results were as follows:

| Hb 9.5 g% | WBC 18,000/mm^3 | P 78 L 21 M 1 E 0 | Platelets adequate |

Chest X-ray showed haziness in right lower zone.

She was diagnosed as pneumonia and was prescribed IV Cefotaxime and Amikacin.

Fever responded after 4 days, after which IV therapy was continued for a total of 10 days. Chest X-ray was repeated on completion of antibiotic therapy for 10 days, which showed a persistence of the radiological lesion as it is, though the child was afebrile, had regained her appetite and well-being and had also gained weight. She was totally asymptomatic. Anticipating that the radiological shadow may take more time to resolve, the pediatrician advised them to wait and watch, without any drug. The chest X-ray was repeated 15 days later, only to find that the radiological lesion still persisted. At this juncture, the pediatrician ordered a Mantoux test and CBC. The Mantoux test was reported 10-mm positive and CBC was normal. Hence, in view of a persistent radiological lesion for a month in spite of antibiotic therapy and a positive Mantoux test, the diagnosis of pulmonary TB was made. The parents did not accept the diagnosis and requested for another opinion.

At the referral center, the child was confirmed to be totally asymptomatic. Physical examination revealed a comfortable child with an impaired note on the right side of the chest anteriorly, in the lower half. There was no other abnormality.

Explanation...

This child suffered from acute bacterial pneumonia and responded well to the IV antibiotics used. Though it is known that radiological lesions may persist for a few weeks in spite of a good clinical response, it should have at least started clearing, after a few weeks. Since this did not happen, the pediatrician started looking for another etiology of pneumonia. He suspected a tuberculous pneumonia because such children are known to give an erroneous impression of having clinically recovered in terms of fever, though their radiological lesion persists. Their clinical recovery is transient, and symptoms recur shortly. However, tuberculous pneumonias are usually subacute in their presentation. Further, though the child may be transiently afebrile as mentioned above, she will not be absolutely alright in all respects. On the other hand, this girl developed acute pneumonia and when she recovered, she was absolutely asymptomatic eating well, playful, active. Therefore, it is unlikely to be tuberculous pneumonia.

Since there is no doubt about this being an acute bacterial pneumonia to begin with, we need to consider reasons for a persistent radiological lesion in acute bacterial pneumonia in spite of good clinical recovery. If the reason for this persistence would have been a complication like a lung abscess or empyema, the child would have been quite symptomatic with spiking fever. Thus, it is likely to be a noninfective lesion.

There is no possibility of an uncomplicated pneumonia leaving behind sequelae that may give rise to a persistent radiological lesion without symptoms. Thus, it may be a lesion that already existed before the development of pneumonia. In fact, the presence of such a lesion may have led to a secondary infection leading to pneumonia. Though the pneumonia was successfully treated, the preexisting lesion may have remained as before. Since, this child has never had an X-ray chest taken in the past, such a lesion could have existed silently. So it is likely to be a congenital malformation. Retained foreign body can also lead to secondary infection and the development of pneumonia; after successful treatment of infection, the foreign body may persist with a segmental collapse. Such a child is likely to suffer from persistent cough even though the fever would have responded to antibiotics. Since this girl was not coughing, such a possibility is unlikely.

CT scan confirmed the diagnosis of **cystic adenomatoid malformation.**

Experience gained…

The differential diagnosis of a persistent radiological abnormality after an apparently reasonable clinical recovery from pneumonia includes a tuberculous pneumonia besides preexisting congenital abnormalities. A detailed history about the general well-being of the child in terms of appetite, activity and playfulness is vital in distinguishing a genuine clinical recovery from a transient spurious one, especially when there is no fever to go by.

CASE 78

■ Clinical and Radiological Persistence

Events...

An 8-year-old child presented with fever off and on for last one month. He complained of a pain on the right side of the chest for the first few days, but thereafter, the pain disappeared. The family doctor ordered an X-ray which suggested pneumonia, so he was treated with antibiotics. However, there was no response in the fever; meanwhile, he had lost 3 kilograms over this month. At this point, he was referred for further management. A physical examination revealed an impaired note on the right side of the chest anterolaterally. His breath sounds were normal, and there were no foreign sounds. A CBC was ordered and the chest X-ray was repeated. His counts were normal, but the X-ray showed a dense shadow on the right side of the chest laterally. In view of persistent clinical symptoms and a possibility of persistent pneumonia, the antibiotics were changed. However, since there was no response even after a week, at this juncture, he was referred to a tertiary care center for further management as a case of persistent pneumonia.

Explanation...

Analyzing the history, this child had developed chest pain on the right side of the chest. This suggests pleural involvement; coupled with fever for a month it denotes a pleuro-pneumonia. Since it did not respond to antibiotics, it may be either a subacute, not bacterial infection or a noninfective pneumonia. An impaired note on percussion without any other physical signs, favors a pleural pathology. Since the pain subsided in a few days though the child continued to be unwell, it meant that the two layers of the pleura had been separated by fluid. However, this did not result in breathlessness; therefore, the pleural effusion must have been small in quantity. Since the child did not deteriorate, it was unlikely to be a collection of pus. In other words, this was neither an empyema, nor a classical allergic tuberculous pleural effusion (which generally presents acutely as a large effusion).

A dense shadow on an X-ray, which does not correlate with a lobar pattern, may be a pleural or a mediastinal shadow. Since this particular shadow was towards the periphery of the lung field, it was likely to be a pleural shadow. Since there was no obliteration of the costophrenic angle, it was unlikely to be an effusion; it almost suggested a space occupying lesion.

Whenever there is a disparity between clinical findings and radiological signs, an attempt must be made to localize the lesion by a lateral chest X-ray. Occasionally, if the lateral chest X-ray fails to delineate the anatomy correctly, one may need a CT scan. Thus, anatomical localization is the first step in any such case, and only then one proceed with the pathological and etiological diagnosis.

The CT scan of the chest showed a localized pleural collection of fluid that suggested an infective pleural pathology, with an attempt at healing. In view of this, a tuberculin test was done which was strongly positive. A pleural tap revealed an inflammatory exudate which suggested a diagnosis of a **localized tuberculous pleural effusion**.

Experience gained…

In this child a localized pleural effusion mimicked pneumonia on cursory evaluation, though the clinical and radiological findings were quite inconsistent with a diagnosis of pneumonia. It emphasizes the need for a good correlation between clinical and radiological abnormalities. Not all shadows seen on a chest X-ray represent pneumonia, since there are many other structures, whose shadows can overlap those of the lungs. The clinician must learn to read X-rays carefully to ascertain the correct anatomy of the disease, embarking on probable etiology.

CASE 79

Clinical Persistence, Radiological Recovery

Events...

An 8-year-old child presented with an acute onset of high fever and mild cough for the last four days. Clinically, there were localizing signs related to the right middle lobe, suggestive of pneumonia. A CBC showed marked neutrophilic leukocytosis and the chest X-ray revealed a middle lobe pneumonia on the right side. Considering it to be acute bacterial pneumonia, he was put on IV antibiotics. Even after 4 days of compliant antibiotic therapy, there was no clinical improvement. Therefore, the counts and a chest X-ray were repeated, to rule out complications like an empyema. While there was a further increase in the neutrophilic leukocytosis, the chest X-ray revealed that the right-sided pneumonia had cleared, but a left-sided pneumonia had now developed. Considering it to be a drug resistant pneumonia, the antibiotics were changed, but to no avail. At the end of two weeks, after two sets of IV antibiotics had failed to demonstrate any clinical improvement, and the left-sided pneumonia had also persisted, he was referred for further management.

Explanation...

It is interesting to note that the diagnosis of acute bacterial pneumonia was made on firm grounds and the treatment started accordingly, but further progress was unusual. The radiological clearance of the right-sided pneumonia, even when the clinical symptoms persisted, was quite unanticipated. Such a clinical persistence with radiological clearance is against the diagnosis of acute bacterial pneumonia. Meanwhile, the appearance of another pneumonia on the left side seemed to suggest a 'recurrent' pneumonia; however, what it actually represented was not an infective pathology, but an acute inflammatory disease of allergic origin. Increasing neutrophilic leukocytosis is a feature of any severe inflammation, though it is commonly seen in acute bacterial infections. Thus, this was not bacterial pneumonia at all, and that is why there was no response to antibiotics. Further laboratory tests confirmed the diagnosis of **Wegener granulomatosis**.

This could be erroneously considered to be a recurrent pneumonia since he presented with a right-sided pneumonia first and later developed a left-sided pneumonia. However, this was not a recurrent illness but the same continued disease with changing manifestations. Such changing lesions in the lungs may also represent an inhaled foreign body that is moving from one area to another after a bout of cough. However, in such a child, cough is the predominant symptom and not high persistent fever. Other changing lesions are those that are allergic in nature as seen in this child.

Experience gained...

In this child, the diagnosis of acute bacterial pneumonia was justified on the basis of its presentation at the onset. However, its progression spelt a clear warning that the disease was anything but pneumonia. This case illustrates the importance of following the progress of any disease; if it strays from its anticipated course, corrective action is called for. Therefore, it is ideal to chart the expected course of events right at the beginning of treatment and watch out for variations, if any, so that appropriate changes can be made at the earliest.

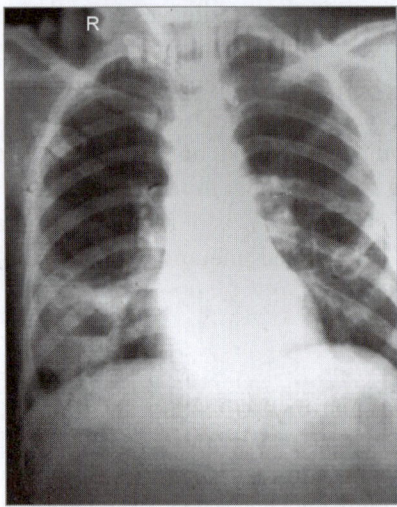

Right middle lobe pneumonia.

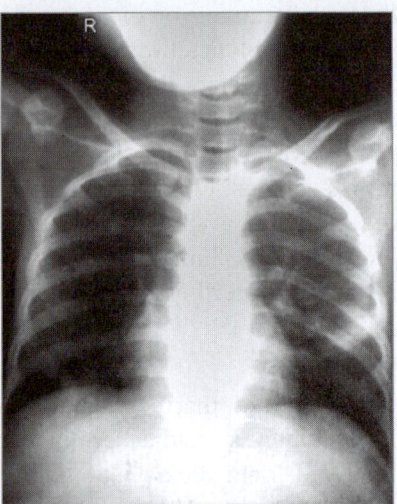

Right middle lobe pneumonia cleared—left lobe pneumonia appeared.

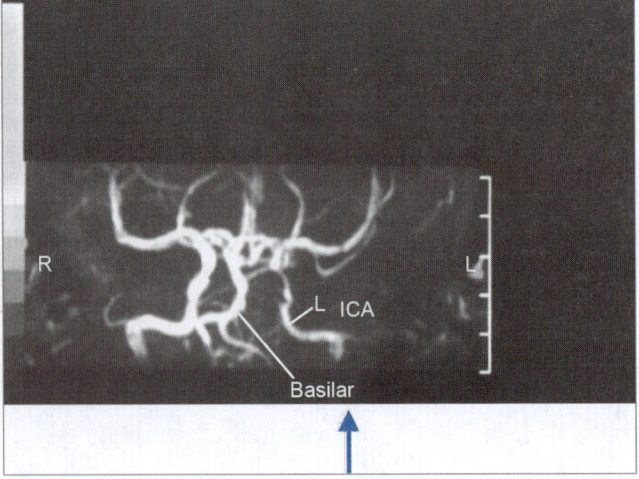

Evolving vascular lesion in the same patient.

Evolving vascular lesion in the same patient.

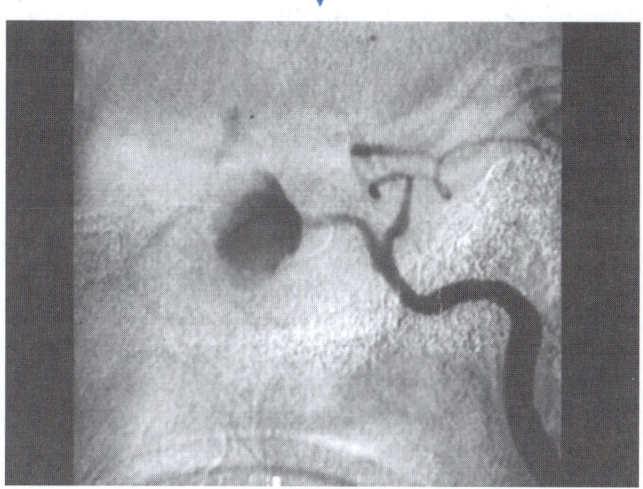

CASE 80

■ Recurrent Pneumonia at the Same Site

Events...

A 3-year-old child presented with high fever and mild cough for the last 6 days. Physical examination revealed signs suggestive of pneumonia in the right middle zone. It was confirmed to be an acute bacterial pneumonia, on the basis of neutrophilic leukocytosis and the chest X-ray showing localized haziness. A dense opacity with an air bronchogram, which is localized to a lobe, is the classical radiological sign of pneumonia. This is exactly what was seen in this child, though sometimes pneumonia can exist without a demonstrable air bronchogram. This child improved on antibiotic therapy as expected. At this point, the parents mentioned that this child had suffered from a similar pneumonia 6 months ago, which was also successfully treated. A review of the previous X-ray confirmed the pneumonia to have involved the same area, then. However, at that time, the X-ray was not repeated to confirm radiological clearance.

Explanation...

On both occasions, the diagnosis of pneumonia is not in doubt. Similarly, on both occasions, the child has been clinically cured. So this is not persistent clinical pneumonia. But it is not clear whether, after the first episode, the pneumonia had cleared radiologically or not. So it could either be a persistence of the radiological shadow in spite of clinical recovery, or it could be a 'true' (clinical and radiological) recurrence of pneumonia. In the former case, the inference would be that there is a persistent structural abnormality like a congenital malformation of the lung or a retained inhaled foreign body. A recurrent pneumonia at the same site is unusual without any underlying local abnormality. Therefore, even though radiological clearance was not documented in this child at the time of the previous pneumonia, he must have had a local abnormality that predisposed to the development of the present pneumonia.

Thus, once this episode of pneumonia recovers clinically, after 2–3 weeks, one must confirm the radiological status. It is expected that the radiological abnormality would persist in this child; in which case, a CT scan would confirm the type of abnormality. Sequestration of the lung can be confirmed by angiography.

Once the abnormality is detected, it may need appropriate surgical action.

This child was confirmed to have a **sequestration of the lung** that was responsible for the recurrent pneumonia.

Experience gained...

Recurrent pneumonia at the same site must be considered to result from a local defect. This case raises the question whether a repeat chest X-ray should be routinely asked for, in a case of pneumonia to demonstrate complete radiological resolution. It may be ideal, though it is not routinely required. If the site of infection is such that it is not accessible to organisms routinely, it is necessary to demonstrate normalcy at the end of treatment (e.g., meningitis, UTI). It may be of interest to note that diagnosis of pneumonia is possible at the level of primary health care purely on clinical grounds, without even the first chest X-ray, as is practiced in ARI control program.

Unlike above discussed cases of *mistaken diagnosis or presence of underlying defect leading to recurrent pneumonia,* the following case scenarios describe pneumonias of different etiology that are treated as acute bacterial infection with antibiotics and as treatment fails, are considered as persistent pneumonia.

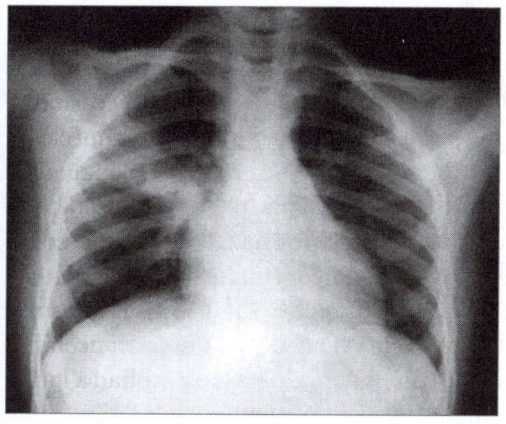

Recurrent pneumonia in right midzone.

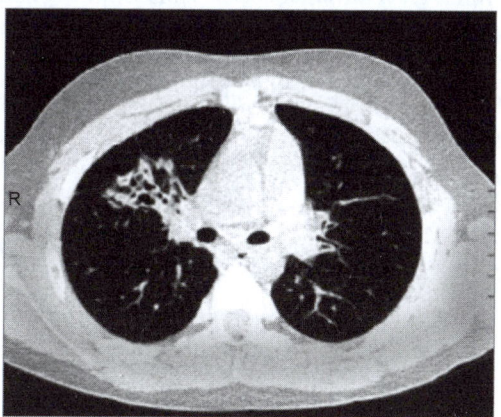

Sequestration.

CASE 81

■ Subacute Pneumonia

Events...

A 10-year-old child presented with fever and cough for 5 days. Though the physical examination was normal, she was treated with amoxicillin. Since there was no response after a few days, a CBC and a chest X-ray was ordered, which showed normal blood counts and a doubtful infiltration in the right upper zone. Considering a drug resistant bacterial infection, the antibiotic was changed to cefpodoxime. At the end of another week, the child continued to be symptomatic, though she had not deteriorated either and hence, the investigations were repeated. The chest X-ray now showed a well-established pneumonia in the right upper zone. As the lung lesion had worsened radiologically in spite of two sets of antibiotics, it was decided to attempt an etiological diagnosis of the pneumonia. So, a lung aspiration was tried, which grew *Staphylococcus epidermidis* sensitive to all antibiotics. However, considering that there could be a discrepancy between *in vitro* and *in vivo* sensitivity, the child was put on Vancomycin, but she did not improve even after another week. At this point, a CT scan of the chest was ordered, which showed a caseating pneumonia with lymph nodes, suggestive of **tuberculosis.**

Explanation...

This child had a subacute infection, with the pneumonia developing over a few weeks and she was never acutely ill. There was no neutrophilic leukocytosis. Moreover, there was no response to multiple antibiotics and even then, she was not deteriorating either. This should have given a clue to a probable different etiology other than acute bacterial infection. A bronchoalveolar lavage could have been an ideal investigatory modality in this case. The lung aspiration that was done in this child must have grown a contaminant from the skin, which compounded the wrong actions.

Experience gained...

> Proper analysis of the history (subacute onset, and slow progress over 2 weeks without clinical deterioration), along with a normal physical examination and blood counts, should have warned against an acute bacterial infection. Failure to respond to two sets of antibiotics demands a change of etiological diagnosis, especially in community acquired infections. In this child, a CT scan made it possible to define the probable etiology as tuberculosis, though BAL would be the best method of proving the etiology of tuberculosis.

CASE 82

■ Nonbacterial Etiology

Events...

A 5-year-old child presented with fever and cough persisting for a month in spite of being treated with multiple antibiotics. She was normal prior to this episode, and had grown well without any significant diseases in the past.

The present illness started insidiously as a fever and cough that got progressively worse over a month. She was diagnosed as pneumonia based on radiological findings. A CBC done on four different occasions showed a mild neutrophilic leukocytosis, while repeat chest X-rays showed progressively worsening lesions bilaterally. In spite of two sets of antibiotics and even anti-TB therapy for the last 2 weeks, she did not show any improvement. Gradually, she started getting hypoxic and was then referred for further management.

Explanation...

This has been a progressive bilateral pneumonia without any local complications, and yet, there has been a therapeutic failure with antibiotics and the child has gradually developed respiratory failure. While the diagnosis of an acute bacterial pneumonia could have been acceptable to begin with, the subsequent course of events should make one suspect a different etiology other than an acute bacterial infection. The usual tendency is to try different antibiotics instead of investigating properly, which often delays the correct diagnosis. In fact, such a delay could have endangered this child's life. Acute bacterial pneumonia is always a localized lesion and hence, bilateral lung involvement demands a search for another etiology, such as viral, fungal, or tuberculous and at times, even parasitic. A bacterial bronchopneumonia is a misnomer and such a term is obsolete.

This child was subjected to a bronchoalveolar lavage that grew *Candida albicans*. With the diagnosis of **fungal pneumonia**, it was imperative to search for an underlying immunodeficiency, since fungal infections are not common in immunocompetent hosts, except in newborns who have been treated in the NICU for various reasons. All immune functions were normal in this child. So, it was presumed that multiple antibiotics could have led to a superimposed fungal infection; even if this was true, the primary diagnosis remained elusive. At this point, it is worth noting that a possible mechanism of introduction of a fungal infection is through the use of nebulizers.

Experience gained...

In case of a suspected infection, the need for an etiological diagnosis is rarely emphasized. It is not even attempted; the excuse given most often is that it calls for invasive procedures and that the bacteriological services available are unreliable. However, an etiological diagnosis must be attempted, at least when the primary treatment fails. It is our experience that, if two antibiotics fail, one must look for an alternate diagnosis as a further trial with newer antibiotics is unlikely to succeed.

Other etiologies met with in cases of pneumonia include cytomegalovirus, toxoplasma, rarely *hanta* virus and *Pneumocystis carinii* (typically in immunocompromised patients). These conditions can be conclusively diagnosed only, if an attempt is made to go for an etiological diagnosis with bronchoalveolar lavage.

A common cause of persistent pneumonia is the development of complications that is not controlled by antibiotic therapy. The following cases illustrate such examples.

CASE 83

■ Complication

Events...

A 2-year-old child presented with high fever and a mild cough for 3 days and was correctly diagnosed to have acute bacterial pneumonia of the right lower lobe. He was treated with IV antibiotics and was expected to improve over the next few days. However, the fever continued and so also his toxicity. Blood counts and the chest X-ray were repeated and they showed a persistence of neutrophilic leukocytosis and the same radiological picture, i.e., a large opacity in the right lower zone. This prompted a change of antibiotics and when that did not work, the child was referred for further management.

Explanation...

It is important to realize that though drug resistance is increasing in the community, it should not be the first consideration in a community acquired infection. A search for other common causes of therapeutic failure is mandatory. Common complications of acute bacterial pneumonia that may be construed wrongly as antibiotic failure include empyema, lung abscess, respiratory failure, and sepsis. Hence, one must exclude such complications before assuming drug resistance (which may actually be hypothetical), and embarking on a trial with second line antibiotics.

This child had developed an *empyema*. It was a fair amount of collection of pus that was overlooked on the repeat chest X-ray. In the AP view, if the pneumonia involves the right lower lobe, it may not be easy to suspect an additional pleural collection. It can only be picked up, if one suspects and especially looks for such a complication, by ordering a decubitus film or sonography. In fact, it should be routine in every case of pneumonia to search for an empyema, if the child does not show initial signs of an improvement within 3-4 days (such as a reduction in the respiratory rate, fever, and toxicity). Empyema is a common accompaniment of acute bacterial pneumonia in infants and young children even when the patient first presents, and therefore, it may be ideal to look for it right at the onset of treatment of pneumonia. If an empyema is diagnosed at an early stage, major surgical intervention may be prevented.

Experience gained...

> If an acute bacterial pneumonia fails to respond to treatment as expected, within 3-4 days, one should search for common complications like an empyema before considering other issues, such as drug resistance. In infants and young children, such complications could exist right at the time of initial presentation and should be looked for. Delay in diagnosing such complications may endanger life or lead to significant morbidity.

CASE 84

■ Complication

Events...

A 4-year-old child presented with high fever and mild cough for the last 8 days. He was correctly diagnosed to have acute bacterial pneumonia, on the basis of neutrophilic leukocytosis and the chest X-ray showing haziness in the right middle zone with an air bronchogram. He was put on IV amoxicillin with clavulanic acid. After 5 days of treatment, since he was not better, the chest X-ray was repeated, and it showed a persistence of the pneumonia, though the CP angle was clear (i.e., there was no empyema). Considering drug resistance, he was treated with IV ceftriaxone. As there was still no response after another 4 days, he was referred for further management.

Explanation...

When routine antibiotics fail in a community acquired pneumonia, it is mandatory to search for complications or consider a change of diagnosis. In this case, an empyema had been ruled out. Infections caused by organisms other than bacteria would have presented with a different clinical profile and progress. Noninfective conditions, such as pulmonary manifestations of systemic vasculitis may be a possibility, and therefore, it may be justified to investigate for the same. However, such conditions are rare and may not be a priority before ruling out other commoner possibilities.

The first step in such a child is to use different imaging modalities to define the anatomy of the lesion, before proceeding to other tests. If the lesion is well-localized, a lateral film is a useful modality. A lateral film is easily available everywhere, at all times, and can be read by the clinician himself; therefore, it has its own utility. A USG may be superior to a lateral film in diagnosing a small pleural fluid collection. As against this, if the lesion is not well-defined, or bilateral, a CT scan may be superior.

In this case, a lateral film was asked for, which clearly showed a ***lung abscess*** with an air and fluid level. The presence of such a level indicates that the lung lesion is/was in communication with a bronchus. Therefore, it is likely to be drained naturally, over time, provided the communication persists. Attempts at chest physiotherapy and postural drainage may help. One may need to continue antibiotics for a longer time for complete resolution. In this case, IV ceftriaxone was continued for the next 10 days, and the child recovered completely.

Experience gained...

This case illustrates the value of lateral film in evaluating chest lesions. The utility of diagnosing a complication like a lung abscess is that it helps us to persist with the same antibiotic, though it may be needed for a longer period. Usually, there is no need to change the antibiotic, though at times, one may have to consider additional anaerobic cover.

It is an age-old dictum that any pus collection in the body has to be drained, as antibiotics alone would not be able to clear the lesion. Typically, in children, one may encounter abscesses in the subcutaneous tissue, brain, lung or liver. While abscesses of a significant size in the first two sites almost always need to be drained, this may not be true in the case a liver abscess, since there is a chance of natural resolution. It is the size and the toxicity of the patient that decides; usually antibiotics are tried, but if the abscess is enlarging and/or threatening to rupture, it may require drainage. At the opposite end of the spectrum is a lung abscess, which almost never needs surgical drainage. This is because it usually drains naturally into the bronchus; chest physiotherapy and postural drainage are useful adjuncts to systemic antibiotics in such cases.

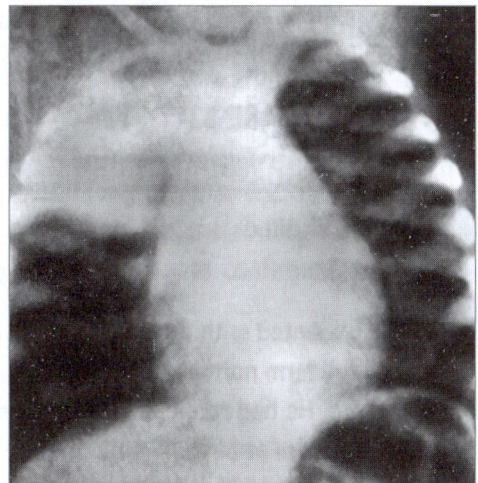

PA film showing pneumonia.

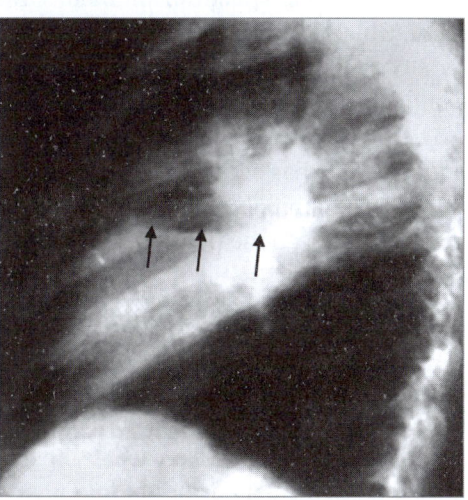

Lung abscess demonstrated clearly on lateral film.

CASE 85

■ True Recurrence

Events...

A 3-month-old infant presented with a persistent pneumonia for the last one month. He was born of a full-term normal delivery with a birth weight of 3.1 kg. He was exclusively breast-fed. He had received BCG vaccine and the first dose of hepatitis B and oral polio vaccines at birth. Apparently, he remained well for the first month, after which he developed fever and cough that was diagnosed as pneumonia on the basis of chest X-ray and blood counts and was treated with broad-spectrum antibiotics. He recovered from that illness, but he had lost some weight, which he never regained. Shortly thereafter, he developed another febrile illness that was subsequently diagnosed as pneumonia again. In spite of a trial with two sets of antibiotics, he improved only partially, and hence, was referred for further management.

There was a family history of consanguinity. The father has been suffering from cough frequently, and has been labeled as bronchitis, though he has never been investigated.

Physical examination revealed a malnourished sick infant with signs of respiratory distress and pneumonia on the right side. There were no other positive findings.

Explanation...

Considering that an exclusively breastfed infant was suffering from a recurrent/persistent pneumonia, it suggested a host immune defect or functional abnormality. Immune deficiency manifesting so early in life has to be T-cell or severe combined immunodeficiency. Since he reacted normally to the BCG vaccine, he had a normal T-cell function. B-cell deficiency would have generally presented after 4–6 months of age, because till then, infants are protected by way of maternally transmitted antibodies. So this was unlikely to be an immune deficiency disorder. Moreover, since he suffered from a recurrent/persistent infection localized to the respiratory tract only, it was likely to be a functional defect localized to the respiratory system. Ciliary dyskinesia is not present so early, so he was investigated for cystic fibrosis. Bronchoalveolar lavage grew *Pseudomonas aeruginosa*, which is indirect evidence in favor of cystic fibrosis. He also had metabolic alkalosis even though he was in respiratory failure and was therefore, expected to show respiratory acidosis. This offered another clue to the diagnosis of **cystic fibrosis**. In this condition, metabolic alkalosis is due to the loss of chlorides through sweat. The diagnosis was confirmed with the demonstration of the classical delta F 508 mutation.

Experience gained...

> Recurrent lower respiratory tract bacterial infection is always a result of some serious underlying cause that must be defined clearly for a better outcome. Diagnosis of cystic fibrosis in such a case can be suspected clinically by history of consanguinity and fatty stools as evident by large foul-smelling greasy stools with oil droplets.

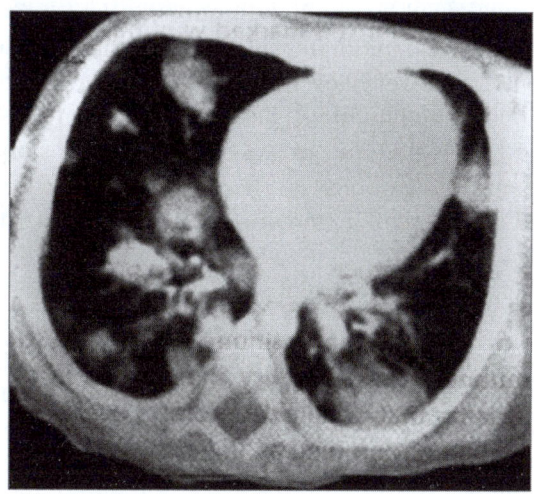

CT scan showing cystic lesions.

CASE 86

■ True Recurrence

Events...

A 12-year-old child presented with fever and cough, off and on, for the last 7–8 years. The initial episodes were easily controlled by antibiotics, but over time, he started taking longer to recover. Eventually, this led to a deterioration of his general health as well as his lung function, so that he had lost considerable weight over time, and had now started getting breathless even on accustomed exertion. He had multiple chest X-rays that showed infiltrations at different sites at different times, each time diagnosed as pneumonia, supported by neutrophilic leukocytosis and a response to antibiotics. There was no history of infections at any other sites. He had received all his regular immunizations in early childhood and had reacted normally to them.

His elder brother had died at the age of 15 years, due to a similar illness. There was no history of consanguinity.

Physical examination showed marked wasting, clubbing of nails, bilateral scattered lung lesions in the form of a few cavities, patchy pneumonias, and bronchiectasis. He was hypoxic in room air.

Explanation...

It is clear that this child had suffered from recurrent pneumonias resulting in extensive involvement of both lungs, leading to progressive respiratory failure. This had to be secondary to a serious underlying cause, such as an immunological (B-cell) deficiency or a functional immune defect—cystic fibrosis or ciliary dyskinesia. An immunological deficiency that results in recurrent respiratory infections is IgA deficiency that usually deteriorates over several years. The family history of an elder sibling having died at 15 years of age favors such a diagnosis. Ciliary dyskinesia may also present with a similar history of recurrent respiratory infections. However, each episode usually recovers well, so that there is no destruction of the lung and the child does not deteriorate progressively. A child with cystic fibrosis who has such a destroyed lung would have presented much earlier in life and would have progressed faster.

This child had **total absence of IgA** in the serum.

Experience gained...

> This child had recurrent pneumonia with a chronic progressive respiratory failure developing over several years. The serious underlying cause that is responsible for this is such that it is compatible with life for many years and has not involved any other system. This offers a clue to an immunological deficiency that affects only the respiratory system primarily, i.e., IgA deficiency. The only other condition that simulates this is ciliary dyskinesia. Typically, IgA deficiency is diagnosed accidentally when an older child presents with ataxia-telangiectasia and has had a history of repeated respiratory infections since early childhood.

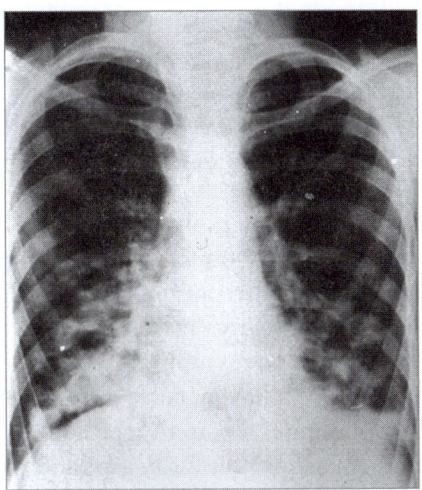

Bilateral basal cavitatory lesions.

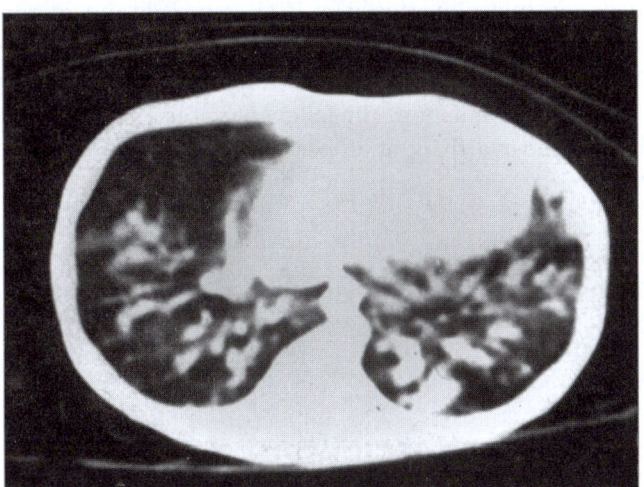

CT showing the same.

■ Recurrent Cough With or Without Wheezing

Preamble

Recurrent cough is a common symptom in office practice. It is often accompanied with noisy breathing that may either be wheezing or misinterpreted as wheezing (when there are nasopharyngeal sounds conducted to the chest). Wheeze may not be noted each time but episodic bouts of cough do suggest such a possibility. Just like a 'cold' can present either as a running nose or a blocked nose, 'running bronchi' can present as cough and blocked bronchi as wheeze. Thus, cough and wheeze may represent the same disease and one may not notice both each time. It is also not easy to clearly differentiate between a recurrent and persistent pathology, unless there is a long enough symptom free period. Thus, recurrent cough may either represent a recurrent infective pathology, such as recurrent viral infections or a persistent pathology, such as asthma. Vomiting is a common accompaniment of cough, especially in younger children. It could either be the cause (as in aspiration) or the effect (of severe cough). Contrary to common belief, aspiration can exist without overt vomiting. If cough is associated with fever, it usually suggests infection. However, if fever appears a few days after the onset of cough, it may not denote infection, especially, if it is low grade and intermittent. It is indicative of allergic inflammation as seen in asthma. The relative prominence of each symptom and their temporal interrelationship gives vital clues. Thus, many diseases mimic one another, and they need a sound clinical evaluation. The following cases illustrate various points of clinical significance that may help in arriving at proper diagnosis.

CASE 87

■ Wheeze Associated Lower Respiratory Infection
Events...

A 2-year-old child presented with recurrent episodes of fever, cold, cough and wheezing since the age of 6 months. Each time, the episode began with a high fever that lasted for about 2–3 days. It was accompanied with cold and cough that went on increasing, followed by wheezing. The wheezing would then settle down within a short time, but the cough usually continued for two weeks, He was often treated with antibiotics, though he always took nearly the same amount of time to get better and the next episode could not be prevented. The results of routine investigations were normal. He remained well in between episodes and had maintained good growth and development. The father had suffered from similar episodes during his childhood. There was no personal or family history of asthma or atopy.

This child was prescribed inhaled steroids for a period of 3 months, but there was no change in the frequency of his episodes.

Explanation...

The history suggests that this child has been getting frequent viral infections as against repeated bacterial infections, because the fever has been self-limiting and the child has grown well in spite of repeated episodes of infection. This is also the typical age group for such an occurrence. Further, if it were to be repeated bacterial infections, there is usually a serious underlying cause for such infections, in which case the child may not thrive so well. This is obviously not a case of tuberculosis as cough and wheezing are rare manifestations of tuberculosis. While in a known case of asthma, viral infections are known to trigger asthmatic attacks, this child cannot be labeled as asthma yet, since each episode starts with fever, and there is no family history of asthma or atopy. This child is typically suffering from wheeze associated viral respiratory tract infection. Since these children have hyperreactive airways, they manifest a prolonged cough following viral infections. Unfortunately, viral infections recur frequently at this age with cross infection amongst children in the play group. Over time, these children may either evolve into classical asthma (in which case the frequency of cough and wheezing episodes may increase and occur without fever) or get better (which is the typical clinical profile of **wheeze-associated lower respiratory tract infection (WALRI)**. Till such time that a definite diagnosis evolves, only symptomatic measures are justified, inhaled steroids are not. Inhaled bronchodilators can be tried in such cases, though they may not work very well, if the diagnosis is primarily wheeze associated viral infection. In this child, inhaled steroids were tried but did not work; in WALRI, they are not expected to, since there is no persistent allergic inflammation as is the case with asthma. Such an illness is common in children at this age; the parents should be reassured, and the child should not be drugged irrationally.

Experience gained...

Many nonatopic conditions, such as small airways of preterm or IUGR babies, neonatal lung damage due to meconium aspiration syndrome or hyaline membrane disease, or respiratory syncytial virus infection in early infancy can lead to hyperreactive airways. Such children present with recurrent cough and wheeze during the first few years of life and then mostly outgrow their problems while atopic children continue to suffer. The prognosis of WALRI is generally good though recent studies have shown that such children may continue to have abnormal lung function even in later life.

CASE 88

Gastroesophageal Reflux Disease (GERD)

Events...

A 6-month-old infant presented with mild fever followed by persistent cough and wheezing for two days. He had suffered from a similar episode a month back, which was diagnosed as pneumonia on the basis of a chest X-ray and he recovered after being nebulized and given antibiotics. There was no history of vomiting or choking while feeding. There was no family history of asthma.

Physical examination revealed a mild tachypnea with chest retractions and rhonchi, without any other localizing signs in the chest. The other systems were normal. Routine investigations did not reveal any significant abnormality, though the chest X-ray was again reported as pneumonitis. Considering it to be a case of recurrent pneumonia, this child was investigated for immune deficiency and cystic fibrosis; the results were normal.

Explanation...

Significant cough and wheezing primarily suggest an airway disease and not pneumonia. This history is similar to the previous case except that this is an infant and fever is not a predominant symptom. Often, a chest X-ray is reported as pneumonia, though what is really seen on the X-ray are linear or granular opacities, which could actually represent small areas of atelectasis (that are common in airway obstruction) or prominent bronchovascular markings (which are nonspecific). One of the common causes of recurrent airway disease at this age is aspiration syndrome, and this child was diagnosed as **gastroesophageal reflux disease**. It is important to note that there may not be any history of vomiting, regurgitation or choking spells while feeding, in spite of significant gastroesophageal reflux and aspiration into the lungs. Thus, a history that is negative for the above symptoms, does not rule out the possibility of GER. Similarly, when GER presents with cough as a major symptom, failure to gain weight may not be prominent. Weight could be an important issue when vomiting is the chief complaint in GER. The diagnosis of GER is not easy and needs a structured radiological evaluation. Of course, the most ideal investigation is continuous monitoring of esophageal pH, but it is cumbersome and not easily available. A radionuclide milk scan may be an alternative that can demonstrate aspiration into the lungs on periodic follow-up scans. However, this is also not commonly available. Therefore, a barium study is what is used most commonly. Ideally, a barium study should be performed under the supervision of either a pediatrician or a pediatric surgeon. The barium should be of the consistency of breast milk, and the quantity should be nearly equal to an average feed of the baby. The infant should be in a neutral position and not in Trendelenburg position, because in that case, a reflux may be visualized, even if it is not significant. Finally, the study should be performed for a period of half an hour, since the reflux may not be evident within a shorter time. Such a carefully performed barium study may pick up the GER in most of the cases. However, if it does not, and there is a strong clinical suspicion, one must attempt the other investigations mentioned above. If they are also negative, or not available, then even in the absence of positive proof, one may be justified in a therapeutic trial. Of course, by then, other esophageal anomalies, such as esophageal stenosis, achalasia or chalasia cardia have been already ruled out by the barium study. Other causes of aspiration syndrome include palatopharyngeal incompetence, swallowing dysfunction in developmentally delayed children and H type of tracheoesophageal fistula.

Experience gained...

> One must attempt to correlate clinical symptoms, physical signs, and the radiological picture before accepting a diagnosis of pneumonia.
>
> One of the most common causes of recurrent airway disease in infancy is an aspiration syndrome.
>
> Absence of vomiting, regurgitation, choking spells while feeding, or inadequate weight gain is compatible with a diagnosis of GERD.

CASE 89

■ Achalasia Cardia

Events...

A 6-year-old child presented with fever, cough and wheezing off and on for the last two years. He also complained of difficulty in swallowing, and vomiting off and on, over the same period. The vomitus was never bile stained. He was repeatedly treated with antibiotics and cough mixtures which resulted in only a temporary improvement at times; the symptoms always recurred within a few days.

Physical examination revealed a poorly nourished, averagely built child with a weight of 15 kg and a height of 109 cm. There were no localizing signs in the chest and the other systems were also normal.

Explanation...

As difficulty in swallowing is an unusual symptom in this child, it may be best to analyze this symptom first. The combination of dysphagia and vomiting suggests an obstruction at the level of the esophagus. Since the complaints have been going on for the last two years without obvious worsening, it is likely to be a slowly progressive or a static obstruction. It could be either congenital or acquired; further, it could be organic or functional. Since this child was asymptomatic for the first 4 years, he seems to have acquired the obstruction over time. It could be a slowly developing mechanical obstruction such as esophageal stenosis or a functional obstruction such as achalasia cardia. The vomiting could have led to repeated microaspiration, which in turn could have resulted in the recurrent episodes of cough and wheezing. Thus, significant vomiting due to dysphagia strongly suggests aspiration syndrome. At this age, it is unlikely to be due to gastroesophageal reflux disease. However, GER in the past may have resulted in reflux esophagitis and resultant obstruction at the lower end of the esophagus. Esophageal obstruction may also result from a space-occupying lesion in the posterior mediastinum. However, it would have been progressive, unlike in this child.

On detailed questioning, the fever in this child was found to be low grade; it may not necessarily suggest infection. It could even be due to inflammation caused by the chemical irritation following aspiration. Further, though this child seems to be underweight, he has a normal height. This suggests that though he has suffered nutritionally due to his vomiting, it must have been an intermittent phenomenon, and having started late at 4 years of age, the height seems to have been not much affected. This also favors a mechanical problem rather than infection. An additional burden of chronic infection would have certainly affected the height.

It is unlikely to be asthma because the significant vomiting and dysphagia cannot be explained.

A barium study proved it to be **achalasia cardia**.

Experience gained...

> While analyzing a group of symptoms, it pays to start analyzing the most uncommon symptoms first, especially when the other symptoms are too common and are shared by many diseases.

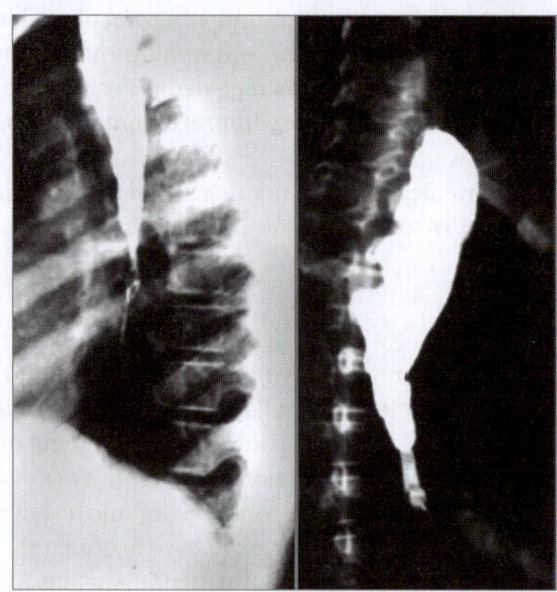

Achalasia cardia.

CASE 90

■ Coarctation of Aorta

Events...

A 10-month-old infant presented with recurrent episodes of cough and wheezing; there were four such episodes over the last 6 months. Each time, he presented with wheezing and was found to be dyspneic. He used to be nebulized with bronchodilators and often treated with antibiotics that seemed to offer temporary relief. After the second attack, he was put on prophylactic inhaled steroids but that did not help either, and he continued to get such recurrent episodes of wheezing.

There was no family history of asthma or a personal history of atopy. Investigations had ruled out aspiration syndrome due to GER or other upper esophageal anomalies.

Physical examination revealed an undernourished infant who had failed to thrive. There were scattered crepitations heard at both bases. He had a firm hepatomegaly. This had been noticed in the past, but was inferred to be a 'pushed down liver' secondary to air trapping, as a result of repeated episodes of wheezing. Similarly, the infant had a marked tachycardia, which had also been documented in the past but was considered to be secondary to his respiratory distress.

Explanation...

It should be a dictum to rule out other causes of wheezing before one label an infant as asthmatic. No doubt this was attempted in this infant by his previous doctors, who had ruled out an aspiration syndrome and only then diagnosed him as asthma. At this stage, one may have reluctantly accepted this diagnosis, and put him on inhaled steroids. But if in spite of compliant treatment with correct techniques, there is a failure of therapy, it is mandatory to reinvestigate and try to find some other explanation for the wheezing. Also, though an asthmatic infant or child may not gain adequate weight, *failure to thrive* is quite unusual in asthma.

Quite often, in such cases, a thorough clinical examination is rewarding. This is exactly what happened in this child. The marked tachycardia and a firm hepatomegaly gave a clue to a probable cardiac disease. In a primary respiratory disease, tachypnea would have been more significant than the tachycardia, and a 'pushed down liver' is not firm. The liver span would also have differentiated between a 'pushed down liver' and true hepatomegaly. So there were enough clues to cardiac disease. Besides these clinical findings, this child also had a cardiomegaly on the chest X-ray. This was again overlooked, because sometimes, chest X-rays of infants are taken in the supine position which can give a false impression of cardiomegaly. One of the most important parts of clinical examination of the cardiovascular system is the palpation of all the peripheral pulses and the measurement of the blood pressure that clinched the diagnosis in this infant. He had a coarctation of aorta that had presented with repeated episodes of left ventricular failure-cardiac asthma.

Retrospectively it was discovered that he had baseline tachypnea in between attacks, though he was reported to be normal.

Experience gained...

Asthma in infancy should be diagnosed only after excluding close differentials. Having done so, therapeutic failure should again prompt a reconsideration of the diagnosis.
There is no substitute for a sound clinical examination.

CASE 91

■ Cystic Fibrosis

Events...

An 8-month-old infant presented with fever, cough, and wheezing, off and on, for the last 4 months. Each time, he was treated with antibiotics and was nebulized with bronchodilators, with a minimal temporary benefit. Over the last four months, he had also failed to thrive; he weighed 4.5 kg now with his birth weight being 2.9 kg. There was a history of vomiting off and on. There was also a family history of asthma.

Physical examination revealed a malnourished, sick looking infant, who had clubbing of his finger and toe nails. He was tachypneic and had scattered crepitations and rhonchi. Other systems were normal.

He had been investigated for GER in view of the history of vomiting, but the tests were negative. So a therapeutic trial was also attempted but it failed to relieve the problem. In view of the family history of asthma, a trial with inhaled steroids was also considered but was not successful.

Explanation...

Failure to thrive and clubbing of nails strongly suggests a recurrent or persistent bacterial infection with suppuration. Recurrent bacterial infections always have some underlying cause to account for the same. This may be an anatomical malformation, or immunodeficiency or a functional defect. This infant obviously does not have asthma, in fact clubbing rules it out completely. Anatomical defects are localized, and immune deficiency disorders present with infections at multiple sites. So both these conditions are unlikely. Similarly, clubbing and progressive deterioration is not a feature of GER disease. This child was confirmed to be suffering from cystic fibrosis.

In India, cystic fibrosis is not as rare as was earlier thought to be. However, it is not easy to confirm the diagnosis. The estimation of sweat chlorides is used as a good screening test. Frankly elevated levels are almost diagnostic, though borderline elevations are seen in conditions other than cystic fibrosis also. This is a test that is technically difficult and therefore may not be easily available; iontophoresis is the only standard method of collecting sweat. However, indigenously manufactured equipment is now available and is believed to be reliable. Molecular diagnosis is definitive, though we do not know all the mutations that exist in the Indian population; the classical delta F 508 mutation is seen in not more than 50% patients in India. Isolation of *Pseudomonas* in bronchoalveolar lavage and metabolic alkalosis in presence of acute respiratory failure, are indirect evidences in favor of cystic fibrosis. Many infants may not present with diarrhea, though laboratory tests would confirm fat malabsorption and on direct questioning, the stools may be reported to be greasy due to the presence of oil droplets.

Experience gained...

> Clubbing without cyanosis is rarely encountered in infancy because chronic infective lung diseases are not common at this age. *Infants* with respiratory infection often wheeze, and thereby simulate hyperreactive airway disease or asthma.

CASE 92

■ Foreign Body

Events...

A 2-year-old child was brought with the complaints of cough and wheezing for the last 2 months. The cough was not only present throughout the day, it also disturbed his sleep. Severe bouts of cough were followed by wheezing, and he would often end up in vomiting. There was no history of fever, nor any past history of a similar illness. There was no family history of atopy. Physical examination was essentially normal.

Routine investigations were normal and treatment with antibiotics and cough syrups did not help the child.

Explanation...

On detailed questioning, it transpired that the cough had started all of a sudden one day while the child was playing and thereafter, it just continued. This gave a clue to the possibility of an inhaled foreign body. Even if this history would not have been available, it was unlikely to be asthma since the cough was not episodic or nocturnal and there was no past history of similar complaints.

A careful review of the chest X-ray revealed a suspicious small area of emphysema in the right middle zone suggesting partial segmental obstruction. Typically, in such cases an inspiratory film appears normal while an expiratory film demonstrates retained air in the segment in which the foreign body is lodged. However, this is usually seen only when a large bronchus is affected.

The foreign body was removed through bronchoscopy and the child recovered completely.

Experience gained...

> Inhaled foreign body is a diagnosis that needs a high index of suspicion. History of a *sudden* onset of cough with or without choking should alert the physician about such a possibility, even if one apparently fails to demonstrate it on a chest X-ray. Small areas of emphysema or atelectasis may be easily overlooked. In case there is a strong clinical suspicion, a bronchoscopy is indicated, especially when no other cause of a persistent or recurrent cough can be determined. These problems are compounded when an asthmatic child inhales a foreign body and presents as an acute exacerbation of asthma. If such a child does not respond to the conventional management of an acute attack of asthma, one may have to suspect an inhaled foreign body.

CASE 93

■ Miliary Tuberculosis

Events...

A 3-month-old infant presented with fever, cough and wheezing for the last one month. He was born of a full-term normal delivery and weighed 3.2 kg at birth. He was exclusively breastfed and had apparently grown well for the first two months. However, he had lost weight over the last one month, ever since his symptoms started.

Physical examination revealed that his weight was 4.1 kg and his length was 58 cm. He had moderate pallor and significant hepatosplenomegaly. He was mildly tachypneic with scattered crepitations in the chest. The chest X-ray was reported as bilateral bronchopneumonia. He was treated with antibiotics and saline nebulization but showed no improvement.

Explanation...

A respiratory disease that has involved both the lungs, in conjunction with hepatosplenomegaly, suggests a disseminated infection. Though acute bacterial infections are known to involve multiple organs like lungs, liver and spleen, as a part of severe sepsis leading to multiple organ failure, this happens over a shorter time frame. This infant has been ill for the last one month and has been slowly deteriorating, so acute bacterial infections are ruled out. So, this could be a chronic infection like tuberculosis or a fungal infection. A severe respiratory infection in a full-term breastfed baby should make one think of cystic fibrosis; however, the hepatosplenomegaly is unusual. Aspiration syndromes are also ruled out for the same reason. Congenital torch group of infections are unlikely, since his birth weight was good, and other common manifestations of congenital infections, such as skin rash, purpura, eye signs and brain involvement are absent in this child.

Noninfective conditions, such as storage disorders would present with asymptomatic hepatosplenomegaly and/or delayed milestones at this age and are therefore unlikely.

Bronchoalveolar lavage yielded *Mycobacterium tuberculosis.* This could represent either congenital tuberculosis or the infection could have been acquired immediately after birth from other contacts.

The infant's chest X-ray showed miliary mottling, which had been earlier reported as bilateral bronchopneumonia. The mother was found to be normal; the placenta was not reported to be abnormal, though it may not have been examined seriously. No contact could be traced on radiological survey of the family. This is not unusual in a young infant who could be infected at the time of delivery by attendants at the maternity hospital.

Experience gained...

> Bilateral lung disease with hepatosplenomegaly in a young infant strongly suggests a disseminated infection, and though uncommon, tuberculosis is still a possibility in our epidemiology. Cystic fibrosis, storage disorders and alpha 1 antitrypsin deficiency are other examples of disorders that may affect the lungs and liver/spleen. However, such involvement is sequential, over an extended period of time, and not over a short time as was seen in this infant.

Recurrent Cough, Cold and Fever in Office Practice

In routine office practice, one often sees children who present with the symptom complex of recurrent cough, cold, and fever. The following cases illustrate how a systematic history and clinical examination can help differentiate the three main causes of this symptom complex— **namely viral infection, asthma and bacterial infection.**

CASE 94

■ Frequent Viral Infections

A 3-year-old child was brought for recurrent cough over the last 1 year. He has been treated with many antibiotics and cough syrups; CBC and X-ray chest has not helped.

Detailed History

This child was apparently alright till two years of age, after which he started getting frequent episodes of cough. Each episode was accompanied with fever to begin with, followed by cold and cough. The fever used to respond to antipyretics and subsided after 3 days. Cold was usually in the form of a running nose, occasionally a thick mucoid discharge. The cough was dry, moderately severe, throughout the day and intermittent at night, and lasted for a few days before subsiding. On an average, after every 4-6 weeks, the child would go through a more or less identical cycle. There was no family history of atopy.

On Examination

Temperature 101°F
Throat—mild congestion
RS—normal

Coryza
No tonsillar hypertrophy
Other systems normal

Analysis

Since each episode of cough and cold in this child begins with fever, he is getting frequent infections. Fever at the onset of the illness every time indicates an infection. The presence of a watery running nose and the fact that the illness has always been self-limiting suggests that this child seems to be suffering from **frequent viral infections**. The clinical examination as on today also suggests a viral infection. This is the age when children often start attending playschool and pick up frequent viral infections. A close differential would be a child with hyperreactive airway disease. However, the differentiating points are the presence of fever each time, the type of cough, and the absence of a family history of atopy. The parents of this child just need to be reassured. As the child grows older, the frequency of these infections will decrease. There is no need for any further investigations.

This is typically a recurrent viral respiratory infection with an involvement of both upper and lower respiratory tract—generalized respiratory infection. In this child, fever and cold/cough subside within a short time of each other. Unlike this, in a child with hyperreactive airways, such a viral respiratory infection presents with a similar clinical profile, but the cough gets worse by the time the fever subsides, and it continues for 10-14 days. This is typically WALRI—wheeze associated lower respiratory infection (As discussed in the preamble, a wheeze may not be present each time, though cough is representative of a similar pathology).

CASE 95

■ Asthma

History

A 4-year-old child is brought for frequent cough, cold and fever. He has a perpetual watery running nose with itching and often sneezing. The cough is dry, more at night, and occurs in severe spasms at the end of which the child often vomits. There are variable periods of cough free intervals, but the nasal symptoms are almost constant. There is no history of breathlessness or wheezing. Sometimes, the illness starts with fever and then the cough escalates; however, most of the episodes are not triggered by fever.

There is a family history of atopy; the father suffers from frequent 'sneezing' episodes.

On Examination

Height 98 cm
Dry skin, flexural dermatitis
Watery nasal discharge
RS—normal

Weight 15 kg
Conjunctival hyperemia
Rest of general examination—normal
Other systems—normal

Investigation

Various reports of CBC showing eosinophils 3–5%, otherwise essentially normal. Chest X-ray is normal.

Analysis

This child has a perennial history of a 'cold' with itching, suggesting allergic rhinitis. A nocturnal cough along with a family history of atopy, suggests a diagnosis of hyperreactive airway disease that is atopic in nature. The occasions when high fever is an accompaniment, viral infections may be triggering the episodes. However, when fever is low grade, occasional, and comes up a few days after the onset of cough, it may not denote infection, but could just be a manifestation of allergic inflammation. In either case, there is no need of an antibiotic. In this child, even though there is no wheezing on clinical examination or a history of breathlessness, cough equivalent asthma is well known. Symptoms in asthma can be typically intermittent or persistent. Clinical findings may be present only during the episodes. The mild eosinophilia is supportive.

The diagnosis of hyperreactive airway disease is largely clinical. In a nutshell, the diagnosis of asthma should be considered in any child who has recurrent cough with or without wheezing, whose symptoms are mainly nocturnal or worse at night, whose symptoms are usually not associated with fever, who has a personal evidence of atopy in the form of allergic rhinoconjunctivitis or atopic dermatitis, and in whom, there is a family history of asthma or other atopic manifestations. It is not necessary to do any further investigations to diagnose asthma. Depending on whether asthma is infrequent or persistent, therapy can be planned accordingly. Infrequent asthma should be treated only symptomatically with the use of bronchodilators as and when necessary, while persistent asthma is treated with long-term prophylactic inhaled steroid therapy.

CASE 96

■ Bacterial Infection Secondary to Adenoid Hypertrophy

History

A 4-year-old child was brought for recurrent cough, cold and fever. He used to get high fever 103-104°F, which did not come down significantly with antipyretics. Along with this, he often used to have a thick purulent nasal discharge. On direct questioning, he used to constantly have a feeling of nose block, even when he did not have a nasal discharge. He also used to snore at night and often slept restlessly. Whenever he developed a cough along with these symptoms, it was typically on lying down. In each of these illnesses, the high fever would continue for 2-3 days by which time some antibiotic would be started, after 36-48 hours of which the fever would gradually subside. Subsequently, if there had been a purulent nasal discharge or cough, these would also resolve gradually over the next few days. However, the nose block and the snoring would persist. There is no family history of atopy.

On Examination (Not during Acute Illness)

Height 94 cm
Adenoid facies
Postnasal discharge +
Bilateral jugulodigastric lymph nodes enlarged, nontender
RS—normal

Weight 14 kg
Bilateral tonsillar hypertrophy
Ears—N

Other systems—N

Analysis

This child clearly has a history suggestive of recurrent, acute, bacterial upper respiratory tract infections. Recurrent bacterial infections always result from some underlying cause, and that is evident in this child in the form of adenoid hypertrophy as suggested by adenoid facies. Persistence of nasal discharge and nasal block well after control of fever suggests extension of the disease into the sinuses. So this is rhinosinusitis. Cough is due to the postnasal discharge, therefore typically manifests on lying down. Examination confirms the diagnosis. The presence of hypertrophied tonsils (which often coexist with enlarged adenoids) adds to the diagnosis.

Typically, the diagnosis of enlarged adenoids is often confirmed by a lateral X-ray of the neck. However, further management decisions are based on the degree of clinical symptoms and not on X-ray appearances.

Comparison/Comment on the Above Three Cases

The above three cases illustrate the most common causes of recurrent cough—asthma, viral infections and upper airway bacterial infections. Though the patient may typically present with similar sounding complaints, viz. frequent episodes of the triad of symptoms—cough, cold and fever, a detailed history can fairly differentiate one from another. The nature of cough is different in all the three conditions. In viral infections, it may be dry or wet, but is throughout the day. In asthma, it is typically nocturnal. Though this cough may be reported to occur on lying down, it occurs a few hours after the child sleeps. As against this, the child coughs immediately on lying down in adenoid related bacterial infections due to a postnasal drip.

Similarly, the nature of the cold is different in all the three conditions—intermittent watery along with fever in viral infections, a perennial cold with itching of the nose in asthma, and an infected thick purulent nasal discharge in bacterial infection. Though fever is a complaint in all the three conditions, once again the specific features differ— self-limiting fever responding to antipyretics in viral infections, occasional fever in asthma, and a hectic fever in bacterial infection.

In other words, in viral infections all the three symptoms, i.e., cough, cold and fever are equally prominent in asthma cough and cold dominate but fever does not. Whereas fever is the most dominant in bacterial infections, cold is equally significant, and cough is relatively a lesser complaint.

The family history of atopy helps; however, it is only supportive, if rest of the history corroborates. Since atopy is so common, a family history of atopy may be coincidental.

During an acute attack, physical examination clearly differentiates these conditions from one another. In an acute viral infection, there is evidence of upper and lower respiratory tract involvement as suggested by congested eyes, nose and throat, besides scattered signs in the chest. In an acute bacterial infection, signs are often localized classically to the throat, while the chest is clear. Exudates on enlarged and inflamed tonsils, congestion of anterior pillar, purpuric spots on the palate and tender jugulodigastric lymph nodes are highly suggestive of bacterial acute pharyngotonsillitis. Asthma may present with prolonged expiration with or without rhonchi, along with nasal congestion.

When seen between episodes, a child with recurrent viral infections looks perfectly normal without any trace of recurrent problems. A child with recurrent bacterial infections does show an underlying cause of recurrence in the form of enlarged adenoids. This is evident by the mouth breathing and adenoid facies, the persistence of enlarged jugulodigastric lymph nodes (though nontender), and hypertrophied tonsils in without any signs of acute inflammation. A child with asthma may show perennial rhinitis as a marker of atopy.

Laboratory and radiological investigations are not contributory in such cases and diagnosis of these three conditions rests primarily on clinical grounds alone.

CASE 97

Recurrent Cold and Fever

Case

A 5-year-old child presented with recurrent cold, blocked nose and fever off and on for the last 6 months. He used to get frequent cold, and cough since the age of 2 years. His mother has had asthma since early life. He has had antibiotics and inhaled steroids locally in the nose but with temporary benefit.

How would you manage his recurrent problem?

Mostly, this child has atopic rhinitis. But the fact that he gets fever off and on may mean either a chronic infection or recurrent infections. While a chronic infection may seem to temporarily respond to antibiotics initially, over time, it would progress. Since this child has an obstructed nasal passage, he is a candidate for recurrent bacterial infections. Since the 'cold' persists for a longer time, it needs to be considered as sinusitis—disease extending to paranasal sinuses. If fever is high and persistent, it must be taken as evidence of infective sinusitis on the background of atopy. Sinusitis can only be confirmed on CT scan—plain X-ray is not reliable. Growth faltering may suggest chronic persistent infection while normal growth is against it. Role of antibiotics in chronic infective sinusitis is not clear and emphasis is on control of atopy rather than antibiotic for infection. The culture of nasal secretions is not ideal because of presence of many commensals and sinus puncture may be invasive for routine use. Long-term antibiotics or prophylactic antibiotics have no role and at best one can consider a single course of amoxyclav for 10–14 days to hopefully eradicate persistent infection. Long-term management of nasal atopy with local steroids, leukotriene inhibitors, such as montelukast and antihistamine need consideration. Atopic rhinitis has many phenotypes; hence, an individual child may or may not respond to the given options. Inhaled steroid is the first option with antihistamine on a SOS basis just to ensure peaceful sleep at night. If not successful, one can add montelukast orally. At times, montelukast alone might work. It is just a chance, and one must try out different options. Control of trigger factors, such as dust, animal dander, molds, pollen, etc. and irritants, such as strong smell and smoke is most important. Food items are rarely the major culprit and should not be restricted without evidence. Allergy tests have limitations, and the best allergen search is based on clinical observation combined with epidemiological knowledge. Similarly, immunotherapy is reserved for the one odd extreme case.

Recurrent Abdominal Pain

Preamble

Amongst recurrent problems in children, abdominal pain is the most intriguing for a clinician. Diagnosis is difficult and often empirical, based on clinical judgment and considered to be correct only after the child experiences sustained relief from pain. Investigatory modalities have a limited role, largely to rule out specific conditions, as there are no diagnostic tests for most of the causes. A general rule that may be followed is that chronic pain restricted to any quadrant should be investigated. However, tests are unlikely to yield any answers in cases of chronic generalized abdominal pain. Of course, acute severe abdominal pain, with or without localization, may necessitate appropriate tests. Following cases illustrate some of the problems.

CASE 98

■ Habitual Constipation

Events...

A 10-year-old girl presented with a history of abdominal pain for the last one year. She was treated with frequent courses of anthelmintics considering parasitic infections to be a common cause of recurrent abdominal pain. She was advised to stop milk and milk products considering the probability of milk allergy. She also underwent a trial with omission of wheat products. After these initial trials failed, she was referred to a surgeon. Chronic appendicitis was suspected, and she was investigated. Routine tests were normal, and the USG was reported as suggestive of appendicitis. She was advised surgery. When she went for a second opinion, she was advised to confirm the diagnosis with a CT scan. The CT scan revealed a few mesenteric lymph nodes in the right iliac fossa and suggested that abdominal tuberculosis be ruled out by doing a barium follow through.

This child complained of abdominal pain that was not localized to any quadrant, was mostly a dull ache, though occasionally, she also had colicky pain. It generally did not interfere with her routine activities. The pain would often be relieved after passing stools. There was no history of any change in bowel pattern, vomiting, fever, loss of weight or appetite. On direct questioning, the parents claimed that she was toilet-trained since early childhood and had normal bowel habits. Her diet mainly consisted of noodles and biscuits; she drank two glasses of milk daily.

Physical examination revealed an averagely-built and nourished child and the only positive findings were fecal masses felt on both sides in the flanks along with a vague tenderness all over the abdomen.

Explanation...

This child has generalized vague abdominal pain, and she is definitely constipated as evident by fecal masses felt on both sides of the abdomen. As she has complained of this pain only for the last one year and has not failed to thrive, it is most likely to be a recently acquired problem. Though amebiasis and giardiasis may present without loose stools, this child has had several stool tests and trials with anthelmintics without any benefit. Therefore, such infections can be ruled out.

This child never had a history of acute abdominal pain that may have suggested an attack of acute appendicitis. Chronic appendicitis is a difficult diagnosis to prove, though localization of pain to the right iliac fossa and demonstration of imaging abnormalities in the same area may favor such a diagnosis. Unless one finds a localized mass in the right iliac fossa, the diagnosis may not be definite. One could easily commit an error of commission or omission by unnecessarily subjecting the child to surgery or by missing the diagnosis. Such a diagnosis must be made cautiously as there is no risk in delaying the diagnosis and thereby, the treatment; surgery should not be considered as a trial.

The finding of mesenteric lymph nodes on a CT scan should be carefully evaluated. Unless the lymph nodes are large in size, they may not be of any significance and at best, may be followed up further for any change in size. Mesenteric lymph nodes do exist in normal individuals, and they may be prominent due to previous repeated intra-abdominal infections.

In school going children who usually look after their own personal habits, the parents are often unaware of the fact that the child is constipated. Further, visiting the bathroom daily does not necessarily equate with the passage of a normal, complete stool. This child is obviously constipated as evident from the fecal masses and the cause of constipation is obviously related to poor eating habits. What this child now needs is systematic and thorough management of her constipation, rather than further investigations or trial with different medications.

The treatment of constipation demands an aggressive approach to avoid long-term morbidity. Bowels must be evacuated daily, and completely, either by the use of enema or laxatives or both. Meanwhile, the diet needs a modification with increased roughage in the diet and avoidance of junk food. Long-standing constipation may result in permanent laxity of the rectal musculature secondary to constant dilatation and stretching by the retained stool. In these cases, the problem may almost seem to defy a solution forever. To avoid such situations, it should be recognized and adequately treated, in time.

Experience gained...

Constipation is a common cause of recurrent/persistent abdominal pain in children and is often overlooked. It needs prompt treatment at the earliest to avoid long-term morbidity.

CASE 99

■ Meckel's Diverticulum

Events...

A 5-year-old child presented with a history of recurrent abdominal pain for the last 6 months. She was apparently well prior to the onset of this problem. She suffered acute attacks of severe abdominal pain that would last for 8–12 hours at a time and would repeat at irregular intervals averaging once or twice a week. There were no other symptoms such as vomiting, change in bowel pattern, urinary complaints, or fever. Physical examination at the time of an acute attack was reported as generalized abdominal distention with generalized tenderness. Once the attack subsided, she was absolutely normal and had no abnormality on physical examination. Several investigations had been carried out that included stool microscopy, urinalysis, abdominal sonography, abdominal X-ray, barium study, CBC and peripheral smear, ESR, radionuclide scan for Meckel's diverticulum and studies for porphyria. None of the tests offered any clue. Each attack was treated symptomatically, though the response was suboptimal and she had to endure significant pain that was difficult to control. She was also subjected to a psychological assessment, but it was noncontributory.

Explanation...

This child has a genuine pain that is so severe. The only abnormal finding during an attack has been generalized abdominal distention. This could be a nonspecific finding though it may suggest a primary intestinal problem. It could be a recurrent subacute intestinal obstruction that corrects itself, such as volvulus with malrotation. This may only be picked up, if the child is investigated during the attack. Intestinal tuberculosis can present with subacute intestinal obstruction, though such an obstruction would not resolve over a few hours each time and would be accompanied with general symptoms of a chronic infection, such as loss of appetite and weight. So it was decided to image her abdomen during an attack and that turned out to be normal. At that stage, the differential diagnosis was extended to include abdominal migraine or epilepsy. However, there was no family history of migraine, nor did she complain of any headache along with abdominal pain. She also did not experience an aura before the attack of abdominal pain to consider abdominal epilepsy. Thus, we were at a loss to diagnose her condition.

Further Progress

One day she presented with acute intestinal obstruction that required urgent exploration. It revealed the presence of Meckel's diverticulum that was missed by the radionuclide scan done earlier. She was obviously cured after surgery.

Experience gained …

This case illustrates how difficult it can be to diagnose the cause of recurrent abdominal pain. When it is severe, it definitely calls for several investigations though they should be prioritized, based on prevalence as seen in office practice. This case also brings forth the limitations of laboratory tests, as almost no test is hundred percent sensitive and specific. One may have to be cautious of both false negatives and false positives. A radionuclide scan for Meckel's diverticulum can be falsely positive in case of an intestinal bleed of any other origin. Many problems unfold over time and one has to wait for such an opportunity.

CASE 100

■ Dyspepsia

Events....

A 6-year-old child presented with recurrent abdominal pain for last 7 months. The pain was a continuous dull ache and localized to the upper abdomen. It worsened a few hours after meals and at times, he would get up from sleep early in the morning, with severe pain. It was accompanied with bloating of the abdomen that made this child uncomfortable. He also complained of a burning sensation in the middle of the chest and had vomited occasionally. The vomitus contained whatever he had ingested. Over time, the pain had gradually worsened in severity and frequency. There was no change in the bowel pattern and there were no other symptoms. Physical examination revealed epigastric tenderness. There were no other abnormal findings. Routine investigations including abdominal sonogram did not show any abnormality. He had no relief with antispasmodics.

Explanation...

This child has abdominal pain that is localized to the epigastrium. Anatomical structures in the epigastrium include stomach, duodenum, pancreas, liver and transverse colon. Pain related to meals is likely to originate from the stomach or duodenum. There has been no hepatomegaly, nor a tenderness extending to the right hypochondrium. Colonic disease would have manifested with a change in bowel pattern and also, there would have been physical signs over other parts of the abdomen, since localized colonic disease is rare in children. Acute pancreatitis is ruled out in this child, as he never had any acute severe attack of pain. Chronic pancreatitis is a result of previous acute attacks that have not resolved completely, and it could have been picked up by abdominal sonography since it presents as a pseudopancreatic cyst. Pain coming up a few hours after meals, burning sensation—'heart burn' and bloating of abdomen suggest involvement of the stomach in the form of dyspepsia.

Ideally, it is necessary to investigate the cause of dyspepsia that may be due to reflux of acid or *H. pylori* infection. Accordingly, triple antibiotic therapy may be necessary to treat the infection, while acid blocking agents alone may suffice to treat acid reflux disease. In routine practice, since tests for *H. pylori* are invasive and serological tests are not reliable, a trial with acid blocking agents is worth it, and only, if it fails, one may have to resort to endoscopy and biopsy for definitive diagnosis.

Experience gained...

Dyspepsia is common in children and diagnosis is mostly clinical as evident by localized epigastric pain related to meals. However, absence of meal related pain does not rule out dyspepsia. Investigations are seldom required, and therapeutic trial is worth.

CASE 101

■ Functional Abdominal Pain

Events...

A 10-year-old child presented with recurrent abdominal pain for last 3 years. The pain was localized to the periumbilical region, intermittent, not severe and had no apparent aggravating or relieving factors. There was no particular pattern to the pain; it would come up anytime. There was no change in bowel pattern or vomiting and he had no urinary complaints. He had a normal appetite and was growing well. He slept well and was active. His play activities were never disturbed because of pain and whenever he was engrossed in watching television, he had no pain. At times he would complain of bloating of abdomen and passage of gas would relieve his pain. Occasionally, he would get an urge to pass stools when he felt the pain and the passage of stools would relieve it. His parents were quite worried, because in spite of several investigations the cause of this pain could not be diagnosed; the child had got no relief even after a trial with many drugs that included antibiotics, anthelmintics, antacids, antispasmodics, digestives, enzymes and diet modification.

A detailed enquiry about his behavior and school performance revealed that he was an insecure child with a disturbed interpersonal relationship, particularly at home. His mother had a dominating personality and expected him to excel in studies as well as other extracurricular activities, which he could not cope up with.

Explanation...

This child has chronic abdominal pain for last three years that has not disturbed his health and activities. So obviously, it is neither a progressive problem nor any serious disease. In general, chronic periumbilical pain is unlikely to originate from any organic pathology. The description of the pain in this child does not fit into any of the classical patterns seen in organic pathologies. Moreover, he has been undergoing a lot of stress at home. Thus, abdominal pain in this child is a somatic feature of an anxiety disorder. He should be treated with behavior modification techniques by a clinical psychologist to reduce his anxiety. He does not need any drug treatment.

Experience gained...

> Diagnosis of chronic abdominal pain is mostly clinical, and investigations are rarely required, especially if the pain is periumbilical or generalized and not localized to any quadrant. Long-standing abdominal pain is often not due to organic causes and may be related to functional or psychological issues. Such children should be referred for psychological assessment and managed accordingly.

CASE 102

■ Inflammatory Bowel Disease

Events...

A 10-year-old child presented with a history of recurrent abdominal pain, loose stools with mucus and occasionally blood, loss of appetite and loss of weight over last one year. Every time, he was treated with antibiotics and metronidazole that gave him temporary relief, but that would last just for a few days. His symptoms would recur again, and again, and would sometimes be quite severe. He would complain of nausea and vomiting in some of the episodes and would also run mild fever. He suffered from repeated mouth ulcers that would come in the way of his eating. Physical examination revealed a sick looking child with marked abdominal distention with generalized tenderness. There was no palpable mass in the abdomen. Stool microscopy was performed several times and was reported as giardiasis on a few occasions. This was treated repeatedly over the last one year without any long-standing relief. In fact, over this period, he had lost 5 kg of weight and was depressed. Several drug trails and dietary restrictions had failed to solve his problem.

Explanation...

This child has a chronic progressive intestinal inflammatory disorder with failure to thrive. He has loose stools with mucus and at times blood, which localizes the lesion to the intestines. Pain suggests an inflammatory disease and significant loss of weight denotes a severe progressive disease. Occasional fever and the occurrence of mouth ulcers off and on, indicate that the disease has spread beyond the intestines and may potentially be a multiorgan disease. This is how one arrives at a probable diagnosis of inflammatory bowel disease. Further classification of this disease would depend upon the results of colonoscopy and biopsy that may help differentiate between Crohn's disease and ulcerative colitis. Though, on clinical grounds alone, severe abdominal pain with diarrhea that is more often than not without blood, and failure to thrive, may favor Crohn's disease. Failure to thrive is not a feature of irritable bowel syndrome, hence that is ruled out. Inflammatory bowel disease is treated with anti-inflammatory drugs and in case of a poor response, with steroids. Besides one needs to offer symptomatic relief with drugs and build up the nutrition of the child. Unfortunately, there are likely to be relapses and one may need long-term treatment. In addition, other psychological issues may come up as a result of chronic illness that may require proper guidance from experts.

Experience gained...

> This type of recurrent abdominal pain is strikingly different from other routine causes, in the sense that failure to thrive is the hallmark of this disease, besides its progressive nature and its severity. This is the type of disease that needs several specialized investigations and a team of experts to treat it effectively. We must recognize this disease early, so as to offer the best possible outcome.

CASE 103

■ Irritable Bowel Syndrome

Events...

A 12-year-old female child presented with history of recurrent abdominal pain for the last six months. The pain was generalized and at times severe, though on many occasions, she would be just uncomfortable. It was worse after meals. It was accompanied by loose stools, at times with mucus, and she would feel better after passing a stool. She had a variable frequency and consistency of stools; occasionally, she would be constipated, though most of the time she passed loose stools. She complained of bloating of abdomen and would pass a lot of gases. She had a normal appetite, though at times she would eat less with the fear of worsening pain. She had not lost weight, and she remained fairly active except at the time of abdominal pain. On detailed enquiry, it was noted that the onset of her symptoms coincided with a change of school. There was no past history of any major illness or a family history of a similar disease. Routine laboratory tests showed no abnormality. She was treated with several drugs including antibiotics and anthelmintics without any benefit.

Explanation...

This child's abdominal pain is certainly related to an intestinal disorder as evident by the bloating of abdomen with gas and relief of abdominal pain after passing stools. There has also been an abnormal frequency and consistency of stools. This is not an infective condition as stool examination never showed any abnormality, nor she improve even after repeated courses of antibiotics and anthelmintics. Though at times there was mucus in stools, there was never any blood or severe griping abdominal pain. She maintained a normal appetite and had not lost weight. Such a clinical profile is against inflammatory bowel disease (Crohn's disease or ulcerative colitis). As the onset of her problem coincided with a change in school, it was always attributed to emotional stress.

This is classically an irritable bowel syndrome that may not be caused by emotional stress but may get aggravated by such stimuli. It results from a hypersensitivity of the intestinal muscle to pain, that may be triggered by a variety of factors either related to diet or emotional stress. There are no laboratory tests to prove the diagnosis. There is no specific treatment for this condition. It essentially consists of a trial with a change in diet, with emphasis on high fiber foods, and taking care of emotional disturbances by proper counseling. Drugs, such as anticholinergics or anxiolytics may be necessary at times.

Experience gained...

> Diagnosis of such conditions is purely clinical, and at best, investigations can rule out other conditions. With a proper history, one may be able to avoid unnecessary investigations and irrational use of antibiotics and anthelmintics.

■ Recurrent Diarrhea

Preamble

Recurrent diarrhea is a common problem in infancy and toddlers, though it can also be present in older children. Its etiology is diverse—it may be a result of an infection, allergy or malabsorption, or multiple factors may be responsible in the same patient. Of course, at times, the fault may not lie with the child at all and yet the child suffers. Thus, it is a real challenge to a clinician to define the exact cause of recurrence. The following cases illustrate various facets of recurrent diarrhea.

CASE 104

■ Recurrent GI Infection

Events....

A 10-month-old infant presents with a history of repeated loose stools and vomiting. He is bottle-fed and has suffered from five episodes of loose stools so far, two of them necessitating hospitalization. His present episode started 3 days back with fever and vomiting; vomiting has now subsided, but he is passing 8–10 stools/day and is running fever. He has been treated with oral antibiotics and antidiarrheals, but there has been no response so far.

Physical examination reveals a malnourished irritable infant, without any signs of dehydration or any other positive findings.

A detailed history of the past episodes and feeding practices revealed that he was never breastfed due to apparent lactation failure. As a result, he was bottle fed, and the bottle was not necessarily sterilized each time. Further, as and when he was offered semisolid food, he used to vomit. So, the mother felt that the solid food did not suit him. As a result, he was largely on a milk diet only. Every time he had diarrhea, the mother was advised to dilute milk and at times, offer only oral rehydration solution without milk.

Explanation...

It is obvious that this infant was at a high risk of gastrointestinal infections right since birth, as he was never breastfed and instead bottle fed. Thereafter, he had continuously faulted nutrition, not only due to frequent infections but also due to wrong advice given by the doctors. It resulted in progressive malnutrition that perpetuated the risk of intestinal infections and this vicious cycle continued. Such an infant cannot be treated with antibiotics alone. The most crucial part of therapy in such an infant is to build his nutrition; only then can he improve. If his nutritional status does not improve soon, he would be at a risk of complications like dehydration, severe electrolyte disturbances and sepsis that may endanger his life. Therefore, this child's management goes beyond mere drug therapy; it involves educating the mother on proper nutrition and hygiene and ensuring improvement on close follow-up.

Experience gained...

> This case illustrates the fact that very often, the causative factors responsible for recurrent diarrhea lie outside the host. However, unfortunately, our attention is mainly focused on the infant in terms of investigations and drug treatment. Unless the basic issues of hygiene and nutrition are looked after, such problems cannot be solved. It is important to recognize these external factors that are responsible for such problems and ideally prevent them, or at least, correct them in time.

CASE 105

■ HIV Infection

Events...

A 6-month-old infant presented with recurrent diarrhea for last 3 months. He was apparently well for the first-three months when he was exclusively breastfed. Thereafter, though he continued to be breastfed, he developed a diarrhea. This was initially considered to be a physiological phenomenon as exclusively breastfed infants are known to pass loose stools. However, this infant got dehydrated and had to be hospitalized for proper treatment. He was found to be febrile and quite sick and was treated with antibiotics and intravenous fluids. He recovered partially but had lost some weight by then. Subsequently, he was advised to continue breastfeeds as the mother was producing adequate milk. Within another week, he returned with severe diarrhea again, and went through a similar course of events. At this juncture, the treating pediatrician thought that he had developed lactose intolerance because the stool examination revealed a large amount of reducing substances and he had also developed a perianal excoriation. So, he was put on a soya milk formula. He used to vomit this formula off and on and lost some more weight.

Explanation...

An exclusively breastfed infant may pass loose stools but he is never sick and dehydrated. To begin with, this fact should have served as a warning that something was amiss. Subsequently, when he was considered to have a bacterial infection, the fact that he was never at risk of an intestinal infection, was overlooked. The subsequent diagnosis of lactose intolerance is also not tenable, as primary lactose intolerance is extremely rare and secondary lactose intolerance does not need a change of milk. If a breastfed infant suffers from a bacterial infection, especially an intestinal infection, it may be due to an immune deficiency or cystic fibrosis. On physical examination, he had an oral thrush that was ascribed to the earlier usage of multiple antibiotics and hence, was ignored. Failure to thrive, oral thrush, and the occurrence of repeated bacterial intestinal infections in a breastfed infant, gave a clue to the diagnosis of HIV infection that was later confirmed.

Experience gained...

> This case was apparently similar to the previous one, in that both the infants were malnourished and had recurrent intestinal infections. However, in this infant, the cause of the recurrent diarrhea lay within the host while in the previous case, it was outside the host (poor hygiene and wrong feeding practices). Thus, it is important to differentiate between these two situations. In routine office practice, a normal immunocompetent host who suffers from recurrent diarrhea due to external factors is common and this should be well-recognized.

CASE 106

Gluten Induced Enteropathy

Events...

A 4-year-old child presented with recurrent diarrhea since the age of 8 months. He was born out of a full-term normal delivery and weighed 3.1 kg at birth. He was exclusively breastfed for the first 6 months and thereafter, while breastfeeding was continued, he was also started on supplementary weaning foods as advised by the doctor. He developed his first episode of diarrhea at 8 months of age along with vomiting and abdominal cramps and was considered to have a viral infection and treated symptomatically. He was correctly advised to maintain the same diet even during the diarrheal episode. However, he did not improve for a long time, though he was never dehydrated. At that stage, he was treated with antibiotics and subsequently, with even metronidazole, giving him the benefit of doubt of a probable infection. While he showed a transient marginal improvement, he never recovered completely and continued to suffer from diarrhea off and on. Gradually, he was getting irritable, and had lost his appetite and some weight also. He used to vomit off and on and would suffer from abdominal pain at times. He had developed an abdominal distention that made him uncomfortable. His stool was examined on many occasions, including a stool culture that did not show any evidence of infection. Nevertheless, he did receive multiple antibiotics.

Physical examination (now, at 4 years of age) revealed a poorly built and a poorly nourished child, who was moderately pale and had a marked gaseous abdominal distention. Other systems were normal. An abdominal sonography confirmed the intestinal distention; there was no other abnormality detected.

Explanation...

This child has been a chronically sick child with stunting and wasting, though he has never had any dehydration, electrolyte imbalance or infection related complications, such as sepsis. Hence, this child does not have any infection and that is the reason why he has never shown a response to several antibiotics. Moreover, this child has been well-breastfed and is not at risk of an infection, unless he is immunocompromised, in which case, he would have gone down rapidly. Stunting and wasting suggest a chronic progressive pathology and are in favor of malabsorption. As the first episode of diarrhea started around the time of weaning, a detailed history revealed that he was first offered wheat cereal at about 8 months of age and it was continued thereafter, all along, as the doctor had advised a normal diet. This gave the clue to a probable diagnosis of gluten induced enteropathy. This was proved by antigliadin antibodies, though other confirmative tests were not possible. Therapeutic trial with a withdrawal of wheat products improved this child remarkably within a few weeks. This was unlikely to be cystic fibrosis as he had no respiratory illness at all, nor did he have any history of consanguinity or a family history of similar illness.

Experience gained...

This child suffered from chronic recurrent diarrhea without manifesting any complications commonly encountered in diarrheal diseases and in fact, over time, he presented with stunting and wasting. This is typical of malabsorption syndrome. Details of the history and the sequence of events related to weaning gave a clue to the probable diagnosis.

CASE 107

Chronic Giardiasis

Events....

A 2-year-old child presented with recurrent diarrhea for the last one year. He was exclusively breastfed for the first 6 months and thereafter, weaned on semisolid food. By one year of age, he had normal family food and was weaned off breastfeeding. This is when he had his first episode of loose stools; they were foul smelling but not frequent. He had occasional vomiting, was irritable and had lost appetite. He had no fever and he otherwise looked well. Initially, he was treated with antibiotics without any benefit and then treated with metronidazole that gave him some relief. Within a week of stopping the drug, he again developed similar loose stools and was proved to have giardiasis for which he was treated again with metronidazole. Such episodes continued off and on, though each time the stool microscopy did not show giardiasis. Considering it to be drug-resistant giardiasis, he was treated with tinidazole and thereafter, nitazoxanide but the recurrence could not be prevented.

Explanation...

This child's diagnosis is not in doubt and in spite of correct treatment, he does not seem to improve. Drug-resistance has been ruled out in this child as the other drugs that have been tried have also failed. This child probably has a continued source of contamination in his environment or needs a longer duration of treatment, as not all children get cured by conventional therapy. It is important to examine other family members, in particular, those who handle his food, if they are harboring a similar infection and transmitting it to the child repeatedly. Simultaneously, this child should be treated with repeated courses of therapy at an interval of a few weeks so as to eradicate the parasite.

Experience gained...

> Even when the diagnosis and treatment is correct, the problem may not be solved due to extraneous factors coming in the way of a complete cure. In such cases, while another coincidental infection may be considered, it is not common. This case also emphasizes the need for individualization of the therapeutic plan in some patients.

CASE 108   Miscellaneous

■ Recurrent Swelling around Angle of Mandible

Case

A 6-year-old child presented with recurrent episodes of swelling around the angle of mandible with fever. The first episode started with high fever and swelling around angle of mandible that was tender on touch, but otherwise not very painful. Fever disappeared within 2 days and the swelling got better over a week after antibiotic therapy. This was diagnosed as bacterial parotitis. Within a week, the swelling recurred on the same side but with minimal fever that lasted just for a day. The swelling was not disturbing the child and took another week to disappear with another antibiotic. Each time there was neutrophilic leukocytosis that prompted the physician to start an antibiotic. A sialogram was performed—there was no blockage of the salivary duct. The same thing recurred a third time, but this time, on the other side. This time a surgeon was consulted who suggested incision and drainage. Incision did not yield any pus, only serosanguinous material. The wound would not heal for the next one month, though the child remained reasonably well.

How do you Manage this Child?

The first time one may have thought of Mumps, but the sudden recovery was a point against. Sudden appearance, disappearance and recurrence suggests noninfective inflammation and hence this is unlikely to be recurrent bacterial infection. Bacterial parotitis would be extremely painful and so also viral parotitis (Mumps). This child did not have significant pain, only minimal tenderness. The fever was short lasting and disappeared much before the swelling reduced. It is not a surprise that the surgeon did not get any pus. In fact, the wound did not heal quickly because noninfective inflammation continued and interfered with healing. Since the parotid involvement was on both sides, it ruled out any local problems like salivary duct obstruction. So, this is immunological recurrent parotitis. Its exact cause is not clear, but it does respond to symptomatic anti-inflammatory therapy, such as ibuprofen. Chances of recurrence do exist but cannot be prevented. Most children will get better by themselves after few recurrences, and it does not call for any tests. Parents need to be counseled, for which physician must be confident about the diagnosis. Mikulicz syndrome may present with involvement of parotids, lachrymal and other salivary glands. By itself, it is considered to be a benign condition, but at times it may be a part of an underlying chronic illness, such as tuberculosis, lymphoma or leukemia. Obviously, this child does not have such a disease.

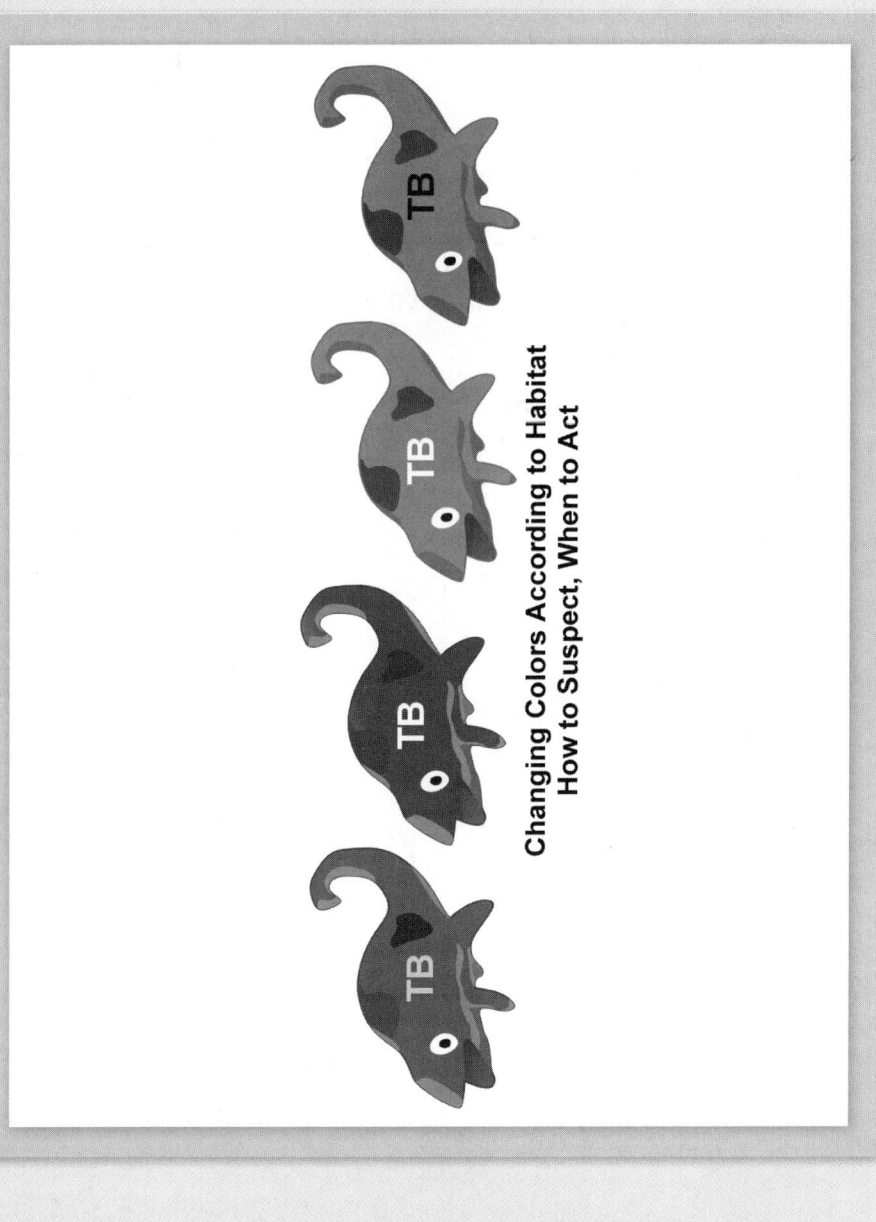

Changing Colors According to Habitat
How to Suspect, When to Act

SECTION 4

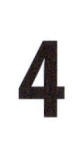

Vagaries in Tuberculosis

■ Host Chooses Pathology and Decides the Outcome

Individuals vary in their response to infection. Given the same infection, its manifestations may differ so widely amongst the population that there is no standard clinical presentation. This is because manifestations of every disease depend on tripartite interaction between the host, organism (or any trigger) and environment. Varied presentations depend upon the different types of pathological reactions that result from a given infection. Thus, at one extreme, the host may simply ignore the infection without suffering from clinical disease, while at the other extreme, the host may succumb to progressive disease. In between lies a wide spectrum of host responses, some of them favorable and others not so favorable. The final outcome of treatment also depends upon the host's ability to respond favorably. Thus, on one hand, even a correct compliant therapy of infection may not guarantee control or cure of the disease, while on the other hand, a clinical disease may get better without specific drug therapy. Therefore, it is obvious that it is the host response that chooses the pathology and decides the outcome.

Streptococcal infection is a classic example of varying host responses, with a resultant wide spectrum of clinical disease patterns. The following are the varied clinical manifestations met with in different hosts:

1. A subclinical infection without manifest disease
2. A typical clinical presentation with throat pain and fever
3. A typical clinical disease getting better without an antibiotic
4. A typical clinical disease getting better only after a specific antibiotic
5. A carrier state as a result of clinical or subclinical disease
6. A carrier state without treatment or in spite of it
7. A complicated disease, such as streptococcal-scalded skin syndrome
8. Postinfective immune complications, such as rheumatic fever and glomerulonephritis.

Science falls short of anticipating the clinical responses of a given host, as there are no parameters that can be assessed to evaluate host responses before, they actually occur. Apparently, all the hosts look similar even when their responses are so different. At best, we know whether the host is healthy or malnourished and immunocompetent or immunodeficient. However, the host immune responses vary a lot even in healthy immunocompetent individuals and also in the same individual at different times, based on the environment with varying exposures to organisms. We may at best detect the organism by relevant tests but we remain ignorant about the virulence of the organism and its sensitivity to antibiotics. While a majority of streptococcal disease is amenable to specific therapy and fatality is rare, sequelae do occur, though they can be further prevented by secondary prophylaxis with penicillin as in the case of rheumatic fever. In other words, the impact of our ignorance of host responses to streptococcal infection is comparatively harmless.

The same may not be true with all infections. When it comes to tuberculosis, the present era shows tremendous variations in this agent–host–environment interaction; no wonder, diagnosis and management becomes a big challenge for the treating physician. This section offers a glimpse into such variations with a discussion on actual cases.

Mycobacterium tuberculosis infection evokes a cascade of immune responses that result in different pathological lesions, with resultant varied clinical manifestations and outcome. It is mainly T-cell immune responses that decide the type of pathology. A B-cell antibody response does not play any significant role in the pathogenesis of tuberculosis. These antibodies are not protective either. At the height of the disease, the B-cell response is at its peak while the T-cell response is at its ebb. As the disease starts recovering, the T-cell response picks up and the B-cell response goes down. Though immune responses are too complex, it may be fair to simplify them for the purpose of easy understanding. However, it must be emphasized that such a simplification may be an exaggeration of simplicity and in reality; it may be much more complex. A T-cell response may be protective (which is equated to the acquisition of 'immunity') or destructive (which is that limb of immunity better known as hypersensitivity). While protective immunity prevents the spread of disease and helps to contain the disease, destructive immunity may lead to local damage that may not be totally reversible and may leave behind sequelae.

It is the relative balance/imbalance between hypersensitivity and immunity that results in varied presentations. The model of leprosy can be largely applied to tuberculosis as both mycobacterial infections share a common spectrum of immune responses.

Hypothetical Model of Immunopathology

Immunity (protective)	Tissue hypersensitivity (locally destructive)	Type of pathology
+++	–/+	Primary infection—no disease
++	+	Primary complex
++	++	Pleural effusion
+	+	Progressive primary complex
+	++	Acute cavitatory disease
+	+++	Fibrocaseous cavitatory disease
+/–	++/+	TBM
–	+/–	Disseminated TB
–	–	Miliary TB

It is evident from the above model that as protective immunity decreases, disease spreads from localized primary complex and pleural effusion to progressive primary complex and cavitatory lesions and further worsening immunity leads to dissemination of infection to distant parts of the body.

The most common test employed in the diagnosis of childhood tuberculosis is the tuberculin test that assesses tuberculin hypersensitivity in a host as indirect evidence of infection. It is clear from the above model that the tuberculin test is most likely to be positive in hosts who exhibit a strong hypersensitivity response, are fairly nourished, and present with acute onset disease. That is how it is always positive in cases of pleural effusion and isolated lymphadenopathy, and often so in cavitatory disease. In other situations, such as progressive primary complex, TBM and disseminated disease, the tuberculin test may or may not be positive, depending upon the age and nutrition of the host. Younger the age, more likely it is, to be negative. In miliary tuberculosis, the absence of a hypersensitivity response on the part of the host reflects in a negative tuberculin test. Thus, a tuberculin test has its own limitations in the diagnosis of TB disease.

It is evident that, if the host exhibits good immunity with or without acute hypersensitivity, the outcome is very favorable as in the case of primary complex and pleural effusions. In such cases, there is complete healing without any sequelae. On the other hand, if the host develops marked hypersensitivity with minimal immunity, as in cases of fibrocaseous cavitatory disease or TBM, the disease may be fatal, but if cured, is highly likely to leave behind permanent sequelae. However, if the host fails to mount either type of immune response, there exists the risk of death, if not intervened in time, but if treated optimally in time, there could be a cure without any sequelae (as is seen in miliary tuberculosis).

It is important to realize that while the host immune response is to some extent governed by its own innate ability, it also depends to a large extent, on the bacterial load. A high bacterial load suppresses immune responses and on successful therapy, this immune suppression is reversed. Occasionally, this reversal of immune suppression may result in a heightened response that may be temporarily harmful and may need proper intervention (cases 126, 127).

Changing Immune Status in Tuberculosis

It is interesting to note that the immune status of the host may change either for the better or for worse, depending upon whether the diagnosis was made early and whether proper treatment was available. Thus, the host may demonstrate a particular type of pathological response depending upon his immune status at that point in time, but if he remains untreated, immunity may get suppressed and he may go on to demonstrate another type of response. Further, with proper therapy, immune status would change again and pathological responses may also change accordingly. Thus, occasionally, one may find different types of pathological lesions resulting from different immune responses, all present at the same time in a host. In other words, one would be astonished to find, mediastinal lymphadenopathy (depicting good immunity) with cavitatory lesion (suggestive of a high degree of hypersensitivity) and also miliary lesions (indicative of poor immunity), **all at the same time, in one chest X-ray** (case 117).

However, what it really means is that these different responses occurred at different times, but stayed on, so that the physician found them all at one time.

Immune-mediated pathological lesions may be transient (e.g. phlycten, erythema nodosum, or small pleural effusion) and such lesions may disappear even without anti-TB treatment. However, they are indicative of an active focus somewhere else in the body that needs proper evaluation (case 119). A primary complex in a host with a favorable immune status may heal without specific treatment, as is seen in many healthy individuals. This is probably the reason why a few patients suffering from tuberculosis did get cured spontaneously, prior to the invention of anti-TB drugs.

Reactivation

It is important to realize that a healed lesion, with or without treatment, still continues to harbor a few dormant tubercle bacilli, that may reactivate under unfavorable situations. Such situations include adolescence, immune deficiency like HIV, severe infections like measles or whooping cough, and immunosuppressive therapy, such as steroid or chemotherapy for malignancy. Such reactivation disease manifests with pathologies that depict the adult type of responses due to pre-existing hypersensitivity. Therefore, they present with infiltrative or destructive disease, and not as lymphadenopathy, that is typical of the primary response of a host who was not previously sensitized. Reinfection represents a newly acquired infection, unrelated to the previously healed infection. However, since it occurs in a previously sensitized host, the pathological manifestations are similar to those in case of reactivation. Thus, it is clearly evident that a primary complex never recurs. If a child who has been successfully treated for a primary complex develops a reactivation or reinfection, a different type of pathological response will be seen viz. hypersensitivity response. This has been earlier referred to as an adult type of a response, but it does occur even in children.

Timetable for the Occurrence of Different Types of Pathologies

Several decades ago, in the 1950s, it was observed that a primary complex with enlarged mediastinal lymph nodes was a common presentation in childhood. Lesions related to such enlarged lymph nodes were commonly encountered, that included air leak syndromes such as subcutaneous emphysema, pneumothorax, pneumomediastinum and hydropneumothorax. Cavitatory tuberculosis was seen only in older children, commonly at adolescence. Urological and bone/joint tuberculosis was also seen in older children. This 'timetable' of yesteryears was based on the fact that exposure to tuberculosis occurred comparatively late in childhood. Over the years, this time table has become totally invalid. Those pathological lesions that were common in older children, are now seen even at younger ages. Thus, cavitatory disease and bone involvement is occasionally seen in infants. In fact in recent years, a large mediastinal lymph node demands a search for lymphoma (cases 110, 111). These changes are attributed to early exposure to tuberculosis and are further modified by a wide coverage of the BCG vaccine. The vaccine induces early sensitization that modifies the type of pathology seen (case 115).

Physical Signs

Physical signs in tuberculosis would then depend upon the type of pathology the host chooses to present with, which is further decided by the host immune response. Thus, a primary complex in the lungs may not produce any physical signs, because the small mediastinal lymph node is not detectable clinically, unless it causes pressure on the surrounding structures. An impaired note on percussion, bronchial breathing and crepitations in an area anatomically localized to a lobe, would suggest a pneumonia that may be the manifestation of a progressive primary complex. Occasionally, obstructive emphysema may be seen resulting from an enlarged mediastinal lymph node pressing over a bronchus (case 109). Rarely, such a mediastinal lymph node may cause segmental atelectasis, though it is difficult to diagnose clinically. Collapse— consolidation in tuberculosis is typically a pathological entity in which the collapse is not clinically evident. Cavitatory disease may be an acute manifestation (case 117) and if so, is not accompanied with fibrosis; such a cavity can heal completely on treatment without any sequelae. On the other hand, a chronic cavitatory lesion typically has a mediastinal shift and localized flattening with depression of the chest wall due to accompanying fibrosis, besides the signs of a cavity. A cavity is clinically detectable only if it is in communication with a patent bronchus, it is large enough and is superficially placed. Therefore, a cavity that is small or is deep seated, may not be detected on clinical examination. In such a case, fibrosis may be the only indirect evidence of existence of the cavity. A large pleural effusion of an acute onset is easy to diagnose clinically by its typical physical signs in the chest. However, a small pleural effusion seen in a partially immune child may present with localized signs posteriorly. In the absence of hypersensitivity, the pleural lesion is restricted to a 'dry pleuritis' without the development of an effusion. Therefore, it needs a careful clinical examination to pick up the small area of a pleural rub. Most of these pleural lesions are primarily the manifestations of a varying degree of hypersensitivity, but at times, the pleura may be involved by way of a direct extension of infection from the adjoining lung parenchyma, that results in the development of a tuberculous empyema. Physical signs do not differentiate it from an empyema caused by any other infecting agent and its diagnosis is possible only on laboratory tests. Miliary lesions hardly produce any physical signs except mild tachypnea. Hepatosplenomegaly may point to disseminated lesions without chest signs.

It is clear that physical signs denote pathology and not etiology. Therefore, the diagnosis of tuberculosis cannot be based on physical signs alone. It also depends upon circumstantial evidence of etiology, coupled with a correlation of the pathology that is anticipated, based on the immune status of the host.

TB meningitis may also have a wide spectrum of physical signs depending upon the host response. Typical disease presents with allergic encephalopathy (seizures) with basal exudates (meningeal signs, obstructive hydrocephalus and lower cranial nerve palsies), increased intracranial tension (boggy fontanelle and a large head), vasculitis and arterial infarcts (hemiplegia and basal ganglion involvement) and venous congestion (drowsiness). However, individual hosts may present with different pathological lesions depending on their immune response. Thus, one extreme presentation would simulate a viral encephalitis, while at the other end of the spectrum would be meningitis without encephalitis. In between, are placed varying combinations of meningeal and encephalitic involvement. At times, the disease may present with one type of manifestation at the onset, and may further evolve into another pattern, depending upon the changing immune status. Older child may initially present with symptoms of meningitis, such as headache and vomiting, and if not recognized and intervened, may go on to produce an encephalopathy and seizures. In such situations, the correct diagnosis evolves over time. In the absence of a typical presentation, the clinical diagnosis may be difficult. While TBM is always secondary to a primary pulmonary lesion, such a lesion is often not detectable. When TBM is a part of miliary tuberculosis, hepatosplenomegaly offers a clue to the diagnosis.

In such cases, CNS involvement is subtle, and the only evidence of involvement may be in the form of a mild abnormality in the CSF.

Amongst extrapulmonary lesions, isolated lymphadenitis is common. There may not always be classic physical signs (matted lymph nodes) suggestive of tuberculosis. Therefore, in case of a significant lymphadenopathy, irrespective of strong clinical judgment, fine needle aspiration cytology should ideally be carried out to confirm the diagnosis. The specimen thus obtained, should also be subjected to staining for acid fast bacilli. Rarely, hepatomegaly may be the only positive finding that offers a clue to the diagnosis of tuberculosis. There are no classical features of tuberculosis on clinical examination of the liver; therefore, the diagnosis may have to be proved on a liver biopsy which will show an infective granuloma.

It is clear from the discussion above that there are no standard, typical physical signs in a case of tuberculosis. The physical signs would change, if the disease worsens, as well as on recovery. Some of the signs may not improve for a long period, thereby indicating sequelae. Some of the sequelae may never disappear. In such patients, it is important to differentiate between the physical signs of activity and those due to sequelae.

Symptoms

Symptoms in tuberculosis mainly result from an immune interaction between the host and the bacteria. But there can also be symptoms that are directly attributable to the development of a structural lesion. **Fever** is induced by cytokine production and hence depends upon the immune status of the host. Thus, generally, younger the age and poorer the nutrition, lower the degree of fever. It is a misnomer that low grade fever with evening rise of temperature signifies tuberculosis. In fact, low grade fever due to any cause may be perceived by the patient only in the evening, due to the normal diurnal variation (physiological increase in the body temperature in the evening). Various patterns of fever are seen in this disease. In fact, the onset and the degree of fever also varies with the type of pathology. An acute onset of high fever is characteristic of a pleural effusion, in a healthy older child (case 112). Progressive primary complex usually presents with moderate fever for a few weeks, while fever in chronic cavitary tuberculosis is variable, but long-standing. The parents may sometimes fail to notice low grade fever. Miliary tuberculosis may even present without fever, especially in an infant. Since fever is an immune response, it may be variable over time, and is therefore, often reported as fever off and on, even without anti-TB therapy. If such a child is treated with antibiotics, one may get a false impression that the infection is nontuberculous, because the fever seems to respond.

But usually in such cases, the fever returns, at times, even while the patient is on antibiotic therapy. For example, an antibiotic trial for an undiagnosed pneumonia may result in a temporary improvement in fever; by itself, this is not against the diagnosis of tuberculosis. Such patients may have to be observed closely for any other symptoms that may denote active tuberculosis. Therefore, the term 'fever off and on' has been aptly described in tuberculosis. It may be of interest to note that on successful therapy, the fever generally abates over a couple of weeks in most of the patients. However, in a few, the fever may continue for a long time, almost to suggest failure of treatment. In these cases, though the fever continues, other parameters do show a definite improvement; this suggests the continuation of the immune response beyond the duration necessary, in spite of disease control (case 120). At times, such an exaggerated immune response may have to be suppressed by steroids. This clearly denotes that immune responses vary in terms of the time frame that they take to shut off, even after the disease is controlled.

Cough, if significant, denotes airway involvement. Pulmonary tuberculosis is primarily a lung parenchymal disease, as the inhaled bacilli get lodged in the lung parenchyma. Together with the enlarged draining lymph nodes, this results in a primary complex. The airway is rarely involved to an extent that it is clinically significant, unless a lymph node ruptures into the bronchial tree. Thus, endobronchial tuberculosis rarely manifests clinically, though it may be evident on bronchoscopy. Hence, *severe cough is not a significant symptom* in most cases of tuberculosis in children, quite contrary to popular belief. However, in the adult type of tuberculosis that is more destructive, cough is a predominant symptom. It is well-known that this adult type of tuberculosis may occasionally be seen in infants and young children also, though mostly it is seen in older children. Rarely, the airway may be compressed by an enlarging mediastinal lymph node and may result in a significant dry irritating cough. Finally, cough with a large amount of expectoration may be typically seen in bronchiectasis that is often a sequela of healed tuberculosis, though sometimes, the disease may be active in such a lesion.

Therefore, it is clear that severe cough is almost always not due to tuberculosis. It is a common mistake to search for tuberculosis in a child *presenting* with severe cough and especially when there are no other symptoms (cases 110, 111).

Loss of appetite is a very nonspecific symptom; there is hardly any disease with a good appetite. Any acute illness would lead to a loss of appetite, which should revert to the baseline once the disease is cured.

Parents of normal children also often complain that their children have a poor appetite. Usually toddlers are not interested in eating well as they are busy trying out their new achievements and they hate to sit and eat. Moreover, eating also depends upon ideal habits that parents often fail to inculcate. Many normal children who eat poorly maintain their weight profile, though they may not gain a lot of weight. Thus, a mere loss of appetite should not be a symptom to search for any disease. However, a recent change in appetite is significant, especially, if it is unexplained.

Loss of weight is recorded in any acute illness and the weight is gained back quickly once the disease is cured. It is the continued loss of weight over time, which may signify a chronic disease. In acute onset tuberculosis, obviously there is no loss of weight. A severely malnourished child may not lose weight due to his pre-existing negative nitrogen balance.

Not gaining weight is not the same as loss of weight, unless it has gone on for a long period. Many children are investigated for tuberculosis since they have not been gaining weight. After the first year, the average rate of growth slows down considerably. Therefore, it often appears that the child is not gaining weight, though it is not actually so. A common mistake is to disregard the 'scale error'; adult scales typically have a least count of one kilogram, and cannot record a difference that is less than that. If not gaining weight is the only symptom, it is not justified to investigate for tuberculosis. If this child really has tuberculosis, over time, either other symptoms/signs will appear or the child will actually lose weight, in which case further investigations are justified. On the other hand, it may so happen that no other symptoms appear and the complaint of not gaining weight is disproved over time. It is only in early infancy that not gaining weight over a month may be of significance, since infants are growing fast at that age, and no gain in weight over a month amounts to a loss of weight. Of course, every other cause must be ruled out, especially a feeding error. On successful treatment, in a child who had lost considerable weight, the weight gain is rapid in the first few weeks. Subsequently, it slows down to gradually reach the preinfection level. Naturally, a malnourished child who had never lost significant weight attributable to the disease, will not show a remarkable gain in weight. However, such a child improves on all other counts, and once the nutrition is also corrected, the gain in weight may be obvious.

Breathlessness is an uncommon symptom of tuberculosis. It is almost restricted to children with a large pleural effusion. Nowadays, tuberculosis rarely presents as a pneumothorax, though one did encounter pneumomediastinum and pneumothorax in the early 70s. This is because large mediastinal lymphadenopathy due to tuberculosis was more common a few decades ago, and that led to air leak syndromes. Nowadays, such presentations are uncommon, probably because sensitization to tuberculosis occurs early in life. Breathlessness is not a *complaint* in miliary disease in *young* children, though mild tachypnea is often a clue to such a lesion. However, slowly progressive interstitial miliary disease in older children may present with gradually developing breathlessness. Even bilateral pulmonary tuberculosis does not manifest with breathlessness, unless it is extensive.

Symptoms referable to any particular system that is affected would need a proper assessment.

History of TB Contact

Diagnosis of tuberculosis, especially in infants and young children, is strongly supported by a history of TB contact. However, it is important to define the contact correctly, in relevance to spread of infection. For this purpose, a contact is defined as an adult suffering from radiologically diagnosed pulmonary tuberculosis within the last two years. While not all pulmonary lesions are infectious, it may be safe to presume otherwise. Though in an individual situation, one may consider close observation without any drugs, such as an older child in contact with an adult with pleural effusion. Lesions such as cervical lymphadenitis in an adult may not be considered to be infectious. It may be prudent to confirm the reliability of the diagnosis made in an adult. A bacteriologically confirmed diagnosis in an adult has an added significance, in that one would also know the drug sensitivity to select appropriate drugs for the child patient.

Laboratory investigations in childhood tuberculosis provide only circumstantial evidence of disease. The gold standard is bacteriological diagnosis, which is difficult, though one must learn to attempt it more often. Gastric lavage may be easy to try out and may be as good as bronchoalveolar lavage. Ideally, multiple samples should be taken to increase the yield of AFB. Lymph node aspiration cytology is a good test whenever available and should be submitted for Z-N staining as well as histopathology.

Issues of tuberculin test are discussed above. It is a test of hypersensitivity and per se does not indicate active disease, nor does a negative test rule out the disease. However, this is the most common test employed in clinical practice in the diagnosis of childhood tuberculosis and hence some practical considerations are worth a discussion. The interpretation of the tuberculin test must take into consideration many factors, such as age, nutrition, immune status, type of pathology and the degree of induration. The younger the age, higher the reaction, more is the possibility of active disease. For the simplicity of clinical application, we suggest the following: Induration equal to or more than 10 mm is considered positive and needs to be interpreted to decide the probability of active disease. In children less than two years of age, a positive test should be taken as active disease. Between two and five years of age, in addition to the positive test, there should be symptoms which are likely to be related to tuberculosis. In children above five years of age, in addition to a positive test and related symptomatology, there should be physical signs suggestive of tuberculosis. The first group may be extended to five years of age if severely malnourished (grade 3 and 4 PEM), for the purpose of interpretation. Such an approach takes into consideration the age and nutrition, that indirectly decides the immune status. Besides these factors, the type of disease also demands a consideration in the interpretation of the tuberculin test. As discussed above, the tuberculin test is almost always positive in pleural effusion and lymphadenitis and if negative, the diagnosis of tuberculosis needs further confirmation. The test is negative in miliary tuberculosis. In tuberculin test negative tuberculosis, the test should become positive after 8 to 10 weeks of successful therapy. Such a reversal to a positive test confirms the diagnosis of tuberculosis retrospectively (cases 110, 111). Besides scientific issues regarding the interpretation of tuberculin test, there are many other technical issues that may upset correct interpretation. They include the source and the strength of tuberculin, the technique of performing the test and also the measurement of the induration. Such individual variations add to the confusion and limit correct interpretation. All such factors make the test less dependable, and hence the emphasis on pursuing a bacteriological diagnosis. The current view is to reserve the test for evaluating contacts of patients rather than using it to make a diagnosis per se. IGRA (Interferon gamma release assay) is also not reliable for diagnosis of tuberculosis as it shares the same limitations as tuberculin test. While culture facilities may not be available everywhere, it is the gold standard for diagnosis of tuberculosis. MGIT is used and results are available in one week. Obtaining samples in children for smear examination has its limitations; further, childhood tuberculosis being mostly paucibacillary, yield on smear is poor. However, smear examination is very much possible at every center and must be tried. For adults, smear examination is a good method of diagnosis. As mentioned above, if not a bronchoalveolar lavage, at least a gastric aspirate or a lymph node specimen is not difficult to obtain. It is just the 'culture' and the right attitude that would improve diagnostic ability.

Routine blood tests are useless and should not be a part of the diagnostic tests for tuberculosis. WBC counts are so variable in tuberculosis, that mere neutrophilic leukocytosis should not be considered as a point against the diagnosis of tuberculosis. A high white cell count with neutrophilic preponderance relates to the degree of inflammation, rather than acute bacterial infection, as it is also seen in allergic inflammation of any etiology. ESR is the least helpful in the diagnosis of tuberculosis as it is high in too many conditions. It is always considered to be of prognostic value but in tuberculosis, there are many other better parameters to monitor prognosis and ESR is rarely required. Only in cases of prolonged fever without a focus, a very high ESR (>100 mm) may suggest tuberculosis, malignancy, or collagen vascular disease.

Other blood tests include **serological tests**. They should never be ordered, and as of now, they have been banned. The reason is simple, clear and unambiguous. The organism *Mycobacterium tuberculosis* possesses multiple antigens, and at present science does not know which antigen denotes active natural infection. It is likely that the antigen depicting active infection may vary according to the site of disease. For example, in hepatitis B infection, we know exactly what each antigen and antibody denote in terms of recent or old infection, active or healed disease and the degree of infectivity. There exists no such knowledge about the serology of tuberculosis and hence, the tests that are available today are obsolete.

PCR is an extremely sensitive but sophisticated test and is not easy to carry out reliably. The test is highly technical and therefore depends upon the expertise of any given laboratory. Being very sensitive, contamination is likely to lead to a false positive result. A compartmentalized test, such as a positive PCR in CSF, may be useful in differentiating TBM from other causes of meningitis. In general, PCR should be carried out by a technically sound laboratory.

Cartridge-based Nucleic Acid Amplification Test (CBNAAT) is highly sensitive and specific for airway secretions collected as sputum, gastric aspirate or bronchoalveolar lavage but not so for other body fluids, such as pleural fluid or CSF. This test has an advantage of quick results in few hours and also gives rifampicin sensitivity pattern. This is the most promising test today and is available in India, though costly at present. However, this test is offered at highly subsidized rates by NGOs working in the field of tuberculosis.

Radiology depicts pathology more than etiology, though circumstantial evidence adds to the possibility of diagnosis of tuberculosis. Fibrocaseous cavitatory and miliary lesions are in favor of tuberculosis in our epidemiology. Detection of mediastinal lymphadenopathy is not easy, as such shadows may be mimicked by other structures, unless it is very large. However, large mediastinal lymph nodes may suggest other causes as well. Prominent hilar shadows are often wrongly considered to be synonymous with tuberculosis. Those shadows may not even represent enlarged lymph nodes. As the right hilar lymph nodes drain the entire right lung and also part of the left, the right hilum is often prominent due to a variety of insults that the lungs have been exposed to. However, left hilar prominence may be significant. An enlarged paratracheal lymph node may be mimicked by an apical segmental collapse of the right lung, or in infants by the thymus. A wide carinal angle may suggest enlarged subcarinal lymph nodes, though one needs perfect positioning and the right exposure to demonstrate it. An increase in the bronchovascular markings is a nonspecific finding; and so is 'pneumonitis'. It should not be considered to depict any definitive diagnosis. A **CT scan** is rarely required to diagnose pulmonary tuberculosis, in routine practice. In fact, when there is a doubt on the plain chest X-ray in the PA view, a lateral chest X-ray is useful for better anatomical localization (cases 110, 111). A decubitus lateral chest X-ray picks up even a small amount of pleural fluid collection. The CT scan may offer additional information about caseating lymph nodes that may favor the diagnosis of tuberculosis. However, radiological interpretation of caseation is subject to individual variations. **Ultrasound** examination of the chest is useful in picking up a small amount of pleural fluid. Abdominal USG is commonly asked for in a case of abdominal pain and the findings often reported include the presence of lymph nodes and some free fluid in the peritoneal cavity. Both are nonspecific findings and unless the nodes are large or the fluid considerable, they may not be given any importance. Abdominal tuberculosis presents with large multiple lymph nodes, and a lymphoma may be a close differential diagnosis.

CSF examination confirms meningitis but not the etiology. TBM presents with a variable pattern of abnormalities that may mimic pyogenic meningitis or encephalitis, and need careful interpretation, with due consideration to the clinical profile and other supportive tests. Similarly, improvement should not be judged only by CSF changes.

Liver biopsy is indicated in a suspected case of disseminated infection where the etiology cannot be proved otherwise, because of a lack of access to any such tissue. It is also indicated in cases of PUO, where no other foci are visible, and no other cause of the fever can be ascertained. In earlier days, when the chest X-ray was negative, miliary TB was diagnosed through a liver biopsy; with the advent of the CT scan, this is rarely needed.

In conclusion, diagnosis of tuberculosis is a challenge. Symptoms and physical signs depend so much on the immune status of the host, that one is faced with a diversity of clinical presentations. Routine laboratory tests are of limited value in confirming the diagnosis. Further, the response to therapy may also be so varied that the clinician should be aware of all such vagaries, so as to offer a correct opinion. In other words, a standard textbook presentation of tuberculosis is good for beginners/undergraduate students to get acquainted with the basics. But for postgraduates and practitioners, greater insights are necessary, as our patients do not seem to read our textbooks before presenting to us!

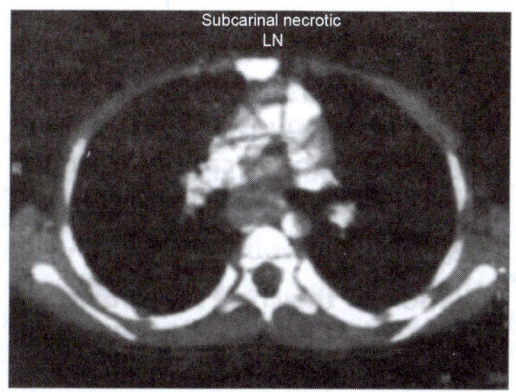

Subcarinal necrotic lymph node.

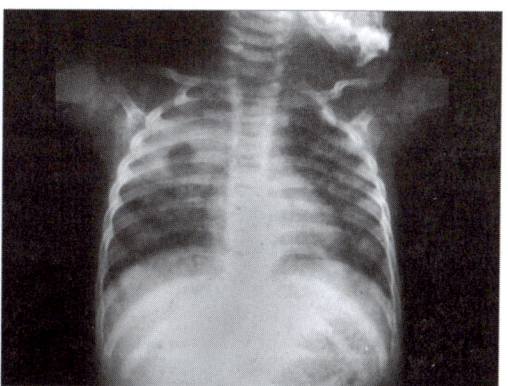

Cavitatory lesion in infancy.

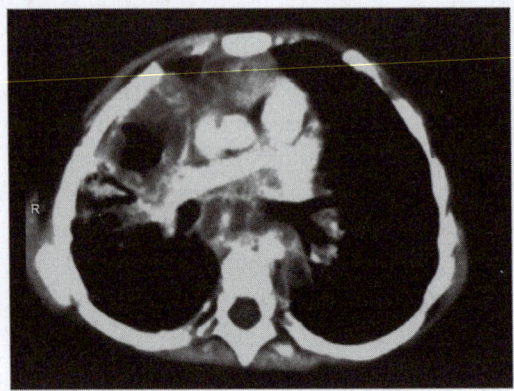
CT scan showing cavitatory lesion.

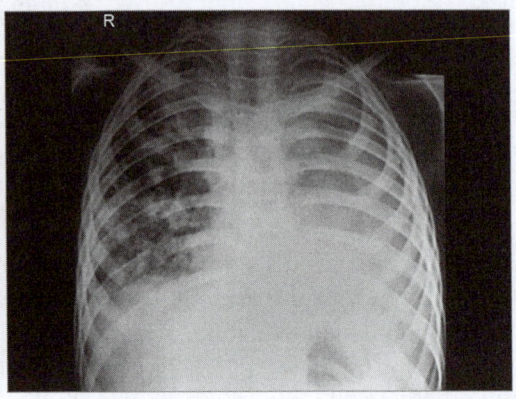
Cavity with pleural effusion on both sides.

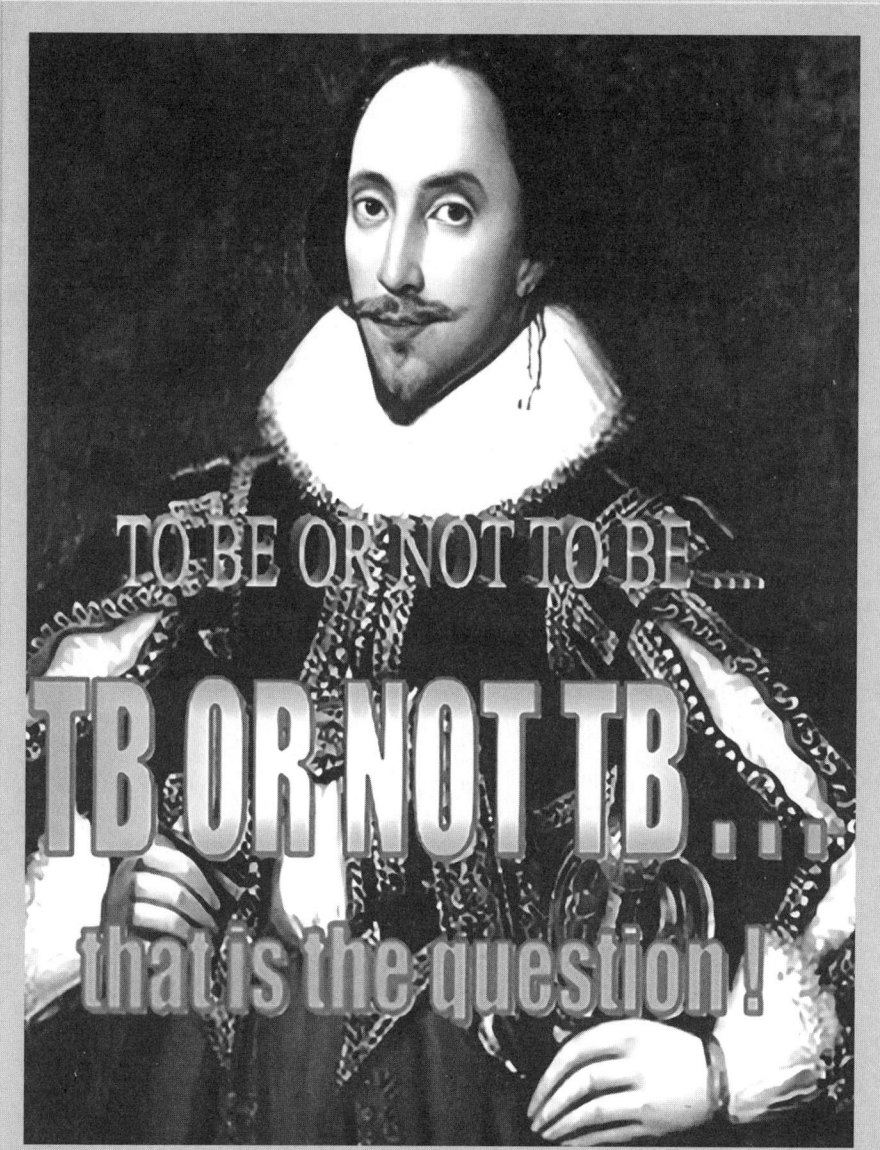

CASE 109

Lobar Emphysema as a Presentation of Large Mediastinal Lymph Node

History

A 3-month-old infant presented with a gradual onset of breathlessness over the last one month. He was born after a normal pregnancy and delivery and was apparently well for the first two months. There was no other significant history. He had gained average weight.

Analysis

This could be a *congenital heart disease;* since cyanosis has not been noticed and complained of it is less likely to be a cyanotic heart disease. Amongst acyanotic defects, it is likely to be a moderately large *ventricular septal defect*. Though *congenital lobar emphysema* commonly presents with breathlessness shortly after birth and is then rapidly progressive, it is known that symptoms can begin anytime up to six months of age. *Congenital diaphragmatic hernia* would either present at birth with respiratory distress or would present anytime thereafter but would not present with breathlessness that is progressive over one month. A *neuromuscular disease* like spinal muscular atrophy could present with progressive breathlessness, but usually the presenting feature would be paucity of limb movements, and only as the disease worsens, respiratory muscle paralysis would be evident. Metabolic acidosis like RTA or inborn errors of metabolism are unlikely because usually, failure to thrive is a striking feature before the infant can present with tachypnea, which is mistakenly called 'breathlessness'.

Physical Examination

Fairly built	*Poorly nourished*	*Generally comfortable*
Weight 4.5 kg	Length 60 cm	Head circumference 39 cm
Temperature normal Peripheral pulses well felt	Heart rate 100/min No cyanosis	Respiratory rate 40/min

Respiratory System

- Hyperresonant note on percussion on left side of chest anteriorly all over
- Markedly diminished breath sounds in the same area
- No foreign sounds
- Other systems normal
- Chest X-ray showed emphysema of the left upper lobe with herniation of the lung on the opposite side.

Analysis

The clinical and radiological findings were consistent with a diagnosis of congenital lobar emphysema. Usually, one would have expected the symptoms to have come up at birth, though on repeated enquiry, the mother was confident that she had noticed the breathlessness only after the age of two months. Therefore, it was almost believed that the mother was wrong, and the infant may have been slightly breathless earlier, but was not noticed. In fact, even if the mother was right and the infant was normal up to two months of age, it meant that he was compensated in the first two months and then started decompensating slowly. This is not against the diagnosis of congenital lobar emphysema, since a few patients may not present at birth, but a little later, in early infancy.

Further Course

This child was taken up for surgery. The left upper lobe was emphysematous as diagnosed clinically and radiologically, but under the emphysematous lobe was hidden a large lymph node that was compressing the left upper lobe bronchus and was the cause of the emphysema. The lymph node was confirmed to be tuberculous on histopathology. A Mantoux test done after the surgery was positive.

Retrospectively, the mother's version that the infant was normal till the end of the second month was correct. This infant must have come in contact with a tuberculous patient probably at the maternity home, since the family screening did not reveal any family member to be suffering from tuberculosis.

Lessons Learnt

This infant had no fever, cough or loss of weight and presented only with pressure signs more than symptoms. This case demonstrates that tuberculosis may present with physical signs without symptoms suggestive of infection, especially in an early phase of the disease, in a breastfed healthy infant. It also proves the fact that a chest X-ray may miss the presence of mediastinal lymphadenopathy. This case has also emphasized that the mother's observations are mostly correct.

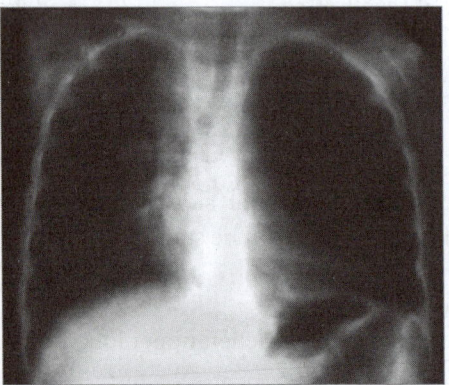

Lobar emphysema—left upper lobe.

CASE 110

■ Missed Mediastinal Lymph Node Enlargement on Routine Chest X-ray

Events...

A 2-year-old child presented with fever for three weeks. Fever was mild-to-moderate and there were no other symptoms. Physical examination did not reveal any localizing signs. Routine investigations were within normal limits. Tuberculin test was negative. Empirical antibiotic trial had failed. Repeat investigations also did not offer any clue. Finally, a CT scan of the chest was ordered that showed mediastinal lymphadenopathy. A trial with anti-TB therapy was considered on the basis of a subacute presentation of a probable infection. At the end of two weeks of treatment, the child recovered and was afebrile. After two months of treatment, the tuberculin test was repeated; it was positive.

Experience gained...

In any undiagnosed fever of significant duration, even if there are no localizing symptoms or signs referable to the chest, it may be justified to look for a possible hidden lesion due to tuberculosis; such a lesion is likely to be picked up on a CT scan. Mediastinal lymphadenopathy and miliary lesions may be easily missed on plain chest X-rays.

Clinically, mediastinal lymphadenopathy can have many different presentations. It may be asymptomatic, or present with only fever as in this case or only cough as in the next case or as hyperinflation as in the first case. Of course, mediastinal lymphadenopathy is not synonymous with tuberculosis and may also be caused by lymphoma or sarcoidosis. Hepatosplenomegaly may offer a clue to the presence of miliary lesions. Negative tuberculin test (as a result of immune suppression) may be compatible with the diagnosis of active tuberculosis. In such cases, at the end of two or three months of successful therapy, the bacterial load reduces leading to immunologic recovery. This, in turn, reverts the negative tuberculin test to a positive reaction. Thus, the restoration of immune competence on successful therapy as depicted by a positive tuberculin test, can be used as a retrospective proof of correct diagnosis.

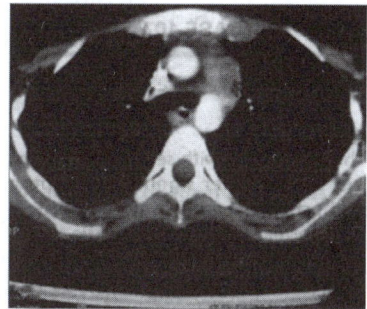

Mediastinal lymphadenopathy on CT scan.

CASE 111

Missed Mediastinal Lymph Node Enlargement on Routine Chest X-ray

History
A 9-year-old child presented with severe hacking cough for the last two months, without fever or any other significant symptoms. The cough was disturbing his sleep and activity. There was no past history of cough. Physical examination was within normal limits. Symptomatic therapy did not help. He underwent routine investigations including a chest X-ray that did not reveal any abnormality. Since the tuberculin test was positive, a trial with anti-TB therapy was attempted. However, even at the end of a month of compliant treatment, there was no relief in symptoms. This prompted further investigations. A repeat chest X-ray showed a suspicious shadow that could have been a mediastinal lymph node. A lateral X-ray of the chest also suggested the same.

Analysis
Prominent cough is an uncommon symptom of TB. Isolated cough is further unusual. A significant cough is a symptom of airway disease, and the airway can be involved in tuberculosis either in the form of compression by a large mediastinal lymph node or as in **endobronchial TB.** Clinically, endobronchial TB would present as tuberculous pneumonia, i.e., there would be the general symptoms of tuberculosis and signs of a tuberculous pneumonia, with cough as an added symptom. It is only on investigation (bronchoscopy) that the endobronchial element would be revealed. Therefore, endobronchial TB is a pathological diagnosis, and cough is not usually the only or major presenting complaint. A severe cough can also be a feature of **tuberculous bronchiectasis**; however, there will be copious expectoration and lots of other symptoms and signs. **Pertussis** can be considered, but it is unusual that the cough has not reduced after 4–6 weeks of its onset. It is unlikely to be **hyperreactive airway disease** because there is no past history of cough. Though a **foreign body** can be associated with a severe cough, one expects to get the history of the initiating event at this age. **Habit cough** is a possibility though it is unlikely to be so disturbing.

Further Course
CT scan of the chest demonstrated a large retrocardiac lymph node that was proved to be Hodgkin's lymphoma.

Comment
In this case, the diagnosis of tuberculosis was based on an unusual presenting symptom and supported by flimsy laboratory evidence. After the age of five years, a diagnosis of tuberculosis should not be made on the basis of Mantoux positivity and symptoms alone; it has to be backed by appropriate clinical signs. In this case, one would have probably pursued the diagnosis of psychogenic cough initially, but later since the severe cough persisted, one would have proceeded with other investigations like CT scan and/or bronchoscopy.

Over the years, there seems to be a change in the epidemiology of tuberculosis, such that large mediastinal lymphadenopathy, which often used to be tuberculous in the past, is now more likely to be nontuberculous. However, Hodgkin's lymphoma may at times be associated with tuberculosis. Hence, a search for a dual pathology becomes mandatory. However, this can be tricky, especially in a child with a positive tuberculin test. Typically, children with Hodgkin's lymphoma are immunosuppressed and are therefore tuberculin negative. However, in those cases with a favorable prognosis who may not be immunosuppressed, the tuberculin test may be positive. Clinically, when a child is being evaluated for lymphadenopathy, if he is tuberculin negative, one is likely to investigate further and probably not miss the lymphoma. However, if he is tuberculin positive, one may first diagnose tuberculosis, and go ahead and start treating. In either situation, it is only, if the child fails to respond, or responds partially, or worsens after an initial response, that the second coexisting pathology is likely to be suspected/investigated for. Therefore, it is always advisable to go for a FNAC, if the node is accessible; at times, excision biopsy may be the only answer.

Lessons Learnt

Severe cough is not a common symptom of tuberculosis except in the presence of airway compression. This case again emphasizes the fact that an enlarged mediastinal lymph node may be easily missed on a plain chest X-ray. Also, a positive tuberculin test may not be taken as proof of tuberculosis, in a case of significant lymphadenopathy, unless there is histopathological support.

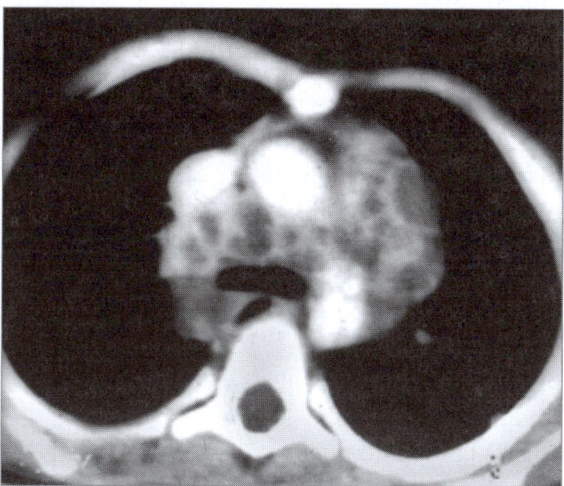

Mediastinal lymph node picked up on CT scan.

CASE 112

■ Acute Onset Pleural Effusion that was TB

Events…

A 10-year-old healthy child presented with an acute onset of high fever one evening, followed by an acute onset of breathlessness within the next 12 hours. He was found to have physical signs of a pleural effusion, which was confirmed by a chest X-ray. Due to neutrophilic leukocytosis in the peripheral blood and the pleural fluid that was aspirated, he was treated as a case of empyema with continuous intercostal drainage and IV antibiotics. Since there was no response to therapy, it was considered to be a drug-resistant empyema and the antibiotics were changed. This was typically a *tuberculous effusion* that responded well to anti-TB therapy. The tuberculin test was strongly positive.

Explanation…

Neutrophilic leukocytosis in peripheral blood and for that matter, even in pleural fluid, is not synonymous with acute bacterial infection. Any acute pathology, be it an infection or an acute noninfective immune-mediated inflammation, elicits a neutrophilic response. In tuberculosis, pleural effusion is an acute allergic inflammation, especially in a healthy child, and may manifest with a neutrophilic response. Pleural effusion is a manifestation of good immunity and hypersensitivity, and hence the tuberculin test is always positive. In fact, a negative test in a case of pleural effusion may prompt one to search for a nontuberculous disease or consider whether technical errors could explain such a test result.

Experience gained…

Tuberculosis as a disease, is traditionally associated with a subacute or chronic clinical presentation. A pleural effusion in a healthy child is one example of an acute presentation. In general, the larger the effusion, more acute the onset; similarly, healthier the child, more acute the onset.

Another example is that of a small infant in whom TB meningitis can sometimes present acutely. However, in such cases, it is the neurological manifestations that are acute; the symptoms of tuberculosis itself (like low-grade fever, irritability, etc.) are not acute, but often subtle, and therefore overlooked.

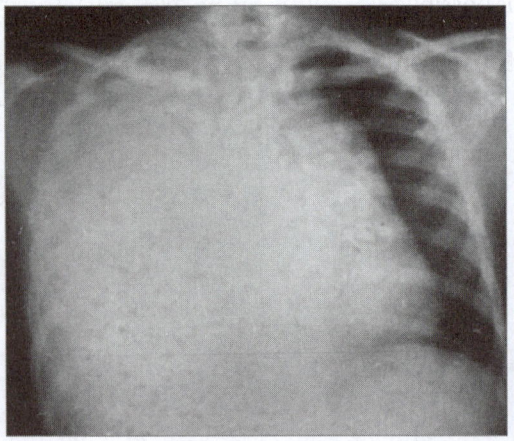

Massive pleural effusion.

CASE 113

■ Localized Pleural Effusion
Events…
An 8-year-old undernourished child presented with low-grade fever off and on for a month. There were no other significant symptoms. Empirical antibiotic therapy had failed. Routine hemogram was normal. Chest X-ray showed a dense haziness on the right lower part of the lung field, which did not correlate with either a lobar or a pleural distribution and hence was considered to be a mediastinal mass. However, a CT scan revealed a **localized pleural effusion**, which was tapped under CT guidance. It suggested tuberculosis and on anti-TB therapy, the child improved. This child had a negative tuberculin test to begin with, that reverted to a positive reaction after three months of therapy.

Explanation…
This child must have started with a small peripheral lung lesion adjacent to the pleura. By virtue of being an 8-year-old, he is likely to have had a previous exposure to tuberculosis. Therefore, he must have developed partial immunity by now. However, due to his undernourished state, he did not elicit a strong allergic pleural response which he would have otherwise elicited had he been a healthy child. In other words, due to his state of partial immunity and hypersensitivity, he mounted a weak allergic pleural reaction which resulted in a low-grade chronic illness. TB effusion in children is a disease with a low bacterial load. Nevertheless, clearance of an effusion probably depends on the stage at which treatment is instituted. In a healthy child, since the presentation is acute, treatment is instituted early; therefore, he clears up completely. On the other hand, this child, being undernourished, presented late as a chronic illness and therefore got onto treatment late. It is natural for the body to try and localize any persistent pathology that it fails to clear, and thereby limit it. This is possibly why a localized pleural effusion developed in this situation.

Experience gained…

> Pleural disease in tuberculosis may present with different types of pathology, depending upon the immune status of the host and the bacterial load. A good immunity in a healthy older child with a low bacterial load, results in a classical large acute onset pleural effusion. A weak allergic response in a not so healthy older child with a low bacterial load leads to dry pleuritis without effusion. In between these two extremes, is the older child who may develop a small or localized pleural effusion. In the case of a high bacterial load in an older child, the infection spreads by direct extension to the pleural cavity and produces an empyema. Thus, this is not an allergic response but a direct bacterial invasion from an adjacent tuberculous pneumonia, as demonstrated in the next case. Rarely, tuberculosis may present with bilateral pleural effusions, as demonstrated in another case. It is worth noting that pleural tuberculosis is a disease of older children, as young children are usually unable to mount an allergic response, and therefore, they are at a risk of the disease spreading. In fact, one should hesitate to diagnose a tuberculous pleural effusion in children younger than five years of age.

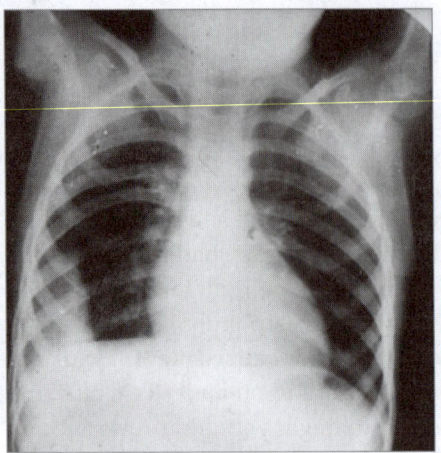
Encysted pleural effusion.

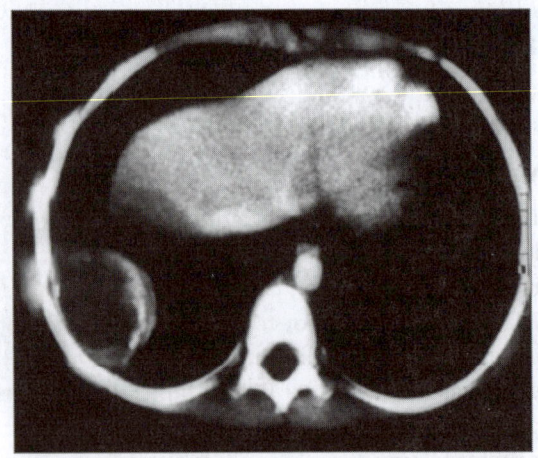
Encysted pleural effusion confirmed on CT scan.

CASE 114

■ Tuberculous Empyema

Events...

An 8-year-old child presented with fever for a month, and chest pain that started within a few days of the onset of fever but got relieved a week after starting antibiotics. A pneumonia was diagnosed, and he was treated accordingly. As the fever did not subside, he was reinvestigated. CBC showed a mild neutrophilic leukocytosis, and the repeat chest X-ray showed a pleural fluid collection, with an underlying pneumonia. The pleural cavity was drained, and the antibiotics changed. The pleural fluid was an exudate with neutrophilic preponderance; Gram stain and culture were negative. As there was still no response to the changed antibiotics, he was referred for further management.

Considering it to be an unresponsive empyema, probably due to inadequate drainage, a sonography was carried out, which confirmed the presence of multiloculated thick fluid with septae. He was subjected to an endoscopy to clean up the pleural cavity; the pleural biopsy showed tuberculosis. Tuberculin test done thereafter was positive.

Explanation...

So this was a case of **tuberculous empyema**. It is rare and difficult to diagnose clinically. Probably the most common reason for an empyema to be unresponsive to treatment, is failure to drain at all, or failure to drain adequately. There may be subtle clues to suggest the diagnosis of tuberculous empyema, such as the relatively 'slow' development of pneumonia/empyema, or the fact that though the child does not improve on proper treatment, he does not deteriorate either. Even then, as in this case, it may not be wrong to continue toeing the line of a bacterial empyema and ensure adequate drainage; the diagnosis of tuberculous empyema is usually stumbled upon.

Experience gained...

A pleural effusion due to tuberculosis is an allergic reaction to a small subpleural focus of infection, in which the parenchymal disease is not evident clinically nor radiologically. The clinical presentation is that of the pleural effusion only. Unlike this, in tuberculous empyema, it is an extension of infection from tuberculous pneumonia, in which the primary clinical presentation is that of the pneumonia, which then complicates into an empyema. It closely simulates an acute bacterial pneumonia with an empyema, except for the fact that it develops rather subacutely and its progress is slow, i.e., there is no significant deterioration over a few days. However, the diagnosis of tuberculous empyema totally rests on bacteriology and/or histopathology of the tissue or fluid obtained. Therefore, this case illustrates the need to attempt an etiological diagnosis—at least in every case of a subacute or chronic infection. Though ideally of course, it should be attempted in every case of infection.

In the above case of tuberculous empyema, one would have found AFB, if one would have looked for it. As against this, in a case of allergic tuberculous pleural effusion, one is unlikely to find AFB.

CASE 115

■ Bilateral Pleural Effusion

Events...

A 6-year-old child presented with low-grade fever and mild cough for the last two weeks. The child had already been treated with amoxicillin—clavulanic acid without any relief. Physical examination showed an impaired note in the subscapular region on the left side of the chest, with diminished breath sounds and occasional crepitations. The chest X-ray revealed pneumonia with an obliteration of the costophrenic angle. Considering it to be a subacute infection, a diagnosis of atypical pneumonia was considered, and a macrolide was prescribed. It did not help, so the child was investigated further. The tuberculin test was weakly positive. A repeat chest X-ray showed bilateral pleural effusions, with atelectasis of a few segments of the left lower lobe. There was no pneumonia. This prompted a consideration of tuberculosis. The child improved on anti-TB treatment and the diagnosis was retrospectively proved with a reversal of the initial negative reaction, to a positive tuberculin response.

Explanation...

What was unusual in this child was **bilateral pleural effusions**, though they are known to occur in adults. This child might have probably developed a small Ghon's focus (peripheral pleuroparenchymal lesion) on both sides. These foci elicited a weak allergic pleural response due to mild hypersensitivity, but as the child was reasonably immune, the disease did not spread to other parts of the lung or other systems but remained localized to the pleural cavity. On the other hand, the focus could be unilateral but the allergic response could be bilateral. It is well-known that a focus of tuberculous infection can elicit an allergic response at a distant site in the body; common examples being the development of erythema nodosum or phlyctenular conjunctivitis. The initial physical signs that were thought to represent pneumonia, were probably due to atelectasis of a part of the lower lobe. This was deemed to be an absorption atelectasis due to pressure exerted by the pleural fluid.

Experience gained...

> This case demonstrates how, at times, children can present with a pathology that is quite uncharacteristic of the usual clinical profile of tuberculosis. Similar examples of other unusual pathologies have been discussed elsewhere. The exact genesis of such unusual pathologies is not clear, though one of the possible contributing factors could be that these children have been sensitized to tuberculosis rather early in life, and therefore their responses are unusual. Such an early sensitization may either be due to exposure to natural disease or may even be due to BCG vaccine. It is well-recognized that manifestations of tuberculosis are modified to some extent in BCG-vaccinated children.
>
> This case also illustrates that in a respiratory disease, different pathologies may simulate one another, due to similar physical signs; thus, atelectasis, consolidation and cavity can be easily mistaken one for the other.

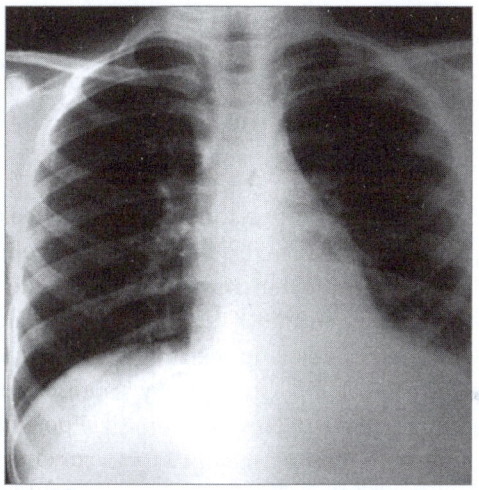
Lower lobe pneumonia on left side.

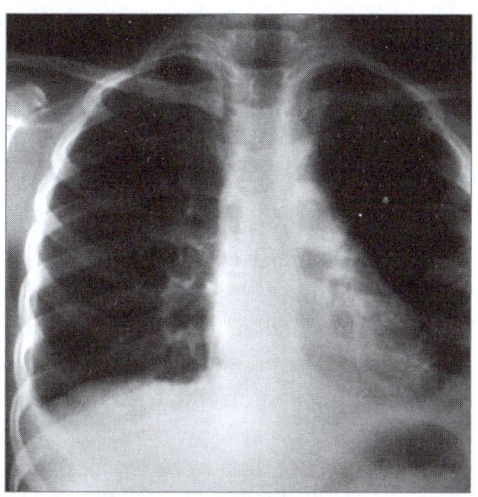
Bilateral pleural effusion.

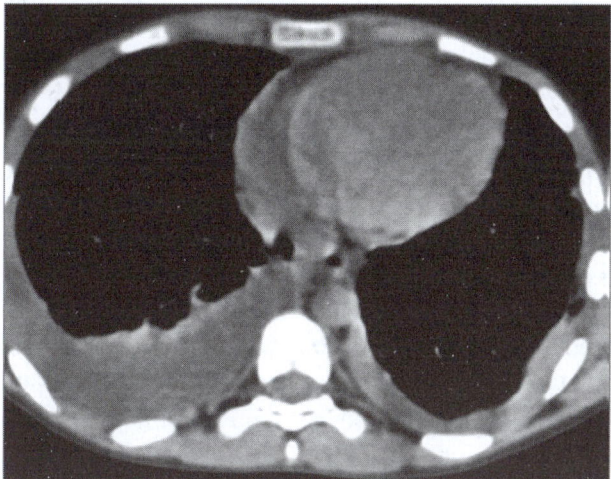
Bilateral pleural effusion confirmed on CT scan.

CASE 116

■ Subacute Pneumonia Missed as Acute Bacterial Pneumonia

Events...

A 6-year-old child presented with fever and mild cough for last one month. His illness started with an acute onset of high fever that was initially treated symptomatically with paracetamol. After four days, since there was no response, he was investigated and was found to have mild neutrophilic leukocytosis though his chest X-ray was normal. Considering it to be an acute bacterial infection, he was put on amoxicillin. After five days of this antibiotic therapy, his investigations were repeated. They once again revealed a neutrophilic leukocytosis, but this time, the chest X-ray revealed an upper lobe haziness. This prompted a change in antibiotics (considering it to be a amoxicillin-resistant pneumonia), and IV Cefotaxime was tried. After a week of further IV antibiotics, as there was still no response in the fever, a needle aspiration of the pneumonia was performed, which led to the growth of *Staphylococcus epidermidis* sensitive to all antibiotics. This led to the decision of trying vancomycin, which also failed. At this juncture, a CT scan revealed a caseating pneumonia with an enlarged lymph node. The diagnosis of tuberculosis was made, and the child improved on anti-TB therapy.

Explanation...

It is due to the mild neutrophilic leukocytosis that this child was mistakenly diagnosed as acute bacterial pneumonia, though it is clear that he developed the pneumonia over ten days (his first chest X-ray was normal). Community acquired bacterial pneumonia presents acutely and the diagnosis is confirmed radiologically early in the course of illness. Subsequently, *Staphylococcus epidermidis* was grown probably secondary to skin contamination; however, it was wrongly considered to be the cause of the pneumonia. Further on, though the antibiogram suggested that the isolated organisms were sensitive to all antibiotics, vancomycin was tried, which is usually reserved for MRSA.

Experience gained...

> This case emphasizes how the diagnosis of tuberculosis must take into account the onset of the clinical presentation of a given pathology. Tuberculous pneumonia does not present acutely. In tuberculosis, what can present acutely with a sudden onset of fever, is a pleural effusion in a healthy child as demonstrated in another case.

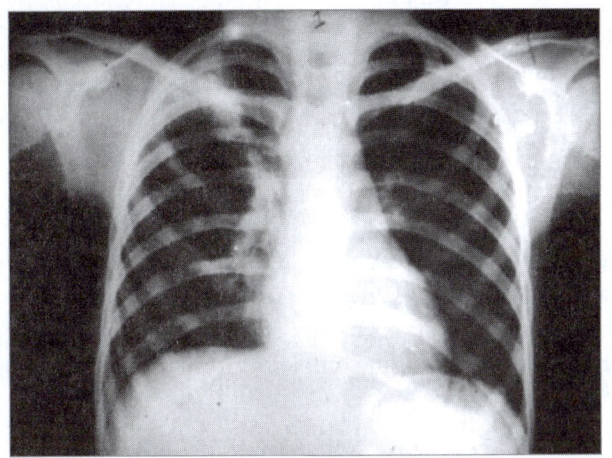
Suspicious lesion in right upper zone.

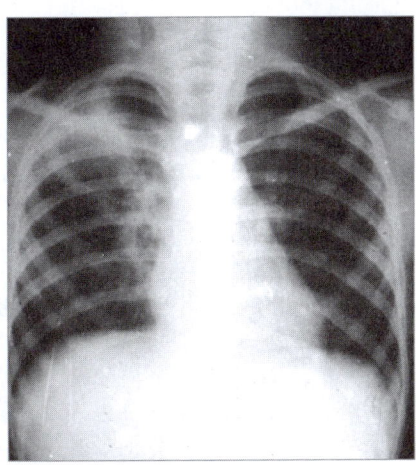
Evolving right upper lobe pneumonia.

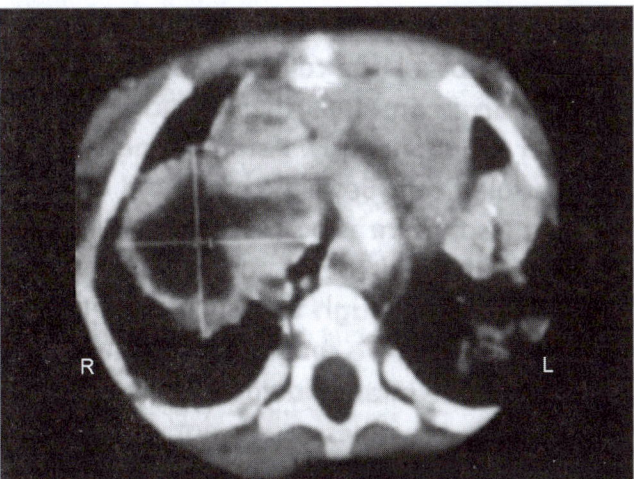
CT scan showing large lymph node with caseation.

CASE 117

Mediastinal Lymph Node, Cavity and Miliary Lesion in Same Child at a Time

History

A 6-month-old infant presented with a history of severe cough for the last six weeks. He had also developed mild breathlessness gradually over the last two weeks, and mild fever for the last one week. He was apparently alright till these symptoms began. He has not gained weight well over the last two months. There was no history of similar complaints from other members of the family, or any past or family history of atopy.

Analysis

This infant's initial and predominant symptom was cough, which indicated that this was an airway disease. Over time, this infant developed breathlessness and fever suggesting that the disease was slowly progressive. It could be either a primary *respiratory* or a *cardiac* disease. *Aspiration* syndromes or inhaled *foreign body* are the common airway disorders seen at this age; they present acutely and do not progress in the above manner, hence unlikely. Both these conditions may present with severe cough and the cough may be persistent, but it does not lead to a slowly developing breathlessness. When they do present with breathlessness (as in aspiration pneumonia or a large collapse/secondary infection in a foreign body), it is of a relatively acute onset. Further, in such a situation the infant may also run significant fever simultaneously. *Asthma* is never diagnosed at this age unless other causes are ruled out. Besides, cough and breathlessness in asthma is an episodic event, and also, there is no personal or family history of atopy in this infant. *Pertussis* or pertussoid cough due to *adenoviral infection* presents with such a severe, persistent cough but such infants are breathless only immediately after the bouts of severe cough or when there is a complication like a pneumonia (in which case, the infant would be quite sick). Thus, while cough in pertussis may be progressive, breathlessness is not. *Cystic fibrosis* is also known to present with chronic cough, but it generally manifests as an acute onset febrile illness with pneumonia. Other causes of airway disease could be external compression by a *mass lesion*. Therefore, a slowly progressive *mediastinal tumor*, including a *lymphadenopathy*, may be a possibility. However, it is unlikely to result in breathlessness. A *left to right shunt* may initially present with cough, and breathlessness may follow. The subsequent development of breathlessness may suggest increasing pulmonary congestion due to the left to right shunt resulting in pulmonary edema. However, in this infant, the severity of the cough seemed disproportionate to the subsequent mild breathlessness. Further, such infants are usually not well even prior to the onset of these symptoms; this infant was reported to be normal. Of course, prior to the development of cough, the symptoms could have been mild and easily overlooked by the parents. Therefore, though this history does not unequivocally suggest a left to right shunt, it cannot be ruled out either.

Mild breathlessness developing slowly in a respiratory condition may suggest **interstitial lung disease**; however, severe cough is not the presenting symptom of primary interstitial lung disease. Similarly, as discussed above, airway diseases do present with significant cough, but are unlikely to result in breathlessness after a month, *unless there has been an extension of the original airway disease into the interstitium*. It is only an infection or infiltration that can spread to the interstitium. Therefore, from amongst the conditions discussed above, the differential diagnosis may narrow down to an **adenoviral** infection with interstitial pneumonia or **lymphadenopathy** due to tuberculosis or sarcoidosis (in tuberculosis, interstitial involvement is known in the form of miliary, and sarcoidosis is also known to involve the interstitium).

Physical Examination

Poorly built poorly nourished	Generally comfortable	
Weight 4.5 kg	Length 65 cm	Head circumference 41 cm
Temperature normal	Heart rate 100/min	Respiratory rate 40/min
No lymphadenopathy		Bones and joints normal
Respiratory system		
Bronchial breathing localized to left mid zone		
Scattered crepitations all over		
Liver span 7 cm	Liver 10 cm +, firm	Spleen 3 cm +
Other systems normal		

Analysis

This child is severely malnourished and hence has a chronic progressive disease. It is obviously a generalized respiratory disease. Scattered crepitations suggest an interstitial involvement or a generalized airway disease, though at this age, generalized airway disease is more likely to present with rhonchi rather than crepitations. Bronchial breathing suggests a consolidation, collapse, or cavity, and therefore, parenchymal involvement. While such an involvement is known in airway disease in the form of a localized area of collapse (due to obstruction by a thick mucus plug), it is unlikely in interstitial lung disease. So, this may be a collapse accompanying an airway disease. Thus, this child has an **unusual combination—** *probable airway disease* as suggested primarily by the history and partly supported by physical signs, *definite parenchymal* involvement denoted by bronchial breath sounds and *probable interstitial disease* as depicted by mild breathlessness and generalized crepitations. A combination of airway and parenchymal disease is known in **cystic fibrosis**, but not interstitial involvement.

The presence of hepatosplenomegaly suggests dissemination of the disease beyond the lung. Therefore, it is likely to be an infective or infiltrative disease, such as **miliary TB** or **sarcoidosis**. Not only is sarcoidosis rare in infants, its classical triad of clinical presentation consists of hepatosplenomegaly, arthritis and uveitis. Further, at this age, accompanying pulmonary involvement is rare in sarcoidosis. Even, if we consider miliary tuberculosis, cough is not a feature to start with, nor is a localized lung parenchymal lesion (as suggested on this infant's physical examination) known.

So at this stage, there is no clear definition of this disease on analysis of the history and physical examination.

Further Course

Chest X-ray showed miliary lesions with enlarged mediastinal lymph node and a cavity. Bronchoalveolar lavage demonstrated AFB. The Mantoux test was negative. The CSF was normal.

Incidentally, the patient also had another chest X-ray that was dated four weeks back, which showed a suspicious right paratracheal shadow. However, at that time it was passed off as a thymic shadow and hence, not evaluated further.

Analysis and Comment

This infant demonstrated multiple types of lesions signifying different types of immune responses. Miliary lesions with hepatosplenomegaly represent immune suppression, lymphadenopathy denotes immune competence and cavity suggests destructive hypersensitivity. Such a combination is indicative of the varying immune status of the patient at different times, as the disease progressed. To begin with, this infant must have had a good immune status when he first contracted his infection. So he developed a lymphadenopathy, which compressed on the airways leading to significant cough. Over time, he developed hypersensitivity, which resulted in the formation of an acute cavity. By then, the infective load must have worsened, resulting in immune suppression, which led to disseminated lesions. Even though the immune status was thus changing over time, those pathological lesions that had developed early in the course of the illness (depending upon the immune status prevailing then), continued to exist. Thus, this infant actually presented with symptoms and physical signs that would not fit in the usual case of tuberculosis but was confirmed to be so.

Lessons Learnt

Different types of pathological lesions that indicate varying immune status at different times may be seen in a given patient, almost charting out the evolution and the progress of the untreated disease thus far.

Regularly maintained growth charts could have picked up a faltering of the weight centiles during the initial stages of the disease, thereby prompting relevant investigations. Had the suspicious right paratracheal shadow been given due importance, it could have been evaluated further by a lateral chest X-ray and a Mantoux test that might have been positive then. Therefore, this case illustrates the need for an aggressive approach while evaluating infants who may harbor a disease that has a potential to progress.

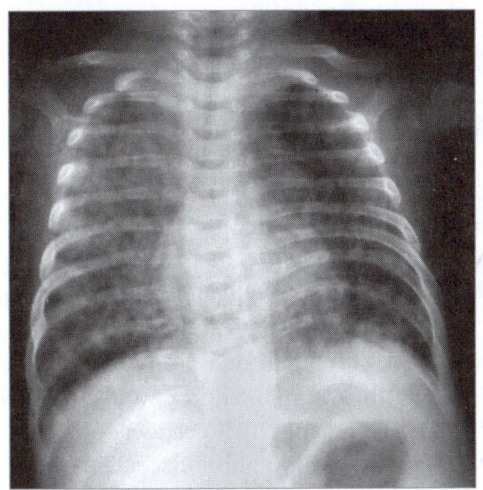

Miliary shadows with suspicious right paratracheal shadow (cavity not seen).

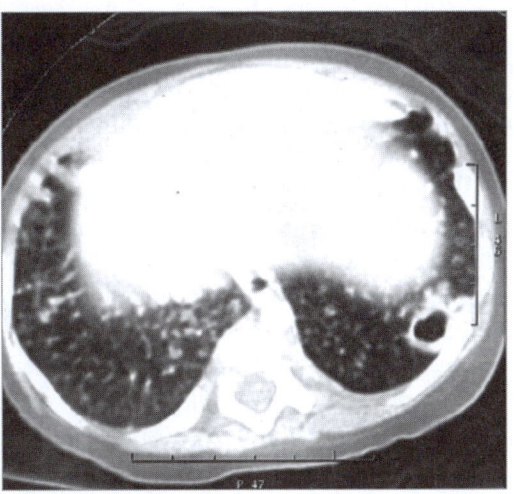

Miliary lesions with cavity.

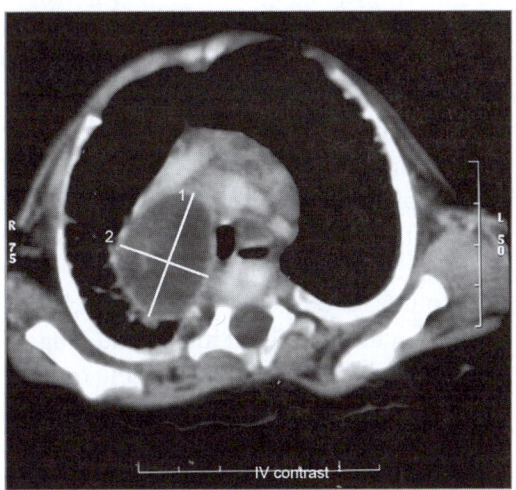

CT scan showing lymphadenopathy in the same child.

CASE 118

Fever, Cough, Breathlessness (TB Lymph Node and Miliary)

Events...

An 8-month-old infant presented with fever and cough for the last six weeks and mild breathlessness for the last one week. The fever was mild to moderate, but the cough was so severe that he would get suffocated and red in the face. He was investigated and diagnosed as mediastinal lymph node tuberculosis on the basis of a Mantoux test reaction of 8 mm and the chest X-ray showing an enlarged right paratracheal lymph node. He was started on HRZ in correct dosages and was asked to follow-up after a month. Within the next few days, he was noticed to be lethargic and was hospitalized for further management. On direct questioning, the mother revealed that the infant's grandfather was diagnosed to have pulmonary tuberculosis two months ago (he stayed in the same house), and an older sib was also suffering from similar complaints.

Explanation...

This infant has a subacute infective illness, as suggested by mild-to-moderate fever for more than 6 weeks, in which cough is the most predominant symptom. Cough indicates primary airway disease and such an infective disease may be pertussis or an atypical pneumonia due to intracellular organisms. Cough in pertussis should have been on the decline by 6 weeks and is not accompanied with prolonged fever. In view of a strong family history of contact, tuberculosis is the most likely diagnosis. Primary involvement of the airways in tuberculosis, is a result of either an endobronchial lesion due to rupture of a lymph node into the airways, or external pressure by a large mediastinal lymph node. In a long-standing chronic disease, airway involvement may result from bronchiectasis. Barring these situations, cough is not a prominent symptom in tuberculosis when it affects the lung parenchyma or the pleura. This child developed breathlessness after five weeks of the onset of his primary complaints, Breathlessness in tuberculosis is rare and is caused by either a large pleural effusion or an interstitial involvement as in miliary tuberculosis. A large pleural effusion is a disease of acute onset in an older well-nourished child and is rare in infants. On the other hand, an interstitial involvement would lead to a gradually developing breathlessness as was reported in this infant. Therefore, this infant must have developed miliary tuberculosis. As his initial chest X-ray did not show any miliary lesions, he was not started on steroids then, nor investigated further for dissemination of infection. This is probably why he has been now brought back with a deterioration in his general condition.

A repeated chest X-ray showed miliary lesions, though the CSF was normal. He was now started on steroids and the same ATT regimen was continued.

Experience gained...

This case illustrates how a functional derangement in terms of mild breathlessness should have suggested miliary tuberculosis, even if it was not supported by chest X-ray. CT scan at this stage would have picked it up. Thus at times, a clinical diagnosis may score over radiological diagnosis. If this infant would have been started on steroids at his first visit, he would have improved earlier. Luckily, in this period, he did not disseminate to the CNS, though he should be still be carefully followed up for the development of neurological disease, even on compliant treatment.

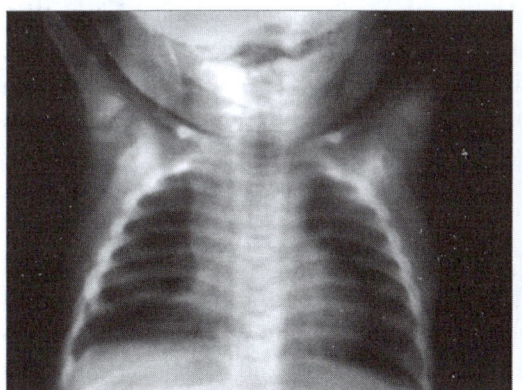

Mediastinal lymphadenopathy
(military lesions not seen in this film)

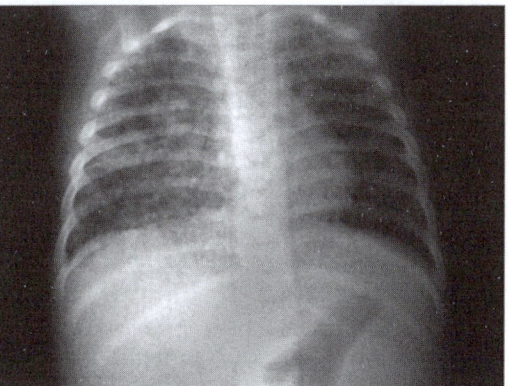

Miliary lesions with lymphadenopathy

CASE 119

Recurrent Arthritis as an Immune-mediated Manifestation of TB

History
A 12-year-old girl presented with a history of ankle joint pain and swelling, and a moderate fever of an acute onset, that lasted for 4 or 5 days and got better on NSAID treatment. After a week, she again developed similar joint pain and swellings, this time affecting both the ankles and also one wrist. The details of the physical findings then, were not available. This time she was investigated. There was mild neutrophilic leukocytosis with eosinophilia and a high ESR, though ASLO, ANA and RA factors were negative. She was again treated symptomatically with NSAIDs for two weeks, but there was no relief in fever, and the joint swellings and pain waxed and waned. She had lost 3 kg of weight over the last four weeks. At this point, she was brought for a second opinion.

Analysis
Though this child seems to have been investigated for suspected rheumatic or rheumatoid arthritis, on analyzing the history, both these conditions seemed unlikely. **Rheumatoid arthritis** would have been persistent; though the symptoms could wax and wane during the day (being at their worst in the mornings), they would not wax and wane over a number of days. Further, there would not have been such a short symptom free period in between two episodes. **Rheumatic fever** is also ruled out because the arthritis in rheumatic fever is typically migratory and the response to NSAID is excellent, unlike in this child where the joint symptoms waxed and waned. Further, rheumatic arthritis is not intermittent as in this case. **Tuberculous arthritis** is usually monoarticular and hence ruled out. Multiple joint effusions are known in tuberculosis but are rare. Therefore, this seems to be a case of **reactive arthritis**, either secondary to some infection or malignancy. The classic example of a reactive arthritis following an infection is that due to Shigella; this arthritis usually resolves a short while after the primary infection is treated. In this case, since the primary disease responsible for triggering the arthritis had not yet been identified and treated, the arthritis had not resolved.

Physical Examination
It revealed a sick child with an arthritis involving both the ankles and the left wrist. In addition, she also had localizing signs in the chest suggestive of a right upper lobe pneumonia.

Investigations
The chest X-ray confirmed an infiltration in the right upper zone. The Mantoux test was strongly positive, and the ESR was high.

Analysis

In view of subacute pneumonia and a strongly positive Mantoux test, she was diagnosed to have tuberculosis. She had developed reactive arthritis in response to the tuberculous disease. She was treated with anti-TB therapy and improved on all counts.

Lessons Learnt

This child clinically presented with a symptom that happened to be an allergic reactive manifestation of tuberculosis, outside the chest. Phlyctenular conjunctivitis and erythema nodosum are other such reactive manifestations of tuberculosis, which are known to occur without obvious clinical symptomatology directly attributable to the tuberculous infection itself. Often, such allergic manifestations may be self-limiting, and may pass off without the child subsequently manifesting the primary disease. Further, such allergic manifestations can be seen not only in tuberculosis but also in many other infections, a common example being streptococcal infections. So ideally, whenever a child presents with such an allergic manifestation, at least an attempt must be made to identify the primary disease. In this child, the primary disease did manifest with some localizing signs in the chest that gave a clue to the diagnosis. The success of therapy proved the diagnosis.

CASE 120

Persistence of Fever for Months in Spite of Radiological Improvement

Events...

A 16-year-old girl had lost 4 kg of weight over a month, without any other symptoms. On direct questioning, she had maintained her appetite and activity. She was investigated, and all her routine laboratory tests were normal, including a chest X-ray and the ESR. So her weight loss was ascribed to her whims of dieting. A month later, she developed fever that settled down with a course of amoxicillin. She remained afebrile for two weeks, only to relapse with a low-grade fever again; this time, she also complained of a loss of appetite. So she was reinvestigated. Her ESR had increased to 104 mm, and this time, her chest X-ray showed extensive bilateral infiltration with cavitatory lesions. Her sputum grew tubercle bacilli sensitive to all routine anti-TB drugs, so she was put on conventional anti-TB therapy. Though she started improving in her appetite and weight, her fever continued. After two months of compliant therapy, her chest X-ray had remarkably improved, though the fever still continued. In fact, now the fever was in the form of high spikes at least two times a day. She received several antibiotics considering secondary bacterial infections, but without any improvement. The fever continued to be high in spite of significant improvement in all other parameters including chest X-rays and ESR. At this point, she was started on steroids, and she started improving. However, on withdrawal of steroids, she started running fever again. Thus, she needed steroid therapy for the next two months continuously, in low doses, that kept her fever under control. After discontinuation of steroids after two months, there was no recurrence of fever.

Explanation...

Significant documented weight loss always needs to be investigated; it usually suggests an occult infection or occult organ failure. Organ dysfunction is unlikely to be occult in 16-year-old; it is more likely in a newborn. Similarly, malignancies in children do not commonly present with only loss of weight—usually there are other symptoms that are obvious, such as pallor in hematological malignancies, localized mass in hepatoblastoma or fever in leukemia, lymphoma and neuroblastoma. Therefore, this was likely to be an occult infection. However, in such cases, one also needs to specifically rule out diabetes and thyrotoxicosis; they also happen to be conditions where routine investigations are normal, and therefore could be easily missed. A low-grade infection like tuberculosis or fungus could also have a normal ESR.

This girl was diagnosed very late after the onset of her disease because it manifested subtly with minimal and nonspecific symptoms.

Tuberculous disease can present with minimal symptoms in two extreme situations—either in the beginning of the disease when it is mild or when the host is overwhelmed by the burden of disease. This second situation is typically seen in an adolescent. This is a host who is immunologically imbalanced by virtue of her age, and when she suddenly gets a large bacterial load which multiplies rapidly over time, it suppresses her immune responses so that there are minimal symptoms. This is the reason why initially she had no fever at all, and when she did develop fever, it was intermittent and mild. Thus, she had multibacillary disease with extensive bilateral involvement of lungs with acute cavitatory lesions—progressive primary complex with breaking down lesions almost simulating a staphylococcal disease. It meant a reasonable protective immunity that did not allow distant spread of the disease, though it was not adequate to contain the disease to a small area locally. Once she was started on anti-TB treatment, her immunity improved and the resultant cytokine response led to a higher degree of fever, though the disease *per se* had started improving. At this point, that the disease had indeed started improving, could be definitively judged by an improvement in appetite, weight and activity, and radiological improvement, in spite of continued fever. This is another example of a paradoxical response. As her immunity improved over time, on one hand there was clinical improvement as well as radiological clearance, but on the other hand the fever persisted.

Experience gained...

Isolated persistence of fever in the face of improvement on other counts does not necessarily indicate failure of therapy, just as isolated remission of fever in the absence of improvement on other counts does not indicate a response to therapy. Persistence of fever in a child who is otherwise improving, may demand institution of steroid therapy for the control of fever as it is an immune-mediated reaction. At times, persistence of fever in tuberculosis may also be due to drugs, especially rifampicin. However, drug fever can only be diagnosed after excluding other causes.

Secondary bacterial infection in tuberculosis is very uncommon.

CASE 121

■ Suspected MDR TB

History

An 11-year-old child presented with fever and cough for the last three months. On investigation, she was diagnosed as pulmonary tuberculosis on the basis of fibrocaseous cavitatory lesions, a strongly positive tuberculin reaction, and acid-fast bacilli seen on Ziehl-Neelsen staining of the sputum sample, though the culture turned out to be negative. There was no history of contact with tuberculosis. She was prescribed 2HRZE/7 HRE. At the end of three months of treatment, she had no fever but her cough continued. She had not gained any weight. The repeat chest X-ray showed no improvement. At this juncture, sputum was collected again, that did not show any AFB on staining or culture, and hence she was referred for further management.

Analysis and Approach

The diagnosis of pulmonary tuberculosis is not in doubt as it was confirmed by sputum examination. The first step in such a case is to confirm compliance of therapy. If compliance is assured, then we may debate further whether the progress in this child would be considered as a poor response to treatment, or one could wait for a few more weeks to gauge the response.

Whenever a child apparently 'fails to respond' to therapy, one needs to be clear as to what one expects, to call it a response. Since this child had a chronic form of tuberculosis, she would be expected to improve only over 2 or 3 months with compliant treatment, in terms of control of fever and cough and also a gain in weight. However, it would not be surprising, if the chest X-ray did not improve by then. Cough in such a child may not be controlled completely as there may be a chance of some irreversible damage. Weight gain depends upon the degree of weight loss due to the disease. If this child was significantly malnourished even prior to the development of tuberculosis (which may be due to prolonged poor nutrition), she may not gain weight in spite of the disease being controlled. Thus, persistence of both these symptoms may not necessarily depict a poor response in this child. Similarly, that the X- ray may not change, was expected.

Since the sputum is negative now, it suggests a bacteriological control and therefore, indirectly confirms drug sensitivity. Therefore, there is not a strong ground to say that she has not responded at all.

On detailed questioning, it was realized that she had stopped the drugs for the last two weeks. Since an optimal response was expected at just about this time, such a drug default may explain the suboptimal response. Hence, it was decided to continue the same drugs expecting an improvement over the next few weeks. Progress in such a child may be judged by sequential anticipation of control of fever, general well-being and improving appetite, followed by a reduction in cough and lastly, some change in the chest X-ray.

As she had defaulted for two weeks only, it may be adequate to prolong her therapy by another four weeks to ensure complete cure. If she had faulted for more than a month, it would have been necessary to restart the treatment regimen afresh, though with the same drugs.

If this child had not faulted, then the question would arise whether this should be construed as drug resistance in view of the so-called poor response. As discussed above, in case she had regained her well-being and appetite and the fever had already subsided, one may consider continuing the same drugs over another month and then judge the further progress. This is especially, so because her sputum had turned out to be negative. Control of cough in such a child may be achieved by chest physiotherapy and postural drainage.

However, if this child did not improve over the next one month, one may repeat sputum examination. Since sputum positivity would be a critical determinant in favor of resistant TB, one must ensure that the sample is collected properly. One could also attempt a bronchoalveolar lavage. In case, the sample does show AFB, it would amount to drug resistance. In that case, one would add two more drugs to the existing regimen, and go by the drug sensitivity report subsequently, to choose the right drugs.

On the other hand, if the repeat sample did not show AFB and the child was not improving, one may have to consider therapeutic failure due to causes other than drug resistance. They include an unfavorable immune status of the host, undetected concurrent illness, or a dual pathology in the form of a coinfection with a fungus.

MDR TB

The diagnosis of MDR TB may be suspected right at the beginning, before starting treatment, if the contact case is known to be drug resistant. In such cases, one must select drugs based on the drug sensitivity of the index case. Otherwise, one may seriously consider drug resistance in an adolescent child with a cavitatory lesion, or a child who has been already treated with anti-TB drugs in the past. In such cases, it is extremely important to attempt a bacteriological diagnosis, even with invasive procedures, if necessary, before starting therapy. However, one should start with a conventional drug regimen, and follow the clinical progress. By the end of three months, clinical improvement or otherwise, coupled with bacteriological results, would guide the further course of action.

In the absence of bacteriological proof of drug resistance, if the clinical improvement is poorer than anticipated, one must first confirm the diagnosis and then look at other factors like compliance, dosages, and adverse host factors. If all such factors are ruled out, one would be justified in calling it drug resistance, and add two more drugs to the existing regimen. As second line drugs are costly and toxic, one may try adding streptomycin and ethambutol to the conventional three drug regimen of HRZ. However, if the child is already on ethambutol and/or streptomycin, one may resort to ofloxacin and/or erythromycin in favor of ethionamide and cycloserine. Ciprofloxacin is not advocated due to its interaction with rifampicin. The drug regimen should extend beyond one year in a child with MDR tuberculosis and even then, the prognosis may be guarded. If the lesion is localized to a small area, surgical removal of the lesion may be considered; if a bulk of the disease is removed, improvement may be enhanced. In routine situations, surgery has no role in the treatment of tuberculosis.

CASE 122

■ MDR TB

Case

A 14-year-old girl presented with fever off and on for last 3 weeks. She had mild cough. She had normal growth and development and was well prior to the onset of this illness. She was diagnosed as primary complex due to tuberculosis, based on persistent symptoms, documented recent loss of weight, chest X-ray showing enlarged hilar lymph node, Mt test +ve and failure of antibiotic trial. However, there was no history of contact and gastric aspirate was negative for AFB. She was started on HRZE for 2 months and she improved in terms of disappearance of fever and had gained 1 kg weight. She was shifted to HRE regimen at the end of 2 months as per standard protocol. Within a week, her fever recurred but she was otherwise well. She was compliant in treatment.

How do you Manage at this Stage?

Review physical examination to assess any change. Repeat chest X-ray and ESR. Repeat gastric aspirate. Till then, continue previous regimen HRZE. It is important to prove MDR status before empirically adding second line drugs. Adding two more drugs while waiting for gastric aspirate results may not be the right action. This is because while drug resistance is a possibility at this stage, the recurrence of fever could be due to an immune reaction that may resolve by itself, or it may also be drug fever.

Further Progress

Chest X-ray and ESR did not show any significant change. Gastric aspirate was negative for AFB; it was also sent for CBNAAT and culture.

Analysis

Standard definition of drug resistance is persistence of AFB at the end of 3 months of therapy. However, failure to demonstrate AFB in gastric aspirate may not rule out drug resistance. Comparatively, CBNAPP is more sensitive in detecting we presents of mycobacteria in any body flood. Besides, it has the added advantage of picking up rifampicin resistant. However, in this case, CBNAPP on the gastric aspirate was also negative.

What is the next action?

It was decided to wait with the same drug regimen and review the child after the culture report comes in. Meanwhile, the child started developing headache and vomiting. Physical examination at this stage showed a drowsy child with meningeal signs that prompted CSF examination which showed evidence of meningitis. This almost meant drug resistance as the disease had spread beyond the lungs. IM Kanamycin and oral Ofloxacin were added to HRZE regimen. By then culture was reported positive, with HR resistance but sensitive to other drugs.

Considering spread to CNS in an adolescent girl, it was decided to add cycloserine and PAS to make it a 6-drug regimen. Last two drugs are bacteriostatic. Steroids were added to treat TB meningitis.

Further Progress

Child continued to deteriorate neurologically though fever was controlled, and subsequent culture became negative. It meant that in spite of drugs acting on the bacteria, the clinical condition worsened. Ultimately, the child succumbed to her illness after several months in a damaged neurological state.

Lessons Learnt

Every attempt must be made to prove the diagnosis of tuberculosis before starting anti-TB treatment and this is most important in case of MDRTB. No test is 100% sensitive and specific and hence smear, culture, and PCR—all tests should be ordered as much as possible. Once diagnosed, compliance must be ensured till the end of therapy and the patient should be monitored thereafter for at least one year for relapse. However, immune complications may continue to endanger life well after control of infection by drugs. Such reactions are not predictable and may not be controlled by steroids, as happened in this child.

CASE 123

■ Extensive Tuberculosis in Infant Poorly Responsive to Treatment

Events...

A 5-month-old infant presented with a history of cough and breathlessness since the age of one month. He was born of a full-term normal delivery with a birth weight of 3.2 kg. He was exclusively breastfed and remained well for the first one month. Thereafter, he developed a cough and gradually, even difficulty in feeding with a 'suck rest suck' cycle. By then, the mother developed fever and cough and was diagnosed as pulmonary tuberculosis with cavitatory lesions.

She was put on four drug ATT–HRZE. The infant was also found to have bilateral lung lesions and was subjected to bronchoalveolar lavage that confirmed tuberculosis. By now, he was hypoxic in room air and required oxygenation through a hood. He was also started on the same drug regimen as that of his mother. While the mother showed a good clinical improvement within 4 weeks, the infant remained symptomatic and continued to require oxygen. At that stage, he was put on oral prednisolone in a dose of 2 mg/kg body weight per day and the ATT was continued. He showed marginal improvement at the end of a month but continued to need oxygen. Prednisolone was continued for another month in the same dosage and thereafter tapered over a few weeks. As soon as it was tapered and withdrawn, he became more symptomatic, and his oxygen requirements increased. By then, he was 5 months old, and had not gained much weight nor had any change in his radiological picture. Hence, he was referred for further management.

Analysis so Far

Diagnosis of pulmonary tuberculosis in this infant is not in doubt as it was bacteriologically proved. Since the mother improved on four drug ATT, it proves that the organisms were drug sensitive. However, in spite of drug sensitive tuberculosis and compliant therapy, this infant had shown no improvement. Though he did show a marginal change while on full doses of steroids, as soon as it was tapered and then stopped, he had deteriorated to his original level. This almost suggests the need of continuing steroids for a longer period. The duration of steroid therapy in tuberculosis would vary in individual patients depending on their immune responses, though the average period recommended is 6–8 weeks, followed by tapering over the next 3–4 weeks. Other causes of a poor response in spite of drug sensitive organisms that can be considered include immune deficiency states. However, it is very unlikely to be so in this infant, as there was no dissemination of disease and there was no abnormal reaction at the site of BCG vaccination.

Physical Examination

Poorly built and nourished Weight 4.8 kg		Irritable and sick looking Head circumference 40 cm
Temp. normal	Length 60 cm Pulse 115/min	RR 45/min
Mild distress		
Mild central cyanosis Systemic examination	No clubbing	No lymphadenopathy
RS–Bilateral crepitations scattered all over		No localizing signs
Other systems normal		

Analysis of Physical Findings

This infant is suffering from tuberculosis as confirmed by bacteriological studies done at the time of diagnosis. Anatomically, bilateral scattered crepitations denote either involvement of small airways or an interstitial disease. Miliary tuberculosis is an interstitial disease and should have resulted in hepatosplenomegaly as a manifestation. Since there is no such finding, the disease in this infant seems to be localized to the respiratory system only. Isolated airway involvement does not occur in tuberculosis and hence, the anatomical lesion must have extended from a primary focus, through smaller airways into the entire lung parenchyma. Thus, this must have been a bronchogenic spread of the disease and not hematogenous. That explains why the findings, though bilateral, are localized only to the lungs. Due to extensive bilateral lung parenchymal disease, this infant is hypoxic. It is necessary to pinpoint the reasons for a poor response to therapy.

Investigations

Hb 11 g%   WBC–12,500/mm^3 P 48 L 42 M 6 E 4   ESR 95 mm
Chest X-ray–extensive bilateral breaking down lesions.
Right from the first X-ray at diagnosis, there are many X-rays which show no change at all.
Mantoux test 8 mm positive
SpO$_2$ on room air—80%   On 5 lit of oxygen SpO$_2$—92%
ABG—pH 7.35   PaO$_2$ 68   PCO$_2$ 39
BAL no AFB seen.
LFT normal

Analysis

This infant has shown no improvement in any of the parameters in spite of compliant therapy for 4 months. Symptomatically, he continues to be hypoxic and has not gained weight. He remains apathetic and anorexic. Physical signs have remained equally bad. There is no change radiologically either. But on the other hand, BAL has been negative that suggests bacteriological control. It means that organisms are drug sensitive, and it is also corroborated by the fact that his mother has improved remarkably with the same drug regimen. This denotes that the host immune system is probably responsible for poor response that may need immunomodulation.

Immunologically speaking, that child has low immunity probably due to a high bacterial load at a very young age but it is not completely immunosuppressed; otherwise the disease would have disseminated to involve other systems. Thus, the disease has remained restricted to lungs only. However, he has developed local tissue hypersensitivity that has resulted in destructive lung lesions. This is consistent with the positive tuberculin reaction in spite of extensive bilateral disease. Unless this local hypersensitivity response in the lungs is suppressed by using steroids, this child may not improve as the anti-TB drugs have done their job. This infant did show a marginal improvement while on steroids, but worsened after tapering and withdrawal of steroids. The duration of steroid therapy will have to be extended in such a case as per the response and certainly would be required for a much longer period.

Management and Further Progress

This infant was put on oral prednisolone in doses of 1 mg/kg body weight in two divided doses and anti-TB drugs were continued. At the end of another 6 weeks, he could maintain adequate oxygenation in room air. He started feeding better, was active and playful, was alert and looked happy. He had no fever or cough. At this stage, his chest X-ray showed no change at all nor was there any significant weight gain.

In such an extensive destructive disease at this young age, what is expected to improve first is the well-being of the infant and his symptoms, rather than physical or radiological signs. This improvement would be followed by a weight gain over a few weeks and thereafter, a change in physical signs gradually. Radiological abnormalities would take a long time to recover and may not revert back to normal.

This infant was advised to continue oral steroids in a single dose on alternate mornings to minimize the risk of toxicity and try to taper off slowly as per the response. Occasionally, such a case may require steroid therapy for the entire length of anti-TB treatment.

Lessons Learnt

This case illustrates how host immune reaction decides not only the pathology but also the progress and outcome of the disease. Science falls short of anticipating and modifying the immune response of the host. At present, steroids, seem to be the only weapon to modulate immune reactions and that may not be always successful.

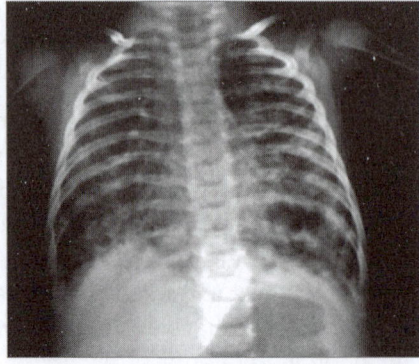

Bilateral bronchopneumonic lesions.

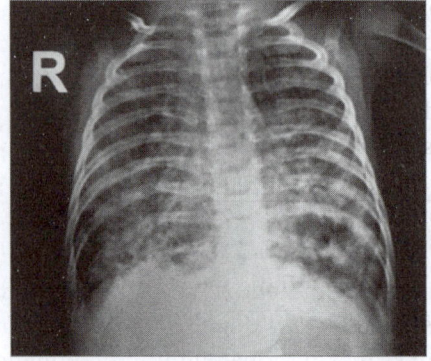

Persistent bronchopneumonic lesions.

CASE 124

Worsening Mediastinal Lymph Node Enlargement on Recovery of Primary Complex

Events...

A 1-year-old infant presented with fever for four days without any other significant symptoms. He had arrived in India two weeks ago and till then, was reported to be normal. Clinical examination did not reveal any abnormality. After symptomatic therapy for another two days, routine laboratory tests like CBC, urinalysis and urine culture were asked for and were normal. Thereafter, a chest X-ray was ordered that showed a small patch of infiltration at the right base. He was prescribed amoxicillin but did not improve. Thereafter, a tuberculin test was done and it turned out to be positive. He had not received BCG vaccination in the past, and was, therefore, diagnosed as tuberculous disease. On anti-TB treatment, his fever improved over the next two weeks. After two months of successful treatment, the parents wanted to get back to USA, so a follow-up chest X-ray was ordered. Contrary to expectation, it showed massive mediastinal lymphadenopathy. That worried everyone and the possibility of having missed a malignancy was strongly debated. Antibiotics were added, considering it to be some bacterial superinfection. However, throughout this period, the child had remained pretty well and had gained weight. A CT scan was asked for, which revealed caseating lymph nodes. A bronchoalveolar lavage yielded tubercle bacilli sensitive to all the drugs. The same drugs were continued, and within the next two weeks, the lymph nodes had started reducing in size. The child remained well thereafter.

Explanation...

This child demonstrated the appearance of newer lesions on successful therapy. This is a phenomenon known to occur during recovery of tuberculous disease. As a result of anti-TB therapy, once the bacterial load goes down, immune suppression caused by a high bacterial load reverts and immune recovery occurs. At times, during such an immune recovery, an excessive CD4 response occurs, that may lead to hypersensitivity manifestations such as lymphadenitis, pleural effusion, or the development of tuberculomas. The site of such new lesions depends upon the presence of subclinical foci that existed prior to the initiation of treatment. The excessive immune response converts these subclinical foci into clinically visible lesions. These are all manifestations of good immunity and hypersensitivity. In other words, an excessive immune response on the part of the host during successful therapy leads to the development of newer lesions, even while the previous lesion is well-controlled. This is a therapeutic paradox. This is not indicative of a drug-resistant infection, as the primary lesion has already been controlled, by the time the new lesion appears. Occasionally such new lesions may need to be suppressed by the use of steroids, if they endanger life, as in the case of a tuberculoma that may lead to seizures, or a large mediastinal lymph node that may embarrass breathing due to pressure exerted on the main airways.

Experience gained…

Appearance of new lesions during successful treatment of the original tuberculous disease is a phenomenon caused by an unnecessary, excessive, CD 4 cell immune recovery response on the part of the host. It is an overenthusiastic immune response, which is not universal, but an individual characteristic of a given host. There is no way to anticipate the same. It typically occurs around 2–3 months after successful treatment of the original disease, as this is the period that is required for recovery of CD 4 cell function and suppression of antibody response. While CD 4 cell function must recover in every patient on successful therapy of tuberculosis, as depicted by a negative Mantoux test reverting to a positive reaction even in miliary tuberculosis, it is the excessive CD 4 response that is responsible for new lesions. Such new lesions should not be mistaken for any other disease.

This case also illustrates the point that the child's clinical condition is of paramount importance while interpreting the results of laboratory tests or imaging studies.

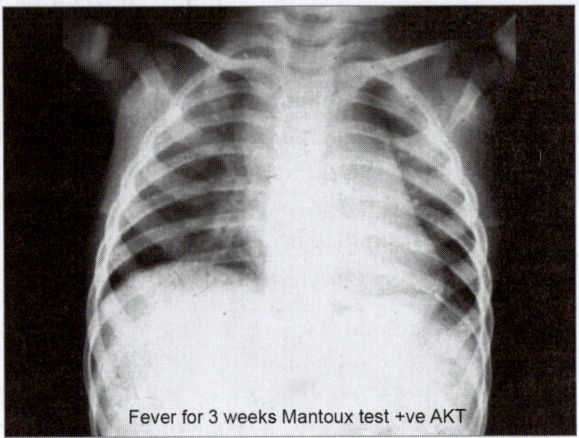

Fever for 3 weeks Mantoux test +ve AKT

Suspicious right lower lobe lesion.

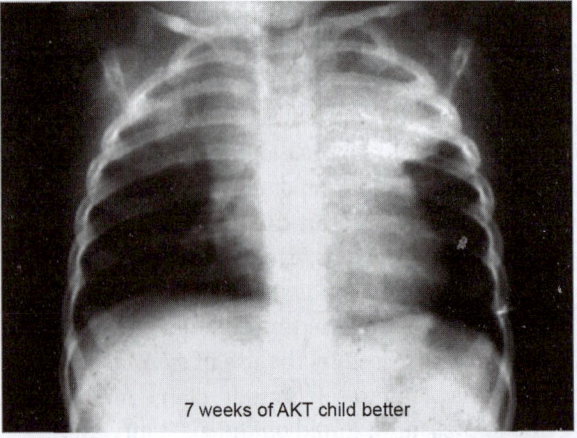

7 weeks of AKT child better

Massive mediastinal lymphadenopathy while on successful treatment.

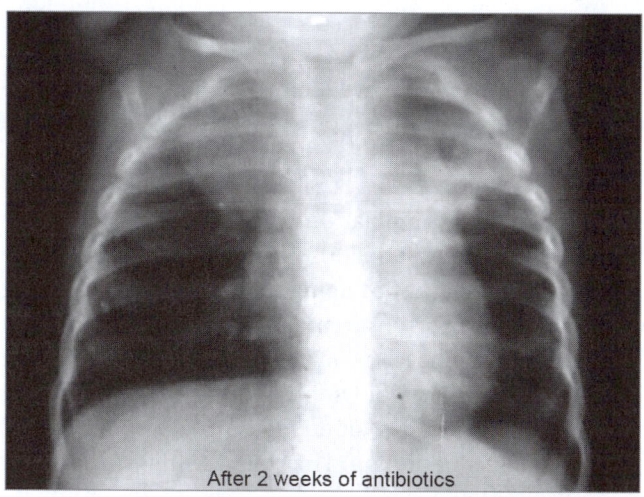

After 2 weeks of antibiotics
Repeat X-ray showing no change.

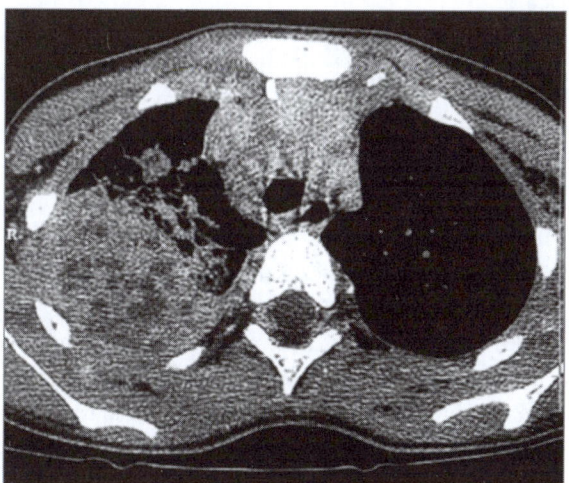

Caseating lymph node with pneumonia.

CASE 125

■ Development of Cervical Lymph Node on Recovery of TB Pneumonia

Events...

A 5-year-old child presented with a similar problem that was discussed in the previous case. This child was diagnosed to have tuberculous pneumonia (progressive primary complex) on the basis of reasonable evidence and was doing well-symptomatically. His repeat chest X-ray after a few weeks had shown some improvement as expected. At the end of three months of compliant successful therapy, he had improved considerably on one hand, but on the other hand, he also developed a large cervical lymph node on the right side. FNAC was asked for, which proved that the lymph node was tuberculous. However, the same anti-TB drugs were continued without any change or addition. The child continued to improve steadily and over time, the lymph node also settled down.

Experience gained...

> It is worth noting that such immune-mediated new lesions occur sometime around 3 months of successful therapy. It has been known that immune recovery takes that much time in most of the patients. Therefore, this is the time to anticipate the development of new lesions; once this period goes through smoothly, no further problems are likely. In this child, one could even have avoided the FNAC, especially since he had otherwise improved.
>
> This is also the time when we expect a miliary TB patient to demonstrate a positive tuberculin test, even when it was negative to start with. Even drug-resistant disease would be clinically suspected by around the same time of therapy; it can be confirmed, if bacteria are found to persist in any body fluid or tissue even after this duration of therapy.
>
> Thus, reassessment of a child who is being treated for tuberculosis, at the end of 3 months of compliant therapy, is invaluable. If the therapy has been successful, this is the time to document it (in the form of radiological improvement or a negative tuberculin test reverting to positive), and also pick up new immune-mediated lesions, if any. If the therapy has been unsuccessful, this is the time to review the diagnosis or suspect drug resistance.

CASE 126

■ Recurrence of Meningitis on Compliant Anti-TB Therapy

Events...

A 2-year-old child presented with fever, convulsion, and drowsiness, and was diagnosed as TBM on reasonable grounds, with the CT scan showing typical basal exudates and hydrocephalus. He did well on treatment and was being followed up. His CSF had returned to normal by the end of the first month of treatment. At the end of three months of successful and compliant therapy, he again developed signs of meningitis and had abnormal CSF. He was reinvestigated for probable coinfection with a fungus or for drug resistance. After other problems were ruled out, steroids were restarted, and he made a good recovery.

Explanation...

It was inappropriate to consider drug-resistant tuberculosis in this child because clinical and CSF improvement had been documented before deterioration—in drug-resistant cases, there would be no improvement at all. Therefore, there was no doubt about the diagnosis or drug sensitivity (At this point it is worth mentioning that the mere absence of fever for 8 to 10 days is not necessarily indicative of a response to treatment; improvement has to be on all fronts consistently).

Routinely, steroids are prescribed for a period of 6 to 8 weeks in case of TBM. This is based on epidemiological observations, that by this time most of the hypersensitivity responses are controlled and thereafter there is no need for steroid therapy. However, this may not be true in every child. An occasional child may need steroid therapy for a much longer duration. There is no test to demonstrate the ideal duration of steroid therapy, since we cannot measure the immune response in patients with tuberculosis.

Experience gained...

> This case demonstrated the recurrence of hypersensitivity in meningitis, once steroid therapy was omitted. Another manifestation of an immune-mediated new lesion in TBM is the development of a tuberculoma.

CASE 127

■ Development of Tuberculoma on Recovery of TBM

Events…

A 6-month-old infant presented with fever for four days, followed by a convulsion and drowsiness. He was diagnosed to be suffering from TBM on the basis of an abnormal CSF and the CT scan showing basal exudates with hydrocephalus, along with an infarct in the region of the middle cerebral artery. He was treated with ATT and steroids, improved, and was discharged after eight weeks of hospitalization, in a stable condition. He continued his treatment regularly at home as advised four oral drugs and tapering doses of steroids. The steroids were omitted after two weeks of going home as advised. After another four weeks, he suddenly developed multifocal convulsions and was readmitted to the hospital. Repeat CT scan showed multiple tuberculomas and this had happened in spite of compliant treatment.

Explanation…

This case illustrates the variability of immune responses in different hosts. Routinely, steroids in TBM are continued for 8 weeks and then tapered, as was done in this child. This is to suppress the local hypersensitivity response in the brain; it is expected to be controlled within 8–10 weeks and hence, the protocol of steroid therapy for that length of time. However, this may not be true in every child. This child must have had multiple silent foci in the brain parenchyma that flared up as his general immunity improved with bacteriological control. This resulted in the development of newer lesions during successful recovery from the primary disease.

Experience gained…

> This case illustrates the scientific limitations in deciding the duration of therapy in individual patients. Usually, duration of therapy is planned on the basis of community studies. Hence, it is mandatory that such patients are followed up closely, during and even after completion of therapy, for some time.

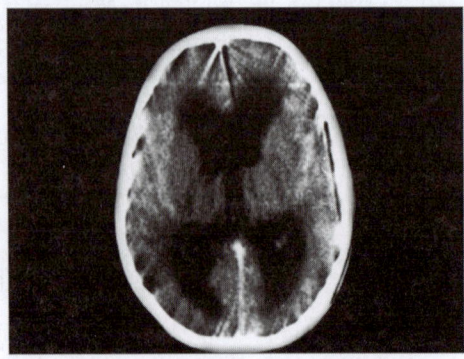

TB meningitis with basal exudate.

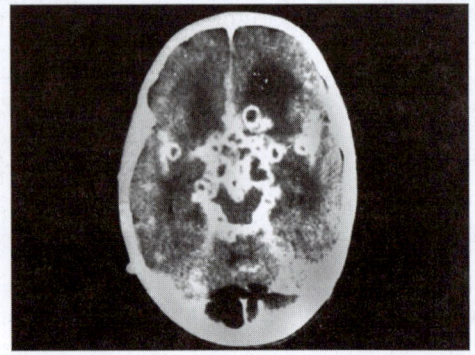

Multiple tuberculous while on successful treatment.

CASE 128

■ BCG Lymphadenitis

Events...

A 1-year-old healthy, well-nourished, infant was brought for a progressively increasing swelling in the left axillary region. The swelling was noticed at around 5 months of age, at which time the pediatrician attributed it to the BCG vaccine and advised no active intervention. However, it has been slowly increasing in size, so now the parents got worried, and came for a second opinion. They were again told that this was BCG lymphadenitis which did not need any treatment. In case there was any reddening of the skin over the swelling or softening, suggesting impending rupture, they should report back since the node may require to be excised. The parents were uneasy and consulted an adult pulmonologist. A tuberculin test was asked for and was positive. A FNAC of the gland suggested tuberculosis, so the gland was excised and the infant put on ATT.

Explanation...

Following BCG vaccination, the development of a local 'primary complex' is the normal physiological response of the body. In other words, there is a primary lesion at the vaccination site and the local lymph node gets involved. Usually, it is the axillary lymph node that gets involved but if BCG vaccine is administered bit higher on the shoulder, draining lymph node may come up in supraclavicular region. In a normal healthy host, the primary lesion heals (BCG scar) and the involved lymph node is too insignificant to be clinically noticed. Therefore, when such a lymph node is clinically visible, it is just an exaggerated reaction on the part of the body, somewhat similar to exaggerated physiological jaundice. As much as exaggerated jaundice in selected situations may justify intervention, BCG lymphadenitis may justify intervention only in few situations. Such a response automatically dies out with time and does not usually need any intervention. The tuberculin test is expected to be positive; similarly, the gland is expected to show histopathological features of tuberculosis, because anyway it is a part and parcel of the local primary complex. Therefore, this cannot be equated to the presence of tuberculous disease and does not need ATT.

Experience gained...

> BCG lymphadenitis is a kind of an exaggerated physiological response that does not need any intervention routinely. There is no role for ATT.

CASE 129

◼ Flaring of BCG Scar as a Manifestation of Immune Disorder

Events…

A 6-month-old infant presented with fever and skin rash for the last six days. There were no other symptoms. Physical examination did not reveal any localizing signs. As symptomatic therapy had failed, he was investigated. The CBC showed moderate neutrophilic leukocytosis with a high ESR. There was no significant anemia, and the platelet count was normal. So there was no specific diagnosis at that point. The next day, suddenly, the BCG scar was noticed to have flared up. He had received the BCG vaccine at birth, and over the next three months, he had gone through the usual sequence of events to develop a scar at the site. The flaring up of the BCG scar gave the clue to a possible immune-mediated disease, in the sense that the disease had rekindled an immune reaction that had occurred long back. After another two days, the infant developed significant lymphadenopathy and mouth lesions and was diagnosed as Kawasaki disease.

Explanation…

It is interesting to note that the BCG-induced immune reaction can get flared up by another unrelated stress to the immune system—seen in this child with Kawasaki disease. We know that the BCG vaccine induces T-cell induced delayed hypersensitivity response. It is a type four immune response. Once a site in the body is sensitized with such a delayed hypersensitivity response, it is likely to demonstrate a flare up at the same site with any other immune stress.

Experience gained…

> When such a response is visible externally, one may get a clue to the recent immune disease which triggered the response. At the same time, we know that phlyctenular conjunctivitis and erythema nodosum are other examples of similar responses to any kind of immune stress, which may actually be nonspecific responses. It is a matter of conjecture, whether one could mistake a similar nonspecific response, for a specific disease process, if it were to occur internally in some organ.

CASE 130

Psoriatic Arthritis Mistaken for TB

Events...

A 6-year-old girl presented with pain around the left shoulder joint. The pain started gradually and went on increasing over a period of one month. It was at its worst in the mornings and improved as the day progressed. By the end of the month, there was also a restriction of joint movements in all directions. There was no history of any other joints being affected; nor was there any history of fever. She was shown to an orthopedic surgeon at this point, who investigated her. CBC was unremarkable and the ESR was 35 mm, while the X-ray chest was normal. MRI of the shoulder joint showed a possibility of infective arthritis (probably tuberculous). On direct questioning, there was no history of any contact with tuberculosis. She was diagnosed to have TB of the shoulder joint and was put on ATT, anti-inflammatory drugs and physiotherapy. Over the next two months, while her pain improved only to a small extent, her movements did not. In view of the unsatisfactory improvement, a confirmation of diagnosis was sought in the form of TB serology, which was positive for both IgG and IgM. The MRI was repeated which showed no change. A month later, with no further improvement on compliant therapy, a second orthopedic opinion was taken. He concurred with the diagnosis and advised to continue the same treatment; however, he gave a guarded prognosis as far as the movements were concerned. About 8 months after starting ATT, the girl developed pain in the right ankle, which was attributed to a fall in the school. Over the next 4 to 6 weeks, she developed progressive pain and swelling of the left ankle, and the right wrist and knee. At that point, a CBC that was repeated was unremarkable, except that the platelet count was 4.89 lacs/mm^3 and the ESR was 60 (which later increased to 100). The MRI was repeated again, and it showed no change. At this point, she was brought for a pediatric opinion.

Explanation...

In this child, the MRI had confirmed arthritis. Though TB of the shoulder joint is uncommon, in the absence of any other obvious cause, in our epidemiology it is not unreasonable to diagnose monoarticular arthritis as tuberculous. Though one expects such patients to run fever, presence of fever denotes inflammation/infection; however, absence of fever does not rule out tuberculous infection. However, if after 2 to 3 months of compliant treatment, there is no improvement, one needs to confirm or revise the diagnosis. In this child, the diagnosis was 'confirmed' by a positive TB serology, which is extremely unreliable and has no place in the diagnosis of TB. Since there is no other reliable method of confirmation other than synovial biopsy in such a case, one needs to consider other possibilities. At that point, one would probably have considered it to be an evolving juvenile chronic arthritis, which was as yet monoarticular. One could only have offered symptomatic treatment in the form of NSAIDs till a diagnostic pattern evolved. Failure of antituberculous therapy may also make one suspect MDR-TB. If so, over time, the disease should have worsened (may be in the form of increasing joint destruction as seen on the MRI) or surfaced elsewhere in the body. Since this did not happen, MDR-TB was unlikely in this child.

When the child was brought to us after a few months, the disease had progressed to involve other joints. She was asked to discontinue the ATT, and a diagnosis of polyarticular JCA was considered. She was investigated in the form of RA test (negative), slit-lamp examination, HLA studies, ANA, and various other antibodies. However, even now, it was difficult to categorize her into any particular subtype of JCA. The rising ESR just confirmed an ongoing inflammatory process. So she was advised naproxen and kept under observation for another 4-6 weeks. Later, on detailed questioning, the mother mentioned that she suffered from psoriasis, and this girl always had a dry skin. So psoriatic arthritis was considered, but even in psoriasis, shoulder joint involvement is the rarest. So a dermatological opinion was taken. At this point, on close scrutiny, 'pitting' of the nails was picked up, and the diagnosis of psoriasis was confirmed.

Experience gained...

Whenever a child presents with monoarthritis, in the first few months, in our epidemiology, it is always considered as an infection like tuberculosis. However, any polyarthritis could also start as monoarthritis, and even remain so for a certain length of time. Therefore, before labeling such a monoarthritis as tuberculous, additional evidence in favor of the diagnosis should be sought, and if not available, the success of treatment should be reviewed after 2 or 3 months. Secondly, when a monoarthritis does evolve over time, but does not fit into any diagnostic pattern, it should serve as a clue that something is amiss.

CASE 131

■ Suspected Abdominal TB

Case

An 8-year-old well-grown child presented with fever, abdominal pain and loose stools with mucus off and on for last 6 months. Fever varied in intensity from mild to moderate. Abdominal pain was generalized and was relieved temporarily after passing stools. There was significant loss of weight and appetite. He was treated with antibiotics without benefit. Prior to this illness, he had been a well-child.

Physical examination showed generalized abdominal distension with mild tenderness without guarding in a sick-looking child. There was no localized mass or local tenderness. Other systems were normal.

Analysis

In view of significant loss of weight, this is a continuous disease with recurrent symptoms. Hence common bacterial infections are ruled out. Moreover, recurrent bacterial infections are not common at this age unless the child is immunocompromised. This child had grown well prior to the present illness and there was no history of repeated infections at any other site(s). Hence, an immunocompromised state is unlikely. So, this child probably has a chronic progressive inflammatory disease which could be due to a subacute/chronic infection or could be noninfective. Intestinal tuberculosis does not present with loose stools; instead, its typical presentation is in the form of subacute intestinal obstruction. This is because tuberculosis primarily affects the submucosal layers of the intestine and not the mucosa. Thus, intestinal tuberculosis is unlikely. Therefore, inflammatory bowel disease is a possibility. Physical examination in this case has not provided any further information.

Case Progression

This child was investigated extensively including an intestinal biopsy and a diagnosis of tuberculosis was established. Histopathology was reviewed by experts and tuberculosis was confirmed. This went against the basic tenet that intestinal tuberculosis does not present with loose stools. However, laboratory diagnosis was considered more reliable than clinical judgment and hence anti-TB treatment was started along with oral prednisolone. Child started improving within a few days and the diagnosis was stamped to be correct. As prednisolone was being tapered over the next 4 weeks and stopped thereafter, symptoms recurred while still on anti-TB drugs. This raised the possibility of MDRTB. At this stage, an intestinal biopsy was repeated and this time experts ruled out tuberculosis and suggested a diagnosis of inflammatory bowel disease. In retrospect, it was steroids that helped to improve this child's symptoms and not anti-TB drugs.

Lessons Learnt

While tests are an important adjunct to confirmation of diagnosis, results may misguide even when reviewed by experts and clinical correlation is vital. Clinicians tend to believe test results more than their own analysis which is based on repeated clinical observations, least realizing that machines and men behind the machines are equally vulnerable to make mistakes as do clinicians. When there exists a discrepancy between clinical judgment and test results, both need to be reviewed and repeated again. In this child, the repeat intestinal biopsy helped to change the original diagnosis, and it now tallied with the clinical profile.

CASE 132

Multiple Recovering Bony Lesions of Hodgkin's Mistaken as TB

Events...

A 15-year-old child presented with a gradual onset of backache over a few days, and thereafter, developed moderate fever. After symptomatic treatment had failed, he was investigated. The CBC was within normal limits and the ESR was high. X-ray of the spine showed a suspicious lesion, so he was diagnosed as tuberculosis. His chest X-ray was normal, and the tuberculin test was positive. After two weeks of anti-TB treatment, his backache had improved though the fever continued.

A few days later, he developed pain and restriction of movements of the left hip joint. X-ray of the hip showed a lytic lesion, but the X-ray of the spine had improved by then. Assuming that the disease had involved another site, the treatment was continued. However, the fever as well as the hip joint problem continued over the next two months, in spite of compliant treatment. As the X-ray of the spine had shown a disappearance of the previous lesion, it was concluded that the therapy was correct, and so, at this point, he was considered for adjunctive steroid therapy. This did lead to a partial improvement in the fever initially, but it was only transient, and the hip joint problem continued. At the end of another one month of steroid therapy with anti-TB treatment, he was put on second line anti-TB drugs, considering drug resistance. Over the next one month, there was still no improvement. Repeated investigations, including an abdominal USG did not reveal any additional information. At this stage (five months after the onset of the first symptom), he was also investigated for collagen vascular disorders, in view of the persistent fever which seemed to be partially steroid responsive, and evanescent radiological lesions. However, these also drew a blank. Another month passed by, and one day, he suddenly developed severe abdominal pain and distention of abdomen. He was noticed to have developed intestinal obstruction, for which surgical intervention was advised. On exploration of the abdomen, large lymph nodes were found; they were confirmed to be due to **Hodgkin's lymphoma**.

Explanation...

When this child initially presented with backache and fever, it was logical to have thought of an inflammatory bony lesion like TB (which is the most common, though other rare infections and inflammatory disorders could also be considered; however, they are less common). However, subsequently, the unusual sequence of events could have prompted the treating physician to consider alternative possibilities. To begin with, after initiating ATT, the fever should have responded before the local symptom of backache, whereas in this child, the fever persisted though the backache had improved. Further, the new lesion noticed in the hip should not have been taken as a 'spread' of the disease. This is so because this child was diagnosed to have 'bony' tuberculosis as against 'joint' tuberculosis. While tuberculosis of the joints can occasionally be seen to affect many joints by way of a reactive allergic manifestation as demonstrated in the earlier case, bony tuberculosis is a local disease and does not spread to distant sites, unless the child is immunocompromised. The development of newer lesions is known in tuberculosis even while the patient is being successfully treated. However, these lesions are not infective but allergic in nature, and therefore are restricted to those tissues that can mount a clinically visible allergic response, such as the pleura, the lymph nodes, and granulomas in the brain (tuberculomas). Further, such lesions develop much later during the course of treatment, usually 2 or 3 months after commencing treatment. This is probably because the basis of such lesions is a change in the immunological status of the patient following successful treatment which takes time. In this child, the new lesion appeared shortly after commencing treatment which had not yet proved to be successful, because though the earlier lesion had cleared, the fever continued. Also, the radiological lesion of TB spine is not expected to disappear within two weeks of therapy. This meant that the disappearance of the old lesion was probably an immune-mediated allergic process rather than successful treatment. Therefore, the differential diagnosis that could have been considered at this point was malignancy or histiocytosis.

Experience gained…

> Immunological manifestations pertaining to a system are similar, irrespective of the etiology that has caused them. Hence, the manifestations themselves, per se, do not offer any etiological diagnosis. Such immunological manifestations may result from diverse etiologies such as infections of different types, malignancies, drugs, immunodeficiency disorders and also autoimmune diseases. It is the course of the disease, and the further evolution of the clinical profile that may suggest a probable etiology. Any unusual presentation or progression must be cautiously evaluated for the correct diagnosis. A malignancy was mistaken for TB in this case and collagen vascular disease in the previous case. When in doubt, care should be exercised not to use empirical therapy, which may increase the difficulty in diagnosis or alter the course of the disease in an unfavorable way.

Extras…

There are very few indications of using steroids in childhood tuberculosis. These are tuberculous meningitis, miliary tuberculosis, and pericardial effusion. (As against a pleural effusion, steroids are used in pericardial effusions because the effusion occurs in a small anatomical space, thereby increasing the risk of cardiac tamponade; hence by using steroids if any additional benefit is accrued, it is welcome). In all these cases, steroid therapy is initiated right from the beginning, simultaneous with the antituberculous therapy. Steroids are never indicated after a few weeks of antituberculous therapy, except in an immunologically mediated new lesion where it endangers life.

CASE 133

■ TB Lymphadenitis Which was Lymphoma

Events...

A 10-year-old child presented with a gradually increasing swelling in the neck since the last two months. There was no history of fever or any other significant symptoms. Considering the diagnosis of tuberculosis, he was investigated. The Mantoux test was negative, the ESR was 30 mm at the end of one hour, and the chest X-ray showed a prominent left hilar shadow. FNAC of the lymph node in the neck, showed an inflammatory lesion suggestive of tuberculosis, and Ziehl-Neelsen stain revealed AFB. With this confirmation, the child was started on 2HRZ/4 HR. Initially, he seemed to improve, as the gland reduced to half its original size over six weeks. However, subsequently, in spite of continued compliant treatment, there was an increase in the gland size and a few more glands appeared around the same area. He also developed moderate fever. At this point, he was referred for further investigations.

Physical examination showed multiple enlarged lymph nodes, firm in consistency, mildly tender and not matted. There was no other lymphadenopathy or hepatosplenomegaly. He was not sick or pale.

Explanation...

In this child, the diagnosis of tuberculosis was confirmed bacteriologically. Therefore, apparently, there was no doubt about the diagnosis. However, there were a few odd features such as the negative Mantoux test and the left hilar lymphadenopathy seen on the chest X-ray. A child with localized cervical lymphadenopathy is almost always Mantoux positive. Secondly, it is rare for such a child to also have associated hilar lymphadenopathy. With a bacteriologically confirmed diagnosis, it is obviously justified to start anti-TB treatment; however, one needs to be careful over the ensuing weeks. Ideally, one should have monitored the progress of the left hilar gland on a repeat chest X-ray at the end of four weeks of therapy, just to confirm that there is no worsening. Further, one could repeat a Mantoux test at the end of two months, expecting it to be positive, if the tuberculosis has been successfully treated. This child did show an improvement initially as expected, but by the end of eight weeks of compliant therapy, the disease seemed to be worsening. The appearance of a new lesion is known during successful therapy as a result of an exaggerated immune response, and it does occur around 2 or 3 months of treatment. However, in such cases, the original index lesion improves, while new lesions appear at another site. In this case, the original lesion worsened, and additionally, some new lesions appeared around the site of the original lesion. In fact, the child's general condition had also worsened since he had now developed high fever.

With a few atypical features to begin with, and the unusual progress subsequently, the diagnosis had to be reassessed. On the basis of the above discussion, it is important to rule out lymphoma. Since tuberculosis is also known to coexist with lymphoma, it could also be a dual disease. This is not multidrug-resistant tuberculosis, as the child did improve over the first two months and then developed a resurgence of the old lesion along with appearance of new lesions. Nor could this be tuberculosis due to atypical mycobacterial infection, in which case the disease would not have improved at all in the first place, rather than improve and worsen later. Atypical mycobacterial disease is difficult to treat, as the organisms are not very sensitive to conventional anti-TB drugs, but it would not have worsened suddenly, as it happened in this child. Lastly it is also unlikely that this child is primarily immunocompromised, with tuberculosis as a subsequent superadded secondary infection. In that case, tuberculosis would not have presented with an isolated lymph node disease (which depicts good immunity).

At this juncture, it was decided to repeat the Mantoux test and the chest X-ray. The Mantoux test continued to be negative, while the chest X-ray was similar to the previous one. Irrespective of these test results, one would have asked for an excision biopsy; with the Mantoux test remaining negative even after 10 weeks of anti-TB therapy, the excision biopsy was mandatory.

Histopathology confirmed the diagnosis of **Hodgkin's lymphoma.** There was no evidence of tuberculosis. In view of the fact that AFB had been documented at the time of the initial FNAC, this could have been a dual disease to begin with. Over time, the tuberculosis probably got controlled.

Experience gained...

> When there is a discrepancy between the clinical presentation of a disease (tuberculous lymph node) and the expected laboratory parameter (Mantoux test expected to be positive), one has to be cautious in making a diagnosis. However, when the gold standard of diagnosis is subsequently achieved (bacteriological proof), one is forced to ignore the earlier discrepancies. At such times, monitoring the further progress of the case is extremely crucial. If it is unusual, one must review the diagnosis again.

INDEX

A

AB-cell antibody response 224
Abdomen 48
 bloating of 209
 distension of 35, 36, 115, 116, 277, 279
Abdominal pain 89, 204, 233, 277
 history of 205
Aberrant immune response 84
Abscess, deep-seated 112
Achalasia 190
 cardia 191, 192
Acidemia, organic 147
Acid-fast bacilli 228
Acidosis 145
 metabolic 32, 118, 119, 146, 147, 150, 237
Acinetobacter 73
Acute appendicitis 9
 attack of 205
Acute bacterial pneumonia 65, 164, 167, 171, 180, 245, 248
 diagnosis of 14, 171, 172
Acute gastroenteritis 9, 87, 88
 causes of 89
Acute rheumatic fever 69
 diagnosis of 71
Acyanotic defects 237
Addison's disease 26
Adefovir 44
Adenoids 54
 enlarged 201
 hypertrophy 201
Adenoviral infection 132, 250, 251
Adrenal failure
 chronic abdominal 26
 non-specific feature of 127
Afebrile 64, 66, 239
Air
 bronchogram 174
 fluid level 4
 leak syndromes 226
Airway 10
 disease 10, 96, 251
  original 251
  primary 254
 involvement, isolated 265
Alkaline phosphatase 116

Alkalosis, metabolic 182, 195
Allergic 171
 encephalopathy 227
 inflammatory disease 11
 laryngitis, acute 118
 manifestation 82
 reaction 245
 response 243
Allergy 12, 213
Alpha-1 antitrypsin deficiency 197
Amikacin 55, 61
Aminoacidopathy 147
Amoxicillin 14, 45, 47, 55, 63, 96, 98, 134, 246, 248, 267
Anemia 59, 91
 acquired hemolytic 122
 dimorphic 108
 hemolytic 122
 microcytic hypochromic 122
 moderate 120, 122
Aneurysms
 diagnosis of 94
 size of 94
Angiogram, pulmonary 34
Anion gap 32
Ankle joint 83
Anorexia 26
Antacids 104, 210
 use of 103
Anthelmintics 210
Antibiotic 14, 43, 46, 120, 210, 203, 223
 irrational use of 47
 long-term 203
 multiple 50
 therapy 63, 64, 94
  continuation of 64
Antibody test, irrespective of 97
Antifungal agent 100
Anti-inflammatory
 agents, symptomatic 83
 drugs 134, 275
Antispasmodics 210
Anti-tuberculosis
 drugs 226, 239, 266, 270, 277
 second-line 36
 treatment 12, 263, 266, 279
Antituberculous therapy 36, 271
 failure of 275

Aorta, coarctation of 193
Appendicitis
 acute 9
 chronic abdominal 205
 diagnosis of 9, 104
Appetite, loss of 207, 229
Arterial infarcts 227
Arthralgia 112
Arthritis 110, 112
 acute 71
 classic triad of 83
 infective 275
 juvenile idiopathic 71
 poststreptococcal
  reactive 110, 111
 reactive 82, 83, 256
 recurrent 82, 256
  reactive 83
 rheumatoid 256
 streptococcal reactive 71
 systemic onset juvenile
  chronic 134
  rheumatoid 132
 tuberculous 256
Ascites 77
Aseptic meningitis, risk of 80
Aspiration syndrome 8, 101, 102, 197, 250
Aspirin 71, 110
Asthma 8, 10, 11, 102, 186, 194, 195, 198, 200, 202, 250
 acute
  attack of 196
  exacerbation of 196
 analysis 200
 bronchial 103, 118
 cardiac 118
 investigation 200
Ataxia 155
 acute onset of 155
 telangiectasia 162, 184
Atelectasis 160
Atopic rhinitis 203
Autoimmune disease 94, 106, 139, 280
Autoimmune disorder 95, 105, 121, 122
 analysis 121, 122
Axillary lymph node 273
Azithromycin 47

B

Backache 107
  severe 15
Bacteria, drug-sensitive 47
Bacterial infections 19, 62, 65, 86, 89, 10, 187, 198, 201, 259, 277
  diagnosis of 25
Barium study 165
Basal cavitatory lesions, bilateral 185
Basal ganglion involvement 227
Basal meningitis, evidence of 153
B-cell
  deficiency 184
  response 224
BCG
  lymphadenitis 273
  scar, flaring of 274
  vaccination 264
  vaccine 274
    coverage of 226
Bernard-Soulier disease 81
Bicytopenia 106
Bile duct 105
Bilirubin, serum 116
Biopsy
  excision 282
  intestinal 278
  pleural 245
Bird flu 108
Bleeding 59, 105
Blood
  culture 46
  pressure, measurement of 193
Bone marrow
  aplasia 105, 123
  disease, secondary 104
  disorders 81
  examination 109
Bone scan 85
Bony disease, generalized 15
Bony lesion, inflammatory 279
Bottle-feeding 75, 88
Bradycardia 30
Brain 280
  abscesses, multiple 21, 22
  damage 21
  parenchyma 272
Breast milk, adequacy of 91
Breastfeeding 91
  exclusive 16, 59
Breathing
  bronchial 227

exercises 63
observation of pattern of 33
sudden cessation of 103
Breathlessness 32, 63, 66, 100, 104, 149, 230, 250, 254
  acute 119
    onset of 31, 118
  gradual onset of 237
  manifestation of 33
  mild 63, 83, 255
  onset of 98, 118
Bronchiectasis 97
  tuberculous 240
Bronchiolitis, acute viral 31
Bronchoalveolar lavage 97, 100, 176, 182, 195, 197, 252, 264
Bronchodilator 96
  drugs 103
Bronchopneumonia, bacterial 177
Bronchopneumonic lesions, persistent 266
Bronchoscopy 102, 196
Bullous rashes 132
Burning sensation 209

C

Calcium, serum 26
Calorie deficiency 91
Campylobacter 83
Candida albicans 177
Capillaria hepatica 129, 130
  analysis 129
  investigations 130
  physical examination 129
  systemic examination 129
  treatment 130
Capillary leak syndrome 24
Cardiac disease 111, 125, 250
Cardiac failure 122
  accompaniment of 105
  refractory 154
Cardiac tamponade, risk of 280
Cardiomyopathy 145, 154
Carditis 71
  treatment of 71
Cartridge-based nucleic acid amplification test 232
Cavitatory disease 225, 227
Cavitatory lesions 255, 233
  acute 259
  chronic 227
Cavity 160, 234, 250, 253
  abdominal 104

multiple 4
pleural 4, 63, 243, 245
Cefadroxil 42, 43
  failure of 43
Cefixime 47
  therapy 45
Cefpodoxime 74
Ceftriaxone 47, 49, 61, 74
Central nervous system 136
  disease 26
  disorder 102
Cephalosporin 47
Cerebellitis, post-infectious 155
Cervical lymph node
  development of 270
  enlargement 95
Chalasia cardia 190
Chédiak-Higashi syndrome 81
Chest
  physiotherapy 180
  ultrasound examination of 233
  wall, depression of 227
  X-ray 4, 10, 19, 36, 53, 64, 66, 97, 164, 171, 174, 196, 239, 240, 256
Childhood tuberculosis 231
  diagnosis of 225
Chlamydia 83, 161, 162
Chloromycetin 47
Chronic abdominal pain 210
  diagnosis of 210
Chronic progressive intestinal inflammatory disorder 211
Chylothorax 4
Ciliary dyskinesia 162, 184
Ciprofloxacin 261
Cirrhosis 116
Classical delta F 508 mutation 182, 195
Clavulanic acid 246
Clay-colored stools, absence of 115
Clostridium difficile 87
Clubbing 34, 195
Coagulation defects 136
Cold 23, 42, 43, 198
Collagen vascular
  disease 12, 25, 82, 132, 280
  disorders 11, 25, 131, 279
Collapse 227
Colonic disease 209
Coma 145
Congenital lobar emphysema 237
  diagnosis of 238
Congestion, venous 227

Conjunctival infection, bilateral 114
Conjunctivitis 83
Consciousness, loss of 125
Constipation 75, 76, 205, 206
Convulsions 26, 115
   multifocal 272
Coronary arteries 94
Cotrimoxazole 74
Cough 8, 42, 43, 96, 97, 184, 191, 201, 229, 240, 254
   control of 261
   episodes of 199
   mild 23
   persistent 189
   pertussoid 250
   recurrent 120, 186, 198, 203
      episodes of 8, 193
   severe 96, 101, 229, 250
   sudden onset of 196
COVID-19 44
Coxsackie 131
Cranial nerve palsies, lower 103, 227
Crohn's disease 212
CSF examination 233
CT scan 29, 85, 183
Cyanosis 34, 195
   central 34, 101, 265
Cycloserine 261
Cyclosporine 78
Cyst, mesenteric 36
Cystic adenomatoid malformation, diagnosis of 168
Cystic fibrosis 16, 149, 162, 184, 189, 195, 197, 250, 251
   diagnosis of 182
Cytomegalovirus 178

D

Death, sudden 125
Dehydration 11
   result of 146
Demarcation 161
Dengue
   fever 24, 132
   shock syndrome 23, 127, 138
      analysis 127, 128
      final diagnosis 128
      investigations 128
      physical examination 128
      systemic examination 128
Dermatomyositis 132
Dextrocardia, presence of 162

Dextrose 144
Diaphragmatic hernia, diagnosis of 4
Diarrhea 20, 88, 92, 146
   acute 88
   antibiotic associated 87
   chronic recurrent 217
   complication of 146
   episodes of 216
   recurrent 213, 215, 216, 218
Diarrheal diseases 88
Drug fever 11
Duodenum 209
Dyspepsia 209
   form of 209
Dysphagia 191

E

Ecchymosis 123
Echocardiogram 94
Echovirus 131
Edema 77
   generalized 78
Efavirenz 44
Electrolyte disturbances 87
Emphysema
   obstructive 227
   subcutaneous 226
Empirical antibiotic therapy 59, 243
   risk of 21
Empyema 63-67, 118, 171, 179, 243, 245
   development of 245
   diagnosis of 67
   management of 63, 68
   stage of 65
Encephalitis, viral 148, 152
Encephalopathy 30, 148, 228
   mitochondrial 153
Endocarditis, bacterial 94, 112
Endothelioma, pleural 28, 29
Enema 76
Enteropathy, gluten induced 216
Eosinopenia 45
Epigastrium 209
Epilepsy 207
Erythema
   diffuse 131
   marginatum 71
   nodosum 131
Esophageal stenosis 8, 190, 191
Esophagus 102
   demonstrate duplication of 165
Exanthematous illness 133
Extrahepatic biliary atresia 115, 116

F

Failure to thrive 90, 193, 237
Fatal disorder 105
Fatty chain abnormality 154
Febrile
   illnesses, recurrent 53
   seizure 7
Feet, mild edema of 105, 122
Fever 11, 15, 42, 50, 64, 93, 96, 121, 131, 162, 184, 198, 203, 223, 228, 239, 254
   biphasic 23
   causes of 15
   central 11
   defervescence of 24
   degree of 97
   early stage of 25
   enteric 45, 48, 51, 52
   high 23, 134
   long duration of 17
   low-grade 93, 242
   mild 149, 150
   mild-to-moderate 254
   moderate 23, 138
   monitor progress of 23
   persistence of 258
   presence of 135
   recurrence of 258
   rheumatic 69-71, 110, 111, 132, 223, 256
   scarlet 132
   spikes of 48
   streptococcal scarlet 132
   sudden onset of 248
   typhoid 48, 49, 50
   viral 24, 42
Fibrocaseous cavitatory disease 225
Fine needle aspiration cytology 228
Fistula, types of 102
Fixed drug eruption 123
Fluid resuscitation 33
Food
   intolerance 89
   poisoning 89
Fracture 108, 109
Functional immune defect 184
Fungal
   infection 99, 131
   pneumonia 96, 100
      analysis 96
      diagnosis of 177
      management 96
Fungi 100, 162

G

Galactosemia 115-117, 151
  analysis 115, 116
  investigations 116
  physical examination 116
  systemic examination 116
Gallbladder hydrops 95
Gastric aspirate 262
Gastritis 127
Gastroenteritis 86, 95, 127
  acute 9, 87, 88
  viral 89
Gastroesophageal anomalies 101
Gastroesophageal reflux 103
  disease 103, 189
Gastrointestinal infection 136
  recurrent 214
Gaucher disease 120
  analysis 120
Ghon's focus 246
Giardiasis
  chronic 218
  drug-resistant 218
Glomerulonephritis 223
Gram stain 245
Granuloma 280
  infective 228
Growth
  failure 56
  faltering 90

H

Haemophilus influenzae 51
Haloperidol 71
Hanta virus 178
Headache 42
  isolated symptom of 18
Heart
  block, congenital 30
  burn 209
  defect 101
  disease, congenital 237
Heat fever 11
Hematological tests 134
Hemiplegia 227
  acute infantile 153
Hemolytic anemia 122
  besides evidence of 122
Hemolytic uremic syndrome 87, 136
Hemophagocytic syndrome 104
Hemophagocytosis 105, 106
Hemorrhage, intracranial 80
Henoch–Schönlein purpura 135

Hepatic diseases 136
Hepatitis 127
  acquired neonatal 116
  B infection 232
  biochemical 105
  syndrome, neonatal 115
Hepatoblastoma 94
Hepatojugular reflux, positive 105
Hepatosplenomegaly 6, 98, 112, 122, 145, 228, 265, 281
Hernia, diaphragmatic 4, 5, 237
Herpes simplex 131
High protein diet 92
Hilar adenopathy 53
Hirschsprung's disease 75
Histiocytosis, symptoms of 99
HIV 162
  infection 215
Hodgkin's disease 121
Hodgkin's lymphoma 142, 241, 279
  diagnosis of 142, 282
Host immune
  reaction 266
  response 223, 227
H-type fistula 186
Hydration 33
Hydrocephalus 153, 271
  obstructive 227
Hydropneumothorax 4, 226
Hyperaldosteronism, secondary 77
Hyperbilirubinemia, direct 115, 151
Hypercalcemia, idiopathic 26
Hyperreactive airway 187
  disease 96, 195, 240
Hypersensitivity 12, 224, 266
  degree of 227
  destructive 252
  manifestations 267
  mild 246
  reactions 131
  recurrence of 271
  response 225, 226
Hypersplenism 81
Hypertension 119
  portal 116
Hyperventilation 150
Hypoalbuminemia 78
Hypocalcemic rickets 108
Hypochondrium 209
Hypoglycemia 30
Hypokalemia 33
  severe 33
Hypoperfusion, evidence of 135

Hypoproteinemia 91, 105
  nutritional 122
Hypothalamic-pituitary axis 17
Hypothesis 3
Hypothetical antibiotic
  therapy 46
Hypothyroidism
  diagnosis of 30
  mild degree of 75
  primary 90
  secondary 90
Hypoxia 101

I

Icterus, mild 105
Idiopathic thrombocytopenic
      purpura 123, 124
  analysis 123, 124
  investigations 124
Iliac fossa 205
Immune
  deficiency 16, 189
  disorder, manifestation of 274
  functions 90
  interaction 228
  mediated disease 274
  reaction 274
  recovery 267
  response 266
    spectrum of 224
  suppression 225
  thrombocytopenic purpura 79
    management 79
    treatment of 80, 81
Immunity 224
  acquisition of 224
  destructive 224
  protective 224, 225, 259
Immunocompetent 223
Immunodeficiency 81, 149
  disorders 280
Immunoglobulin 113
Immunological deficiency 184
Immunopathology, hypothetical
      model of 224
Immunosuppressive therapy 226
In vitro sensitivity 49, 176
Infections 13, 223, 275, 279
  acute bacterial 12, 17, 59, 62, 175, 176, 242
  bacterial 10, 19, 59, 62, 65, 86, 89, 162, 187, 198, 201, 259, 277

chronic 142, 277
community acquired 179
complications of 13
congenital 90
disseminated 6
drug-resistant 87, 267
enteroviral 132
evidence of 77
extra-intestinal 89
intra-abdominal 206
intracellular 96
local 15
parasitic 130
persistence of 49
post-splenectomy 81
proof of 67
recurrent bacterial 201, 203, 219
severe 226
subacute 176, 277
tuberculous 246
uncontrolled 77
viral 23, 42-44, 62, 127, 138, 146, 198, 199
Infective illness, subacute 254
Infiltration, small patch of 267
Infiltrative disorder 94
Inflammation 94, 101, 275
   degree of 11
   severe 171
   symptoms of 107
Inflammatory bowel disease 211, 277
   diagnosis of 211
Inflammatory disorder 279
   noninfective 134
Infliximab antibody 94
Influenza 24
Intercostal drain 63
Interferon gamma release assay 231
Interstitial disease 251, 265
Intracranial hemorrhage 80
   sign of 79
   symptoms of 79
Intracranial tension 17, 227
Intussusception 20, 87
Irritable bowel syndrome 212

J

Jaundice 95, 115
Joint
   disease, evaluation of 134
   minimal swelling of 69
   sacroiliac 84
   shoulder 275
   swelling 110
   tuberculosis of 226, 279
Jones criteria 71

K

Kanamycin 55
Kartagener's syndrome 162
Kawasaki disease 112-114, 132, 274
   atypical 93, 95
   diagnosis of 113
   manifestation of 94
   typical 95
Kawasaki syndrome 113
   diagnosis of 94
Kerosene aspiration 161
Ketoacidosis, diabetic 119
Kidneys 92

L

Lactic acidosis 153
Lactobacillus 73
Lactulose 76
Lamivudine 44
Large mediastinal lymph node 254
   presentation of 237
Leptospirosis 112, 132
Lesions 19
   compressive 107
   cystic 183
   fibrocaseous 55
   gangrenous 136
   interstitial 98
   multiple types of 252
   nodular 131, 140
   progresses 108
   space-occupying 191
Lethargy 26
Leukemia 79, 82, 105, 107-109, 219
   acute
      lymphatic 109
      lymphocytic 15
Leukocytosis
   mild neutrophilic 256
   moderate neutrophilic 274
   neutrophilic 12, 25, 99, 166, 171, 176, 232, 242, 248
Leukopenia 45, 134
Levofloxacin 55
Limbs
   lower 108
   movements, paucity of 33, 237

Lipoid pneumonia 161, 163
Liver
   biopsy 130, 233
   cell failure 116, 145, 151
   cirrhosis of 116
   disease 117, 123
   span 105
Lobar emphysema 237
   congenital 237
Long QT syndrome 125
Low-pitched bronchial breath sounds 160
Lung
   abscess 180, 181
   aspiration 100
   biopsy 100
   damage 64
      neonatal 188
   disease
      bilateral 197
      interstitial 251
   lesions 12
      destructive 266
      interstitial 99
   lobes of 164
   parenchyma
      disease, bilateral 265
      inflammation of 100
      involvement 33
   sequestration of 174
Lymph node 206, 254, 267, 273, 280
   disease, isolated 282
   enlarged
      mediastinal 226, 252
      paratracheal 232
   jugulodigastric 202
   large 249, 279
      cervical 270
      mediastinal 254
      paratracheal 10
      retrocardiac 240
   mesenteric 205
   multiple enlarged 281
   small mediastinal 227
   subcarinal necrotic 233
Lymphadenitis 281
   cervical 230
Lymphadenopathy 226, 241, 250-252, 255, 281
   cervical 114
   isolated 225
   large mediastinal 121
   massive mediastinal 268

Index

Lymphocytosis 45
Lymphohistiocytosis, hemophagocytic 106
Lymphoma 121, 219, 281

M

Macrolide 96, 97
Maculopapular rash 131
Malabsorption 213
    manifestation of 87
    primary 88
Malaria 6, 46, 52, 93
Malignancy 94, 99, 105, 131, 134
    chemotherapy for 226
    mediastinal 82
Malnutrition 53
    secondary 91
Mantoux test 48, 53, 153, 167, 252, 256, 265, 282
    positive 257
Mass
    lesion 250
    mediastinal 85
Measles 226
Meckel's diverticulum 207
Mediastinal lymph node 55, 240, 250, 267
    enlargement 239, 240
Mediastinal lymphadenopathy 67, 98, 239, 255
    detection of 232
    presence of 238
Mediastinum 84
    positive 191
Megakaryocytes, part of 79
Meningeal signs 153, 227, 262
Meningitis 127, 175, 271
    bacterial 21
    recurrence of 271
Meningococcemia 131, 135
Mental retardation 26
Metabolic derangements, secondary 31
Metabolic disorders 115, 116, 127, 146-148, 152, 154, 155
Metabolism, inborn errors of 115, 144, 145, 150
Methyl prednisolone 94
Metronidazole 59, 86
Microbiological tests 55
Migraine, abdominal 207
Mikulicz syndrome 219
Miliary lesions 250, 252, 253, 255
Miliary tuberculosis 197, 225, 251, 254, 265, 280
    diagnosis of 99
    part of 228
Milk allergy, probability of 205
Monoarthralgia 71
Monoarthritis 71
    recurrent 82
Mononucleosis, infectious 132, 133
Mucosal bleeds 80
Multidrug-resistant tuberculosis 36, 282
Mumps 219
Muscle weakness 21
Myalgia 108
Mycobacterial disease, atypical 282
Mycobacterium tuberculosis infection 224
Mycoplasma 43, 84, 96, 97, 161, 162
    antibodies 96
    pneumoniae 97
Myocarditis 127
    viral 154

N

Naproxen 276
Nasal discharge 201
Nasal secretions, culture of 203
Nasogastric tube 101
Nebulizers, use of 177
Nephrotic syndrome 77
    complications of 78
    management 77
Neurological disease, development of 255
Neutrophilic leukocytosis 12, 25, 99, 166, 171, 176, 232, 242, 248
    basis of 174
Nevirapine 44
Nimesulide 42
Nitazoxanide 218
Nodules, subcutaneous 71
Non-nucleotide transcriptase inhibitor 44
Non-steroidal anti-inflammatory drugs 82
    treatment 256
Norfloxacin 72
Nucleotide reverse transcriptase inhibitor 44

O

Obstruction
    intestinal 20, 279
    mechanical 191
    primary biliary 115
    recurrent subacute intestinal 207
    subacute intestinal 207, 277
Ofloxacin 262
Oligoarthritis, acute onset asymmetrical 84
Organ dysfunction 258

P

Pain 210
    abdominal 89, 204, 233, 277
    acute severe abdominal 204
    bony 108
    chronic abdominal 210
    colicky 205
    functional abdominal 210
    generalized abdominal 104
    nocturnal 84
    original abdominal 104
    recurrent abdominal 204, 207, 209-211
    severe abdominal 9, 279
    throat 223
Palatopharyngeal incoordination 8, 102, 103
Pallor, moderate 119
Pancreatitis 127
Pancytopenia 106
Parainfluenza 24
Paralytic ileus 20, 146
Parasites 100
Parenteral broad spectrum antibiotic 98
Parotitis
    bacterial 219
    viral 219
Penicillin prophylaxis 70, 81
    long-term 69, 121
Pericardial effusion 280
Pericarditis 112
    constrictive 35
Peripheral smear 6, 122
    examination 109
Peritoneal tap 77
Periungual desquamation 95, 114
Pertussis 96, 240, 250, 254
    initial diagnosis of 142

Pharyngitis, acute 110
Pharyngotonsillitis, bacterial acute 202
Phenobarbitone 71
Phenotypes 203
Phenylketonuria 152
Plasma, freeze samples of 145
Plasmodium malariae 78
Platelets
　adequate 167
　function defects, feature of 135
　functional disorders of 123
　transfusion 80
Pleural cavity 4, 63, 243, 245
　dry 12
Pleural effusion 66, 98, 121, 122, 160, 225, 234, 248
　acute onset 242
　bilateral 243, 246, 247
　evidence of 122
　large 227, 254
　localized 170, 243
　massive 28, 29, 242
　small 98
　tuberculous 7, 28, 118
Pleural fluid 12, 66, 242
Pleuritis 112
Pleuroparenchymal lesion, peripheral 246
Pleuropneumonia 121
　acute bacterial 121
Pneumococcal vaccine 81
Pneumocystis carinii 162, 178
Pneumomediastinum 226
Pneumonia 14, 67, 100, 118, 160, 161, 167, 171, 175, 176, 181, 182, 227, 229, 245, 249, 269
　acute bacterial 65, 164, 167, 171, 180, 245, 248
　bacterial 67
　bilateral 97
　clinical diagnosis of 160
　community acquired 180
　complications of 14
　development of 245
　diagnosis of 164, 174, 175
　drug resistant 171
　etiology of 100, 161
　left-sided 171
　lower lobe 165, 247
　middle lobe 14
　mimic 160
　persistent 160, 162, 166, 169, 175
　presence of 14, 98
　radiological diagnosis of 160
　recurrent 149, 161, 162, 171, 174, 175, 184
　sign of 166
　subacute 176, 248
　tuberculous 14, 167, 270
　uncomplicated 168
　viral 164
Pneumonitis 10, 149, 233
Pneumothorax 98, 118, 226
Poliomyelitis 33
Polyarthralgia 71
Polyarthritis, acute onset of 110
Polyethylene glycol 76
Polyuria 26
　history of 27
Porta hepatis 105
Prednisolone 71, 77, 78, 264
　short course of 50
Progressive primary complex 225, 270
　manifestation of 227
Protease inhibitor 44
Protein
　deficiency 91
　energy malnutrition, severe 91
　estimation 12
　supplements 92
Proteinuria 78
Proton-pump inhibitor 103
Pseudomonas 73
　aeruginosa 182
　isolation of 195
Psoriasis 276
　diagnosis of 276
Psoriatic arthritis 275
Pulmonary tuberculosis 229
　diagnosis of 167
Pulse 31
　oximeter 101
Purulent nasal discharge 201
Pus
　cells 86
　collection of 169, 179, 181
　development of 104
　localized collection of 104

R

Radionuclide scan 34, 207
Raised intracranial tension
　evidence of 120
　sign of 153
Rash
　drug-induced 133
　purpuric 131, 132
　vesicular 131
Reactivation disease 226
Recurrent abdominal pain 204, 207, 209-211
　causes of 208
Reiter syndrome 83
Renal disease, chronic 56, 119
Renal failure, end stage 119
Renal tubular acidosis 32
Respiration 31
　deep 119
Respiratory disease
　chronic 34
　primary 193
Respiratory distress 83
　acute 66
　sign of 182
Respiratory failure
　acute 119
　chronic progressive 184
Respiratory infection 96, 195
　acute 96
　bacterial 43
　recurrent 54
　viral 199
Respiratory muscle paralysis 33
Respiratory rate 237
Respiratory system 98, 121, 237, 265
Respiratory tract infection
　lower 183, 187
　upper 201
Reticuloendothelial system disease 120
Rheumatic fever 69-71, 110, 111, 132, 223, 256
　acute 69
　management 69
　recurrence of 71
Rickettsial disease 131, 139
Rickettsial infection 25, 112
　diagnosis of 139
Riley-Day syndrome 17
Ritonavir 44
Rituximab 78
Routine blood tests 232
Rubella 132

S

Salmonella 47, 49, 51, 84
　typhi 51, 52
　　growth of 52

Sarcoidosis 99, 251
Scurvy 107, 108
Seizures 125, 227, 228
Sensorium 153
Sepsis 32, 87, 145, 216
　　early 30
　　sign of 30
Severe abdominal pain 9, 279
　　acute onset of 9
Severe cough 96, 101, 229, 250
　　recurrent bouts of 10
Shigella 84
Shock, sign of 23
Shoulder joint 275
　　involvement 276
Sibling's death 154
Sickle cell disease 82, 108
Sinus puncture 203
Sinusitis 54
　　chronic infective 203
Skeletal muscle weakness 145
Skin
　　biopsy 140
　　rash 131
　　　　life-threatening 132
Slit-lamp examination 276
Sonogram, abdominal 151
Spinal muscular atrophy 237
Spine 84
Spironolactone 77
Splenectomy 81
Splenohepatomegaly 120
Staphylococcal exfoliative toxin
　　　　syndrome, phase of 132
Staphylococcal scalded skin
　　　　syndrome 131, 132
Staphylococcal toxic shock
　　　　syndrome 132
Staphylococcus epidermidis
　　　　176, 248
Sterile
　　abscess 67
　　empyema 67
　　pyuria 95
Steroids 26, 83
　　inhaled 8
　　resistant nephrotic
　　　　syndromes 78
　　therapy 271
　　withdrawal of 258
Stevens-Johnson syndrome 131,
　　　　132, 137
Stiffness 120, 125
Stomach 209

Stool
　　culture 58
　　microscopy 58
Streptococcal infection 71, 110,
　　　　141, 223
　　acute 111
　　drug-resistant 25
Streptococcal scalded skin
　　　　syndrome 223
Streptococcus pneumoniae 97
Stress 92
Sweating, absence of 17
Swelling 120
　　recurrent 219
　　　　episodes of 219
Syncope
　　benign 126
　　neurocardiogenic 125
Systemic inflammatory
　　disease 112
　　disorder 133
Systemic lupus erythematosus 134

T

Tachypnea 32, 33, 101, 149, 193
　　mild 189, 230
Tacrolimus 78
T-cell response 224
Tenderness 107-109, 120
　　generalized 207
　　mild 277
Tenofovir 44
Tension pneumothorax 118
Tetracycline 25
Thalassemia major 7
Thoracostomy 64
Thrombocytopenia
　　causes of 81
　　mild 45
Thrombocytopenic purpura 135
Thrombocytosis 99
Thyrotoxicosis 11
Tissue hypersensitivity 224
Toxic epidermal necrolysis 131, 132
Toxic shock syndrome 132
Toxicity 78
Toxoplasma 178
Tracheoesophageal fistula 101,
　　　　103, 149
Tuberculin
　　hypersensitivity 225
　　strength of 231
　　test 225, 240, 241, 246, 273
　　issues of 231

　　negative 225, 239, 241
　　positive 241
Tuberculoma 267, 280
　　development of 271, 272
　　multiple 272
Tuberculosis 12, 46, 55, 66, 99, 131,
　　　　142, 153, 219, 223, 225,
　　　　227, 228, 230, 242, 243,
　　　　245, 246, 254, 259, 264,
　　　　265, 281
　　abdominal 205, 277
　　allergic reactive manifestation
　　　　of 257
　　cavitatory 226
　　childhood 231
　　diagnosis of 53, 228, 230, 231,
　　　　233, 240, 248, 263
　　endobronchial 240
　　extensive 264
　　immune-mediated
　　　　manifestation of 256
　　intestinal 207, 277
　　investigations for 54
　　multidrug-resistant 282
　　mycobacterium 197, 232
　　post-primary 54
　　proof of 241
　　pulmonary 229
　　reactive manifestations of 257
　　uncommon symptom of 230
Tuberculous disease 257, 267
　　presence of 273
Tuberculous effusion 66, 67, 242
Tuberculous empyema 245
　　development of 227
Tuberculous meningitis 227,
　　　　272, 280
Tuberculous pleural effusion 7,
　　　　28, 118
　　localized 169
Tuberculous pneumonia 14, 167, 270
　　recovery of 270
Tumor
　　hypothalamic 17, 18
　　mediastinal 250
Typhoid
　　diagnosis of 47
　　fever 48, 49, 50
　　　　multidrug-resistant 46

U

Ulcer, nonhealing 140
Ulcerative colitis 212
Ulna, fracture of 108

Index

Upper airway inspiratory
 obstruction 33
Upper lobe lesion, persistent 166
Urea cycle defect 149
Urethritis 83
Urinalysis 119, 267
Urinary tract infection 73, 119
Urine
 culture 77, 119, 267
 freeze samples of 145
Urolithiasis 145
Urticarial lesion 143
Uveitis 95

V

Valvulitis, echocardiographic 71
Vancomycin 65, 248
Varicella 131
Vascular purpura, sudden
 development of 135
Vasculitis 140, 227
 systemic 112, 123

Ventricular septal defect 237
Vertebral crack fracture 15
Vertigo 125
Vesiculobullous skin rashes 137
Video assisted thoracoscopic
 surgery 64
Viral encephalitis 148, 152
 diagnosis of 152
Viral fever 24, 42
 hemorrhagic 131
 management 42
Viral infection 23, 42-44, 62, 127,
 138, 146, 198, 199
Vision problems 17
Vitamin
 C, large dose of 108
 dose of C 108
Vomiting 86, 191
 acute onset of 145
 drug-induced 127
 history of 8
 prolongation of 87
von Willebrand disease 81

W

Wegener's granulomatosis 19,
 99, 161
 diagnosis of 171
Weight, loss of 115, 229
Weil Felix test 139
Wheezing 8, 186, 187, 189, 191,
 193
Whooping cough 226
Widal test 51
Wilms' tumor 94
Wiskott–Aldrich syndrome 81

Y

Yersinia 83

Z

Zidovudine 44
Ziehl–Neelsen stain 260, 281
Zinc 89